W0113567

"This book provides multidimensional connections between group analysis, psychoanalysis, social studies and anthropology. The application of the concept of the tripartite matrix in group analysis is highly relevant to our attempts to understand the complexities of our time. The transcultural clinical examples help the reader to build an encompassing perspective of group work and its social psychodynamics. This new collection of chapters will be useful and stimulating for anyone interested in how groups work, and how they can be used in order to enhance processes of therapy for the members of them."

– **Domenico Agresta**, *Clinical and Community Psychologist, Psychotherapist, Group Analyst. Formerly Trustee of the Gordon Lawrence Foundation (GLF), now a Founder Member of "Social Dreaming International Network" (SDiN)*

"This new book enriches our understanding of the social unconscious and the tripartite matrix in Group Analysis. It will be extremely useful to individual and group psychotherapists in many schools of thought. The international selection of contributing authors are master chefs, who have prepared an intellectual feast that is appetising, filling, and nourishing for both senior colleagues and their students!"

– **Richard Beck**, *Former President of the International Association for Group Psychotherapy & Group Processes (IAGP), Senior Lecturer at Columbia University, Honorary Member, Italian Society for Psychosomatic Medicine*

"This new co-creation is an amalgam of deep clinical experience and social and psychoanalytical theory. The multicultural orientations and international 'locations' of the contributors plus their intersectional sensitivities make this book essential for relational clinicians and relational theorists more generally. We are compelled to think more deeply and in new ways about socially unconscious processes in persons and among persons, within their various and numerous groupings."

– **Stavros Charalambides**, *CGP, Psychoanalyst, Director of Institute for Relational and Group Psychotherapy Ltd (Greece), Certified Group Therapy Supervisor (Yalom Institute USA), International Association for Relational Psychoanalysis & Psychotherapy (IARPP) Board of Directors (elected). Co-chair of the Special Interest Group for Couples, Families, Groups*

"The theory and concept of the tripartite matrix in Group Analysis link social theory and psychoanalysis. Authors from the East and the West, and from the North and the South reveal the fecundity and fertility of working with the social unconscious in persons, groups, and societies, enabling a deeper exploration of topics ranging from intersectionality to addiction. Of lasting value to social scientists and clinicians in private practice and in public settings!"

– **Helgis Torres Cristófaro**, *PhD, Clinical psychoanalyst for individuals and groups. Former director of the Open University for Environment and Peace Culture (UMAPAZ) and former senior member of the São Paulo City Council for Sustainable Development and Environment (CADES)*

"A fundamental manual for psychologists, psychotherapists, psychoanalysts, group analysts and for all those who seek a clearer and more complex vision of individual, group and social functioning. S.H. Foulkes was revolutionary in broadening the focus of psychoanalysis. In this new work on the tripartite matrix and the social unconscious, Hopper and his international colleagues expand the field of Group Analysis. They improve our ability to interpret those unconscious phenomena that structure and define our human realities."

– **Alfonso D'Auria**, *Psychologist, Psychoanalytic Psychotherapist, Group Analyst in private practice in Rome. Full Member of the Group Analytic Society International (GASI), Former member of the Management Committee of the Italian Association of Group Analysis (IL CERCHIO) and the Confederation of Italian Organizations for Analytical Research on Groups (COIRAG)*

"This compilation of contemporary developments in the theory and practice of Group Analysis illustrates the application of principles of diversity, equity, and inclusion to clinical work. Under the baton of Earl Hopper, experienced authors from many countries articulate with exceptional clarity the concept of the Tripartite Matrix, the social unconscious and related concepts. Entirely relevant for all who are interested in social and political sciences and various group practices!"

– **Heloisa Fleury**, *President of the International Association for Group Psychotherapy & Group Processes (IAGP). Editor-in-Chief of the Brazilian Journal of Psychodrama. Co-Editor of Psychodrama in Brazil (2022) and author of many books, chapters and articles in Brazilian and international scientific journals*

"No one has contributed more to the internationalisation of group analysis than the esteemed Dr Earl Hopper, trained not only as a sociologist and psychoanalyst, but also as a group analyst. In this hugely important book, Hopper has assembled a rich community of forward-thinking colleagues from many countries who have created inspiring chapters which investigate a variety of topics ranging from envy to addiction to the inability to mourn. This collection will become an essential text in all of our libraries."

– **Professor Brett Kahr**, *Senior Fellow, Tavistock Institute of Medical Psychology, London. Honorary Director of Research, Freud Museum, London*

"Earl Hopper and his international colleagues surprise us with their nuanced approach to understanding socially unconscious processes in terms of the concept of the tripartite matrix, thereby linking group analysis, psychoanalysis, and social sciences. This original work helps develop the theories of Foulkes and other foundational thinkers. We are given many insights into a variety of cultural worlds. Let us hope for a translation of this important book into the German language."

– **Beatrice Kustor**, *PhD, Group Analyst and Psychotherapist. Member of the Institute of Group Analysis Heidelberg and of the Group Analytic Society International (GASI). Founder of the German and Polish group. Editor of the German Group Analysis*

"This new book in the series on the social unconscious in society, groups and persons is an inspiration to all who are interested in the social nature of humanity. Earl Hopper and a selection of international colleagues contribute to our further understanding of this phenomenon both theoretically and empirically as well as clinically. It is a 'must-read'"

– **Uri Levin**, *Clinical Psychologist, Group Analyst, and Organizational Consultant in private practice in Tel Aviv*

"Group Analysis is a field in which the individual, interpersonal and social meet, firmly grounded upon interdisciplinary and transdisciplinary concepts, such as the social unconscious. In collaboration with a set of distinguished international colleagues, Earl Hopper continues to develop the theory of the tripartite matrix, and applies it to both research and clinical practice. Given that 'All groups are microcosms of their contextual society and its many organizations and institutions', this new collection of papers will contribute to further elaboration of socially unconscious constellations, both our own and those of others."

– **Konstantinos Liolios**, *MD, Psychiatrist, Psychotherapist, Group Analyst. Chair of the Analytic Group Section of the International Association for Group Psychotherapy and Group Processes (IAGP)*

"Freud states, 'It is a very remarkable thing that the unconscious of one human being can react upon that of another, without passing through the conscious. This deserves closer investigation…'. And this is precisely what Earl Hopper and his colleagues continue to do. The conceptualisation of the Tripartite Matrix involves the interplay of socio-group-personal organisation that provides a creative specification of possibilities for the exploration of the personification of co-created roles, especially in clinical settings. This work will be of interest to group analysts, sociologists and hopefully psychological therapists in general."

– **Del Loewenthal**, *Emeritus Professor of Psychotherapy and Counselling, University of Roehampton, London, U.K.*

"The theory and concept of the social unconscious continue to be developed by Earl Hopper and our international colleagues. Essential for both psychoanalysis and group analysis, this extends the cornerstone concept of psychoanalysis – the unconscious – and returns it in a more complex form, which is open to other types of knowledge, and allows us better to understand the Human Being of the future."

– **Isaura Manso Neto**, *MD, Psychiatrist, Training Group Analyst and current president of the Portuguese Society of Group Analysis and Group Analytic Psychotherapy. Former member of the Management Committee of the Group Analytic Society International (GASI)*

"These reflections and analyses of Earl Hopper and his international contributors are grounded in years of clinical experience with individuals and groups. 'Before you can inspire with emotion, you must be swamped with it yourself', Churchill once said, perhaps somewhat curiously for an Englishman. An honest and authentic integration of clinical practice and hermeneutics, of the study of social phenomena and heuristics, this book represents contemporary Group Analysis at its best. Few savants can navigate as lightly and comprehensively among the domains of psychoanalysis, sociology, political sciences, and epistemology."

– **Roberta Mineo**, *Academic. Scholar of group dynamics. Friend*

"The study of the Social Unconscious is flourishing. It is a further step towards understanding the foundational dynamics that drive us as war breaks out and global upheaval deepens. I would like to pay tribute to the continuing efforts of the editors and authors of this and the preceding volumes of this series."

– **Professor Kaoru Nishimura**, *International Christian University, Japan. Editor-in-chief, FORUM, International Association for Group Psychotherapy and Group Processes. Board Member, Japanese Association for Group Psychotherapy*

"This book fills a gap in the theory that underpins the connections among group analysis, sociology, social psychology, and psychoanalysis. The Editor and contributors focus on the group, society, and the individual in the context of transgenerational processes. As a radical step forward for the work of all group therapists and social scientists, this book will become a standard text for colleagues and students alike."

– **Gerhard Wilke**, *Member of the Institute of Group Analysis, UK. Hon. Fellow of the Royal College of General Practitioners. Hon. Fellow of the International Association for Group Psychotherapy and Group Process (IAGP)*

The Tripartite Matrix in the Developing Theory and Expanding Practice of Group Analysis

The Tripartite Matrix in the Developing Theory and Expanding Practice of Group Analysis explores the social unconscious in persons, groups and societies in terms of the "un-acknowledged" restraints and constraints of our social and cultural groupings.

In this context, Earl Hopper and an international team of contributors elucidate the theory and concept of the tripartite matrix as a tool for the deeper understanding of the human condition and for clinical work in various settings. They consider topics ranging from envy to intersectionality, and from addiction to the inability to mourn.

The Tripartite Matrix in the Developing Theory and Expanding Practice of Group Analysis will be of great interest to group analysts, psychoanalytical group therapists, psychoanalysts and psycho-dramatists, as well as to social scientists more generally. Its extensive bibliography will be of particular value to students.

Earl Hopper, PhD, is a Psychoanalyst, Group Analyst and Organizational Consultant in private practice in London. He is a Fellow of the British Psychoanalytical Society, an Honorary Member of the Institute of Group Analysis, an Honorary Member of the Group Analytic Society International and a Distinguished Fellow of the American Group Psychotherapy Association. The Editor of the New International Library of Group Analysis, he is a renowned teacher, trainer and consultant in the United Kingdom and many other countries.

The New International Library of Group Analysis
Series Editor: Earl Hopper

Drawing on the seminal ideas of British, European and American group analysts, psychoanalysts, social psychologists and social scientists, the books in this series focus on the study of small and large groups, organisations and other social systems, and on the study of the transpersonal and transgenerational sociality of human nature. NILGA books will be required reading for the members of professional organisations in the field of group analysis, psychoanalysis, and related social sciences. They will be indispensable for the "formation" of students of psychotherapy, whether they are mainly interested in clinical work with patients or in consultancy to teams and organisational clients within the private and public sectors.

Recent titles in the series include:

Psycho-social Explorations of Trauma, Exclusion and Violence
Un-housed Minds and Inhospitable Environments
Christopher Scanlon and John Adlam

Sibling Relations and the Horizontal Axis in Theory and Practice
Contemporary Group Analysis, Psychoanalysis and Organization Consultancy
Edited by Smadar Ashuach and Avi Berman

From Crowd Psychology to the Dynamics of Large Groups
Historical, Theoretical and Practical Considerations
Carla Penna

A Psychotherapist Paints
Insights from the Border of Art and Psychotherapy
Morris Nitsun

Group Analysis throughout the Life Cycle
Foulkes Revisited from a Group Attachment and Developmental Perspective
Arturo Ezquerro and Maria Cañete

The Tripartite Matrix in the Developing Theory and Expanding Practice of Group Analysis

The Social Unconscious in Persons, Groups and Societies: Volume 4

Edited by
Earl Hopper

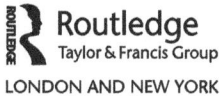

LONDON AND NEW YORK

Designed cover image: Getty | ricochet64

First published 2024
by Routledge
4 Park Square, Milton Park, Abingdon, Oxon OX14 4RN

and by Routledge
605 Third Avenue, New York, NY 10158

Routledge is an imprint of the Taylor & Francis Group, an informa business

© 2024 selection and editorial matter, Earl Hopper; individual chapters, the contributors

The right of Earl Hopper to be identified as the author of the editorial material, and of the authors for their individual chapters, has been asserted in accordance with sections 77 and 78 of the Copyright, Designs and Patents Act 1988.

All rights reserved. No part of this book may be reprinted or reproduced or utilised in any form or by any electronic, mechanical, or other means, now known or hereafter invented, including photocopying and recording, or in any information storage or retrieval system, without permission in writing from the publishers.

Trademark notice: Product or corporate names may be trademarks or registered trademarks, and are used only for identification and explanation without intent to infringe.

British Library Cataloguing-in-Publication Data
A catalogue record for this book is available from the British Library

ISBN: 9781032546391 (hbk)
ISBN: 9781032546384 (pbk)
ISBN: 9781003425915 (ebk)

DOI: 10.4324/9781003425915

Typeset in Times New Roman
by codeMantra

Contents

Acknowledgements

In acknowledging the help that the authors of the chapters that comprise this book and I as the Editor of it have received from so many mentors and colleagues, one age-old adage is particularly apt: "On the shoulders of giants we stand!" Our friends and family have been supportive in so many ways, but for a book of this kind, they must accept that even if we do not thank them individually, they will know who they are. I am grateful to Haim Weinberg for his editorial assistance with several chapters in this volume. On behalf of both the contributing authors and myself, it is a great pleasure to thank once again my personal assistant and secretary Céline Stakol for her meticulous preparation of each chapter for publication and for her patient "negotiations" with each author and our publisher. I am also pleased to acknowledge the support of the Trust for the Study of Social Trauma which continues to facilitate the New International Library of Group Analysis.

Editor and Contributors

Earl Hopper, PhD, is a psychoanalyst, group analyst, certified group psychotherapist, and organisational consultant in private practice in London. He is a fellow of the British Psychoanalytical Society, an honorary member of the Institute of Group Analysis (UK), an honorary member of the Group Analytic Society International, and a distinguished fellow of the American Group Psychotherapy Association. A supervisor and training analyst for several organisations in the UK and a member of the Faculty of the Post-Doctoral Program at Adelphi University, New York. A former president of the International Association for Group Psychotherapy and Group Processes (IAGP), and a former chairman of the Association of Independent Psychoanalysts of the British Psychoanalytical Society. The author and editor of many books and articles in psychoanalysis, group analysis and sociology, he is the editor of *The New International Library of Group Analysis (NILGA)* for Routledge.

Dr Anne Aiyegbusi is a group analyst and forensic psychotherapist. After retiring from a National Health Service Executive Director of Nursing role, she now works part-time as a principal psychotherapist and group analyst within the NHS. She is the director, consultant nurse, and psychotherapist at Psychological Approaches CIC where she provides training and consultancy mainly to forensic and criminal justice system services. A member of the Board of Trustees of the Institute of Group Analysis, with special responsibility for anti-discrimination and intersectionality. She is a Board member for the Forensic Psychotherapy Society. She has published a number of peer-reviewed papers and book chapters, and has co-edited and co-authored several books. She is currently writing a book about forensic psychotherapy and racial trauma.

Dr Kavita Avula is a licensed clinical psychologist. She specializes in the study of international psychology, unconscious bias, and the dynamics of large groups. She is the president of Therapist Beyond Borders, an organization that helps institutions to recognize and counter the many forces of oppression, staring with the top tier. Dr Avula serves as a senior supervisory psychologist at The KonTerra Group, a humanitarian organization that offers critical incident response, staff care and resilience services. She has offered group facilitation and trauma healing in the face of natural disasters and conflict in many different countries. She serves on the Large Group Team at the National Group Psychotherapy Institute of the Washington School of Psychiatry.

Avi Berman, PhD, is a clinical psychologist, psychoanalyst, training analyst and a group analyst. He is a member in Tel-Aviv Institute of Contemporary Psychoanalysis and The Israeli Institute of Group Analysis. He is the initiator and co-founder of the Israeli Institute of Group Analysis and its first chairperson. He is the head of group psychotherapy track in Tel Aviv University's psychotherapy program (within the psychotherapy program of the Sackler School of Medicine). He is the author, co-author, editor and co-editor of many books and articles in psychoanalysis and group analysis.

Penelope Busetto, MA, is a writer and PhD student in the Psychology and English Departments at Stellenbosch University in Cape Town. She is engaged in interdisciplinary research into the history of psychiatry and psychoanalysis in South Africa. In 2021, she completed a fellowship in the Department of Global Health and Social Medicine at King's College London. She is a member of the South African Psychoanalytic Initiative. Her novel, *The Story of Anna P. as Told by Herself,* won the 2014 European Union Literary Award.

Nabil Elkot, MD, PhD, CGP, is a consultant psychiatrist in Cairo. A Board member of the Evolutionary Psychiatric Association, and the Egyptian Association of Group Therapies, and a member of the American Association of Group Psychotherapy. He specialises in working with people living with HIV/AIDS and those living in conflictual areas with UNDP and UNHCR. He was a research visitor at the Free University, Berlin, Germany in 2017. He has experience with mass media, and has a weekly TV programme focusing on mental health.

Dr Helga Felsberger is a clinical and health psychologist in private practice and in the outpatient service in Vienna. She graduated in Psychology and English and American Studies at the University of Salzburg. A training psychoanalytic psychotherapist and training group analyst at ÖAGG (Vienna, Austria) and SGAZ (Zürich, Switzerland), she is an adjunct professor at Webster Vienna Private University. She specialises in "MBT – Mentalization-based Treatment" and "PIP - Psychoanalytic Parent and Infant Psychotherapy". She is married and a mother of two sons.

Frances Griffiths is a group analyst. She has held various leadership positions within the Institute of Group Analysis (UK), and is a former Chair of its Board of Trustees. She is a former member of the Management Committee of the Group Analytic Society International. In recognition of her past contribution to education, she was awarded a Schoolteacher Fellowship at the Lucy Cavendish College at Cambridge University. She currently co-conducts a group for headteachers, and a group for the recently bereaved.

Revaz (Rezo) Korinteli, PhD, is a psychiatrist, Jungian analyst and certified group psychotherapist in private practice in Tbilisi, Georgia. He is a professor at Ilia State University Tbilisi, Georgia, Past-President of Georgian Association of Analytical Psychology and President of Georgian Group Psychotherapy Association. He is a fellow of the American Group Psychotherapy Association and a Board member of the International Association for Group Psychotherapy and Group Processes. His professional interests include the study of the social unconscious and transpersonal psychology.

Marina Mojović, MD, is a psychiatrist, psychoanalytic psychotherapist, group analyst, and organizational consultant in Serbia. She is a member of the Group Analytic Society International, the International Association for Group Psychotherapy and Group Processes, the European Society of Psychoanalytic Psychotherapy, the International Society for Psychoanalytic Studies of Organizations, and the Organization for Promoting Understanding of Society. She is a training group analyst, and supervisor in the Group Analytic Society-Belgrade. She is the founder of the Society's Psycho-social Section and Training – Koinonia-Art, co-founder of its Section for Large and Median Groups, of the Reflective Citizens (RC) Method and Training, of the Belgrade Social Dreaming Training, and of the International Reflective Citizens Koinonia (IRC). She teaches internationally on the topics of trauma and social-psychic retreats.

Richard Morgan-Jones, Graduate and post-graduate education in Anthropology, Theology and Education at Cambridge, Oxford and Exeter Universities in the UK. A registered member of British Psychoanalytic Council (BPC). He is a supervising and training psychoanalytic psychotherapist of the British Psychotherapy Foundation. A former chair of the Brighton Association of Analytical Psychotherapists (now Psychotherapy Sussex). He is a director of Work Force Health: Consultancy and Research. He is a member of the International Society for the Psychoanalytic Study of Organizations, and a member of the Organization for Promoting the Understanding of Society. He is a visiting professor at the Indian Institute of Management Ahmedabad, and at the Higher School of Economics Moscow. He is a consultant to the Association of Psychoanalytic Coaches and Business Consultants for developing group relations in Russia. He is the author of many publications in the field of mental health in clinical and work settings.

Leyla Navaro, MA, is an individual, couple and group therapist in private practice in Istanbul. A former member of the faculty and supervisor at Bogaziçi University (2002–2020), and a former Board member of the International Association for Group Psychotherapy and Group Processes. She is the author of several books and chapters analyzing gender differences in forceful emotions such as envy, jealousy, competitiveness, desire, passion, anger, and the use of power.

Dieter Nitzgen, MA, is a group analyst, a training group analyst and supervisor for the Institute of Group Analysis in Heidelberg and the German Society of Group Analysis and Group Psychotherapy (D3G). He is a former member of the Association of Freudian Psychoanalysis (AFP), the former Head of the department of Psychotherapy of Rehaklinik Birkenbuck, a former Foulkes Lecturer and the former editor of *Group Analysis*.

Gila Ofer, PhD, is a clinical psychologist, training psychoanalyst and group analyst. A co-founder and past president of The Tel-Aviv Institute of Contemporary Psychoanalysis and a founding member of The Israeli Institute of Group Analysis. She serves on the faculties of these institutes and of the Post-Graduate School for Psychoanalytic Psychotherapy, Tel-Aviv University. She is a former chair of the Group Analytic Section and board member of the European Federation for Psychoanalytic Psychotherapy, and later a conjoint member of the Board as the coordinator of Eastern European countries. She presents and teaches in Israel, Europe and the United States. She is the editor of the EFPP's *Psychoanalytic Psychotherapy Review,* and the review editor for non-English books of the *International Journal of Group Psychotherapy.* She is the author and editor of many books and articles.

Kai Ogimoto is a certified clinical psychologist and licensed psychologist in Japan. He is an associate professor of Sagami Women's University in Japan. He practices psychoanalysis and psychotherapy as a candidate of the Contemporary Freudian Society (New York). He also practices group therapy. He has co-authored several books and articles in Japan and elsewhere.

Carla Penna, PhD, is a psychoanalyst and group analyst in Brazil. She is a member of the Psychoanalytic Circle of Rio de Janeiro, past-president of the Brazilian Group Psychotherapy Association and past-president of the Group Analytic Psychotherapy Society of the State of Rio de Janeiro. A member of the Group Analytic Society International and a member of the Analytic Group Section Committee of the International Association for Group Psychotherapy and Group Processes. She has published two books and several articles, especially in the study of the social unconscious and the large group.

Tomas Plaenkers, PhD, psychoanalyst and psychologist. Member of the German Psychoanalytical Association and the International Psychoanalytical Association. Training analyst at the Frankfurt Psychoanalytical Institute. Consultant member of the IPA China Committee, and member of the IPA Asia Pacific planning committee. His main fields of scientific work are clinical and social psychoanalysis. In addition to his many clinical and social-psychological publications, he is the manager of the Freud-Chinese-Translation-Project (FCTP), a pilot project on translating Freud's *Lectures on Psychoanalysis* from German into Chinese.

Mona Rakhawy, MD, is a psychiatrist, psychotherapist and trainer and supervisor in psychotherapy. She is a professor of psychiatry at Cairo University and on the adjunct faculty at the American University in Cairo. She is a member of the Board of the International Association for Group Psychotherapy and Group Processes (IAGP), and a chair of CAOA. She is a chair of the board of trustees of Rakhawy Institute for Training and Research. She has co-founded and is president of the Egyptian Association for Group Therapies and Group Processes.

Dr Jelica Satarić, MD, is a psychiatrist, individual psychotherapist, and group analyst in private practice in Belgrade. She is a member of Serbian Medical Chamber, Serbian Psychiatric Association, Serbian Psychoanalytic Society of Psychotherapists and Group Analytic Society Belgrade. She is the president and a training group analyst of GAS Belgrade and member of coordinating and supervisory bodies of its Psychosocial Section. She is a member of Group Analytic Society International. She is a co-founder and convener of the Reflective Citizens (RC) Method and Training in Serbia, and the co-founder of the International Reflective Citizens Koinonia (IRC).

Joseph (Yossi) Triest, PhD, is a training psychoanalyst, clinical psychologist and organizational consultant. He is a former president of the Israel Psychoanalytic Society. He is the current chair of the "Freud and Followers Unit" at the Tel-Aviv University Psychotherapy Program, and on the faculty at the Tel Aviv University Sackler Medical School. He teaches and supervises at the Israeli Psychoanalytic Institute and at several schools of psychotherapy. He is involved in Group-Relations as developed by the Tavistock Institute (London) and OFEK (Israel), and has co-directed the Program for Organizational Consultation and Development. He is a co-founder and co-director of the "Center for Research of the Psychoanalytic – Systemic Approach". He has also founded and co-directed the "Triest-Sarig Clinic" which offers psychotherapy and psychological services for adults and children to a variety of communities in Tel Aviv.

Martin Weegmann is a psychologist and group analyst in the UK. He has worked in a range of areas: substance misuse, personality disorder and complex needs and is the author of several books and articles. Martin's latest book project is "Novel Connections: Between Literature & Psychotherapy".

Introduction[1]

Earl Hopper

My Introduction to *The Tripartite Matrix in the Developing Theory and Expanding Practice of Group Analysis*, the fourth in the series of volumes concerning the social unconscious in societies, organisations, and persons, in the context of the New International Library of Group Analysis, is also an introduction to both the theory and concept of the social unconscious, and a review of the perspective developed and advanced in the preceding three volumes (Hopper & Weinberg 2011, 2016, 2017). The study of the social unconscious is at the core of group analysis, which is based on psychoanalysis, sociology, and the study of group dynamics. This underlying orientation has crystallised in creative ways in several academic settings, sometimes within small groups of colleagues rather than within formal departments of generally recognised disciplines. These "constellations" have gone under various names, for example, "personality and culture", "mind, self and society", and "personality in nature, society and culture", but it is axiomatic in each of them that the unconscious mind of a person is always both a socially unconscious mind and a neuro-physiologically unconscious mind, as well as a psychologically unconscious mind.

Were it not for the way that traditional mainstream psychoanalysts continue to study the personality without taking into account the social context over time, and the way that traditional mainstream sociologists and other social scientists continue to study society without taking into account the personalities of the members of it, we would no longer need to stress the importance of the *social* in the study of the unconscious mind, and the importance of the *unconscious* mind in the study of society and culture. However, these bifurcations are embedded in the training systems of many Institutes of psychoanalysis and psychotherapy (Davies, 2018), as well as in many Institutes of group psychotherapy and group analysis (Dalal, 2022). This is partly a matter of the way in which people in authority tend to select their students in terms of their own image (Mills, 1956). However, it is also a function of fundamentalism in response to the diffuse prevalence of trauma in the helping professions.

My own ideas about the social unconscious have been developed in several publications, which contain extensive bibliographical references, for example, Hopper (1981, 2003a,b, 2012, 2018a,b, 2022a,b,c). Political journalists tell me that I should not fear the continuing repetition. I have decided to take them at their word.

DOI: 10.4324/9781003425915-1

A definition of the concept of the social unconscious

The concept of the social unconscious refers to the social, cultural, communicational, and technological "arrangements" of which people are "unaware". "Arrangements" is a kind of euphemism for the structures and properties of social systems and their various manifestations, such as, in the case of societies, their specific institutions and organisations, and, at a more abstract level of analysis, their various sub-systems, such as the political, economic, and educational. It is important to specify the social systems in question because social systems vary with respect to these arrangements. "Unaware" is a euphemism for unconscious processes in their entirety. As in the traditional concept of the biologically based unconscious, the social unconscious, with respect to the external world and the internal representations of it, involves the non-conscious and the dynamic unconscious of the repressed, as well as that of the split-off and the denied and/or disavowed. It also involves the pre-conscious.

It is noteworthy that in contrast to this concept of the social unconscious, the classical concept of the *collective unconscious* refers to those arrangements that are more directly derived from and based on the human species and the human organism. The structures of societal social systems are neither as constant nor as universal as the singular structure of the human species. There is no direct analogy between the relationship of the species and the unconscious mind of persons, and the relationship of particular social systems and the unconscious minds of the participants in them. This is not to suggest that the social unconscious is less "deep" than the collective unconscious. However, while the collective unconscious is primarily about the universal id, the social unconscious is primarily about the local ego, ego-ideals, and local super-ego.

Borrowing a distinction from classical genetics, I would suggest that while the collective unconscious is about *genotypes*, the social unconscious is about *phenotypes*. This biological analogy is not perfect. Phenotypical phenomena are exceedingly complex and have their own aetiologies. This analogy implies that while we are unable to alter the basic structure of our species, and will not be able to do so for at least the foreseeable future, we can, with increased awareness, alter the external world through political processes.

It is an unfortunate challenge to the clarity of these distinctions that modern Jungians use the concept of the collective unconscious in much the same way that modern group analysts use the concept of the social unconscious, although it is generally acknowledged that Jungians give more importance to what Foulkes called the "primordial level" than modern group analysts tend to do. Actually, it is not entirely clear whether in his references to the "collective unconscious", Foulkes was thinking in terms of the classical Jungian concept of the collective unconscious or Mannheim's (1929) concept of the collective unconscious by which Mannheim meant the intertwining and overlapping realities of both the social and the psychological, as seen, for example, in ideology as an expression of false consciousness and alienation as a universal social and personal defence against the pain of insight into various forms of helplessness and other patterns of anxiety (Mies, 2022; Scholz, 2022).

This problem of "one term/multiple meanings" is not entirely different from the problem caused by the various ways that the "social unconscious" was used by figures such as Burrow (Pertegato & Pertegato, 2013) and Fromm (1970). Burrow used the term in the classical Jungian sense with its emphasis on the species and the organism, although he later used it in order to emphasise the internalisation of the external world. Fromm used the term in order to emphasise that in his opinion, a society is not merely *like* a living organism but actually *is* one. In other words, he based his thinking on the idea that the society and the person were homologous and not merely analogous.[2]

Bion's basic assumptions, which are often regarded as an example of the social unconscious as a property of the external world, can be understood in terms of both the classical Jungian concept of the *collective unconscious* and the group analytic concept of the *social unconscious*. Genotypically, basic assumptions are universal patterns of defence against universal psychotic anxieties rooted more in the species and the organism than in particular social systems and the variable life experience of the persons within them. Phenotypically, basic assumptions reflect the constraints and restraints of the external worlds that are typical of particular social systems.

As I have often argued, in order to study the social unconscious, several concepts, with slightly different nuances and embedded in slightly different theories, have been adumbrated in various ways (Hopper, 2003a): in terms of interpersonal relations, the shared unconscious (Hobson, 1974), the associative unconscious (Long, 2013), the interpersonal unconscious (Scharff & Scharff, 2011); and in terms of cultures, values, norms, and beliefs, the cultural unconscious (Spector, 1992), and the normative unconscious (Layton, 2020). Some concepts focus on particular entities, e.g., the *societal* unconscious, the *family* unconscious, the *organisational* unconscious, and the *group* unconscious (Bion, 1961). More problematic are applications of this hybrid conceptualisation to larger groupings with more ambiguous boundaries and status as entities, e.g., *racial* unconscious, *ethnic* group unconscious, and *class* unconscious. These various specifications of the concept of the social unconscious are very similar in their heuristic intent.

Concerning the theory of the social unconscious, it is exceedingly important to acknowledge the contributions of the 19th-century French sociologist Emile Durkheim and his younger colleagues and students, which greatly influenced the work of sociologists such as Bourdieu (2000) and the psychoanalytical group psychotherapist Kaës (2006). I would say that Durkheim was attempting to develop a kind of sociology of persons that was analogous to the later attempts of Freud and some of his associates to develop a psychoanalysis of societies. The importance of the work of Durkheim was acknowledged by de Maré (1972). Shortly before he died, Malcolm Pines admonished me for not acknowledging the work of Hans Loewald, for example, his *Psychoanalysis and the History of the Individual* (1978), which was a good example of being able to think in terms of the external world of which persons were unconscious without eschewing the significance of basic psychoanalytical ideas.

I am also pleased to acknowledge the recent work of Frie (2022), as well as that of Dajani (2017), Gonzales (2020), and Rao (2022). It seems to me that it will soon be appropriate to refer to a new "constellation" at the San Francisco Center for Psychoanalysis (PINC) similar to the one that developed in the late 1920s and early 1930s in Frankfurt, the contributions to which continue to shape group analysis and relational psychoanalysis in general. Although most relational psychoanalysts are unaware that the antecedents of the relational perspective can be traced to Frankfurt and to group analysis, the social unconscious has become an essential element in their way of thinking and working. Even contemporary Kleinian psychoanalysts in London have begun to acknowledge the aetiological importance of sociocultural-political restraints and constraints of specific social systems of which the participants in them are in varying degrees unconscious.

From collective minds to social fields to social systems

Shifting from thinking about the social unconscious in terms of collectivity, the concept became embedded in what Kurt Lewin (1951) called "field theory". Although field theory also originated in the late 1920s and the 1930s in Germany, Lewin did not publish in English until after World War II. The more one thinks in terms of a wave theory of cause and effect rather than a particle theory, the more likely is it that one will be sensitive to the study of forces that do not require physical contiguity. A field theory in group analysis can be defined in terms of various metaphors for an electro-magnetic field and for social-psychological-biological "spaces". Recent developments in field theory in psychoanalysis are beginning to take account of this perspective (Penna & Hopper, 2022). There is little doubt that the more one's life experience is universal and cosmopolitan rather than "local", the more likely is it that a person will be sensitive to variations in properties of a field by which he is restrained and constrained.

In the context of field theory, the social unconscious refers to several interconnected elements and dimensions of persons and their groupings:

1   Sociality: for example, prolonged dependency, language, and internalisation;
2   Relationality: for example, interaction, interpersonality, and transpersonality;
3   Transgenerationality: for example, institutions of socialisation and social control such as the family and education sub-systems;
4   Collectivity, plurality, and groupings of people: for example, social classes, ethnic groupings, and racial groupings, who are in varying degrees conscious of themselves as constituting a grouping, usually in contrast, if not opposition, to another grouping. (This is different from social categories of people in terms of any variable of interest, but who lack "consciousness of kind".)

Although the development of general systems theory preceded the development of general field theory, it is also true that thinking in terms of social and relational fields contributed to thinking in terms of systems, and in terms of social systems in particular (Hopper, 1975). As Foulkes observed as early as 1948, although not all social entities are groups or should be called "groups", all social entities are social systems of various kinds, for example, societal social systems, organisational social systems, family social systems, group social systems, and so on. Like all "living human systems" (Agazarian & Gantt 2000), social systems can be defined as a set of variables in which a change in any one of them can be explained by changes in one or more of the other variables in the set. In social systems, these variables pertain to sub-systems directed towards solving fundamental problems associated with work and love. Social systems vary with regard to a number of features, which can be conceptualised as dimensions of them, for example: complexity and simplicity (in terms of role differentiation and specialisation); cohesion and incohesion; dynamism and staticism; stability and instability; and closure and openness.

Although perfectly closed systems are extremely rare, perfectly open systems are a contradiction in terms. Nonetheless, as a consequence of the porous or osmotic nature of their boundaries, social systems are always "contextual". This is the basis for the existence of barometric events, parallel processes, isomorphism, and equivalence. Such processes are not random, but reflect enactments based on the need to repeat experiences in various spaces, particularly when it is felt that it is safe to do so.

Individual persons can also be seen as social systems. However, they are rooted in organismic individuality. With respect to the sociality of their internal worlds, a person can be understood as a kind of "group of one", meaning one organism but a multitude of internal representations of both more significant and less significant others. Foulkes understood that persons are not the same as individual organisms. The *person* is located in the context of transgenerational processes, and transcends biological conception and death. In fact, Foulkes (1990) eventually used the term "open system" in order to emphasise the social nature of a person's internal world.

The social unconscious of persons as social systems is often illustrated by the well-known set of concentric circles. As many circles as deemed to be necessary and desirable can be used in order to represent phenomena such as the nuclear family, the extended family, the neighbourhood, the school, the community, the wider society, the world, and the cosmos. Usually, the body/psyche is put at the very centre, and the cosmos at the very outside, but in so far as it is believed that each individual human being is holy and made in God's image, it can be the other way around.[3] These circles can be drawn with interrupted lines in order to emphasise the porous nature of these social entities and their spheres of influence.

The person as a dynamic open system can be represented as shown in Figure 0.1.

In *The Introduction to Group-Analytic Psychotherapy: Methods and Principles*, S.H. Foulkes (1948) used a set of concentric circles in order to indicate the specialisations of our disciplines as shown in Figure 0.2.

It is worth recounting that Eric Dunning and I once discussed such diagrams with Norbert Elias, who did not like concentric circles with individual human organisms at the centre of them, because they were what he called "ego-centric", and did not convey the nature of persons and perhaps even of organisms who were interdependent and socially "constructed" from the beginning. In other words, such diagrams did not acknowledge that what I have called the "society-ego" is as primary as the body ego, with which it is intertwined and to which it is not reducible,

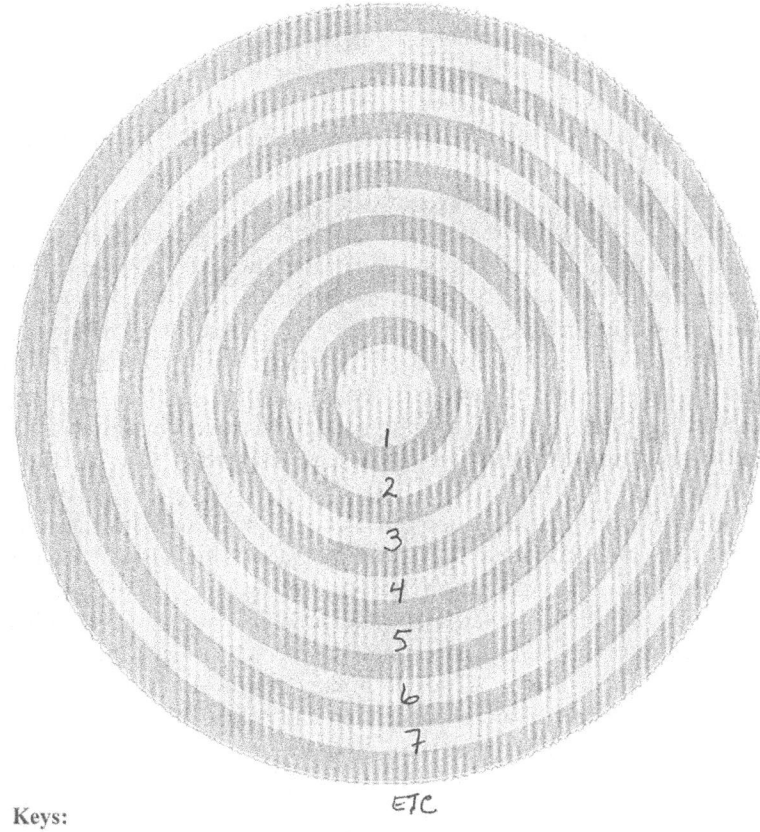

Keys:

1. Body/psyche
2. Nuclear family
3. Extended family
4. Neighbourhood
5. School
6. Wider community
7. Particular organisation/institution such as occupational setting
8. Wider society
9. World
10. Cosmos

Figure 0.1 The Person as a Relatively Open System in the Context of Various Elements in the External World as Represented by Concentric Circles.

and vice versa. The theory and concept of the social unconscious are at the core of the innermost circle of such a set of concentric circles, and contradict the insight that these spatial diagrams are intended to give.

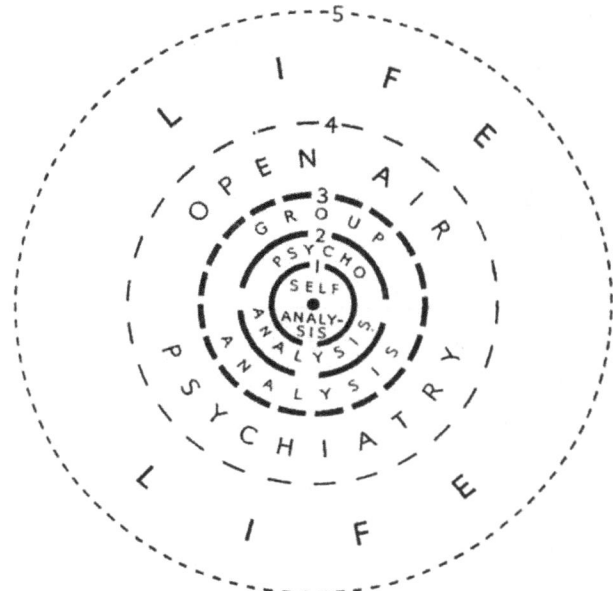

Figure 0.2 Persons and Their Groupings with Reference to Specialised Therapies.

Time and space

In my own clinical work, I have emphasised the importance of the location of communication in terms of time and social psychological space. Space is considered in terms of "Here and There", and time is considered in terms of "Then and Now". "Here" could be extended to include other relationships, and "Time", to include transgenerational processes. These cells of the time/space paradigm indicate the internal worlds of persons in the context of the group as a co-constructed interpersonal and transpersonal entity. However, they also indicate the collective worlds of the members of a particular social entity as shown in Figure 0.3.

Working in the Time/Space paradigm is particularly relevant to the analysis of transference and countertransference processes in the context of socially unconscious phenomena. It is important to recognise that situations can be repeated in the Here and Now of transference and countertransference, not only in individual work, but also in group work. The Here and Then can be repeated in longer term slow-open groups because all the members of the group will have shared collective history. The repetition of the There and Then requires more empathic imagination and shared narratives.

David and Jill Scharff added to this paradigm of time and space the cell of "If and When". This allows for the consideration of the ability and willingness to exercise the transcendent imagination, which is how I continue to define mature hope.

A spiral can be used in order to illustrate the dynamic nature of social systems. This emphasises the variability of the starting point in social, personal and

		Space	
		Here	There
Time	Then	1	2
	Now	3	4

Figure 0.3 Hopper's Time/Space Paradigm of the Preoccupations of Patient and Therapist in Their Clinical Work.

organismic life, and openness to the environment. Foulkes and Anthony (1957) used the spiral in order to describe groups as social systems in which internal process/motion was in a dynamic relationship to the process/notion of the environment. However, in order to emphasise the *developmental* aspects of these dynamic connections, Pichon-Rivière used the concept of a dialectical spiral (Losso, de Setton & Scharff, 2017).

The paradox that social systems are both "inside-out" and "outside-in" can be illustrated by the Mobius strip, as illustrated in Figure 0.4.

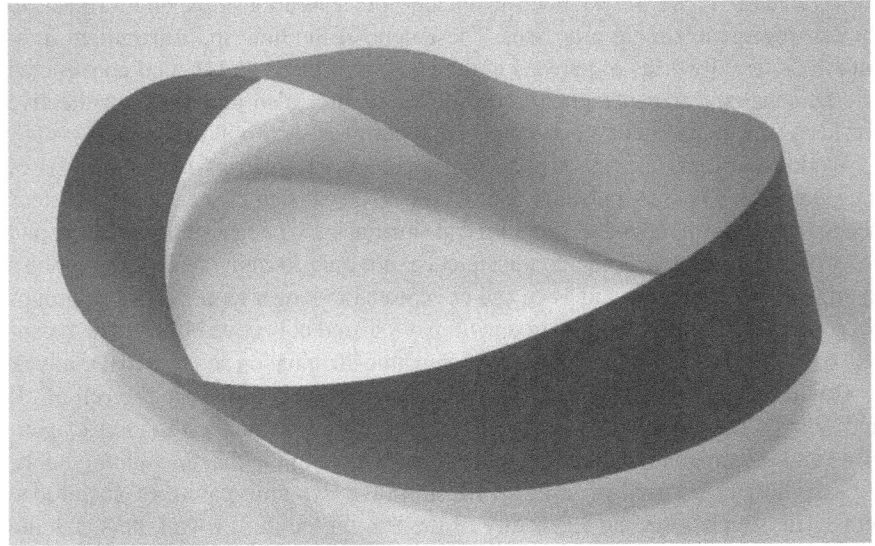

Figure 0.4 A Mobius Strip.

The Mobius strip conveys the dynamic nature of what is outside becoming inside and vice versa, which acknowledges the simultaneous nature of projection and introjection. During the 1960s, in seminars with Foulkes, we began to discuss these images.

As Ogden (2005) has reminded us: "The analyst is responsible not only for remaining receptive and responsive to the truth of what is occurring in the consulting room, but also to what is happening in the outside world" (p. 12). I would add that what occurs in the consulting room is always a reflection of what is happening in the outside world, whether we are aware of it or not! Many Independents in the British Psychoanalytical Society like to recount Little's (1985) iconic memory of a scientific meeting of the British Psychoanalytical Society during the blitz as a "noisy evening with bombs dropping every few minutes and people ducking as each crash came... Donald Winnicott... finally stood up and said 'I should like to point out that there is an air raid going on', and sat down". Little was struck by the fact that no notice was taken of Winnicott's interjection, and that "...the meeting went on as before!" Of course, these external explosions were experienced in terms of a variety of interpersonal explosions, but I have often wondered whether unconsciously the meeting was deeply affected by these explosions, which left their mark on the culture of the society for many decades (King & Steiner, 1991).

I also recall more recent scientific events in the context of the Group Analytic Society International and the Institute of Group Analysis (UK) concerning gangs, terrorism, and terrorists, in which several senior members of these organisations responded to the politicised discussion of these emotive topics by drawing attention to the enactment of angry and chaotic feelings and processes, and to the personification of them within the reflection groups, especially the large groups. These somewhat ritualised interpretive interventions had little effect on the proceedings. Particular individuals seemed to be exceedingly vulnerable to the suction power of the roles that were co-created in the groups.

In other words, it is often hard to know what is "inside" and what is "outside" of any particular group. Moreover, it is hard to know where the boundaries are, and to understand more generally how the land lies. Freud was undoubtedly correct in his famous but ironic aside that "out of this world, we will not fall", but he may not have realised the extent of the challenge that this set for future generations of psychoanalysts.

The social a-priori

In group analysis, it is axiomatic that the *social* takes precedence over the *organismic*, and, thus, over the *psychic* as well. This "social a-priori" applies to the maturation, development, and/or change of all social entities and to the members of them (Nitzgen & Hopper, 2017). As Foulkes (1990) asserted in one of his basic statements about the epistemology of group analysis:

> [We] must reverse our traditional assumption, shared also by psychoanalysis, that the individual is the ultimate unity, and that we have to explain the group from inside the individual. The opposite is the case. The group (the

community) is the ultimate primary unit of consideration, and the so-called inner processes in the individual are internalization of the forces operating in the group to which he belongs.

(p. 212)

The social a-priori is at the core of why the study of the social unconscious is so closely related to the study of trauma. While classical psychoanalysis continues to privilege drive theory, the essence of which is the Kleinian theory of the death instinct, innate malign envy, and the primacy of projection, the theory of the social unconscious privileges trauma rather than the death instinct. Helplessness is at the core of the human condition, not innate malign envy as a representation of the death instinct. In fact, I regard envy as an emergent defence against the anxieties of helplessness. Moreover, helplessness is a function of failed dependency in a significant relationship (Hopper, 2022a, 2003b).

The study of trauma also leads to the hypothesis that in the beginning, the external world is internalised on the basis of disappointment that the figures on whom we depend have failed to satisfy our needs and live up to our expectations. Of course, internalisation is associated with taking in mother's milk, but this is a very simplistic idea. Fairbairn and Ferenczi realised that the psychological reason for building up an internal world is that we need to gain more control of our objects and take responsibility for them. We also internalise our objects in order to protect them from aggression both from other people and from our own objects. It is difficult to over-emphasise the importance of mourning and its vicissitudes, both personally and collectively (Penna, 2015).

Yet another reason why trauma is important in connection with the social unconscious is that Freud was not entirely correct that in the beginning, the ego is a body ego. In fact, in the beginning, the ego is a society ego every bit as much as it is a body ego. Guntrip distinguished the ego of adaptation, a concept that Bion also used, from the ego of agency, which is more or less by definition both a body ego and a society ego. The ego of agency focuses on thinking and making creative use of traumatic experience, and, therefore, develops the capacity for symbolisation, self-reflection, and taking the point of view of the other.

The organisation of Volume 4 and the contributions to it

Volume 4 is organised into four sections. The first section concerns the theory and concept of the tripartite matrix. While recognising the importance of thinking in terms of fields and social systems, Foulkes and his colleagues shifted from the basic notion of collectivity to the concept of the *matrix* in general and subsequently to the concept of the tripartite matrix more specifically. The tripartite matrix of any particular grouping refers to its socio-cultural-personal organisation. No more and no less! The famous Borromean knot is a perfect icon for the tripartite matrix of any human grouping or living human social system, indicating the intertwined connections among their sub-matrices, in which tensions are difficult to disentangle from cohesions. In a significant development of the previous work of Nitzgen and Hopper (2017), Dieter Nitzgen, in Chapter 1, "The Cornerstone, Once More", outlines the development of the concept of the tripartite matrix. He reminds us that Foulkes first introduced the theory and concept of the *foundation matrix* of the contextual society, later the *dynamic matrices* of the specific group and their sponsoring organisations, and only towards the end of his life the *personal matrices* of the participants in it/them. The social unconscious is a function of the three sub-matrices as an intertwined whole, and can be discussed only in terms of the gestalt of selected facts and factors of it.

In Chapter 2, "The Tripartite Matrix in Foulkesian Group Analysis", Earl Hopper describes the tripartite matrix in terms of its three overlapping and inter-penetrating matrices. There is always an interface between each of these "realms", each of which can be considered as a system in its own right or as a sub-system of the whole. He also considers various dimensions of the tripartite matrix, for example: patterns of interpersonal relations, values and norms, beliefs, communication, styles of leadership, followership and bystandership, and technology. Hopper presents two illustrations of his clinical work in the context of the tripartite matrix as-a-whole.

In Chapter 3, "Improvised Vocality of Verbal Communication in Groups: A Contribution to the Conceptualisation of the Tripartite Matrix in Group Analysis", Helga Felsberger elaborates the dimension of verbal communication through the specification of vocality and its vicissitudes. She considers the vocality of groups of seriously mentally ill patients and of groups of people who are marginalised within the wider society, whose voices are muffled and unheard. Clinical work with such populations contributes to their integration into the society, and, thus, is also a political process.

Section II concerns the personification of co-created roles in the foundation matrix and in the dynamic matrices of various groupings. In Chapter 4, "Personification and Polarisation within the Foundation Matrix of Israel: A Case Example", Yossi Triest describes the unconscious impact of the new technology on our psychic lives. Such technology consists of tools and equipment as the Internet, the smartphone, and social media in general. He uses the suggestive notion of the I-Group, which is more than merely a group of people who are connected through the media. He illustrates this phenomenon with a clinical case who he regards as having the head of a person but the body of a crowd, by which he means a person who has been sucked into a role in a group who has become aggregated.

In Chapter 5, "Nikola Tesla and the Social Unconscious of Serbs: The Dance of Science with Poetry, and of the Earthly with the Heavenly", Marina Mojovic and Jelica Sataric write about Nikola Tesla, who was a Serb-American scientist who worked for Thomas Edison, the famous American inventor. Tesla was never fully recognised for his genius, in and by the "West". This was in marked contrast to how highly and almost universally he was celebrated in Serbia, whose values and cultural tropes he personified.

In Chapter 6, "Sex, Custom and Madness: A Case Study of the Personification of the Tripartite Matrix of South-Africa by a South-African Psychiatrist", Penelope

Busetto examines concepts of social and physical evolution in 19th-century anthropology, and their significance in the early development of psychoanalysis. They were imported into psychiatry and social psychiatry in South Africa, supported by more general thinking about races and the so-called primitive "Black mind", and then used to legitimise such thinking. These processes were personified by Laubscher, a well-known psychiatrist who was regarded as modern and scientific.

Section III concerns personification in clinical work. In Chapter 7, "Transference, Countertransference and the Social Unconscious: The Bastion in Clinical Figurations in Tripartite Matrices", Carla Penna draws on the work of several exceedingly important but often neglected South American psychoanalysts such as Pichon-Riviere, Bleger, and Racker. The group bastion is a feature of the tripartite matrix as-a-whole, as illustrated in the context of clinical work in contemporary Brazil. The group bastion is a manifestation of a collective transference (Hopper, 2007).

In Chapter 8, "Recognizing Codes of Superiority in Clinical Work: Social Unconscious, Racism, Sexism and other Elements of Intersectionality", Kavita Avula illustrates the personification of roles in the dynamic matrices of professional organisations in our field in the United States, but which have considerable parallels with such organisations in other countries, such as England. She focuses on the intersectionality of race, sex, and gender, but also refers to social class. Avula illustrates how relational styles of thinking and working with countertransference and transparency can help ameliorate the unconscious restraints and constraints of transgenerational prejudice and discrimination.

In Chapter 9, "The White Mirror: Face to Face with Racism in Group Analysis", Anne Aiyegbusi discusses her innovative concept of the White mirror in which both the conductors of groups and other participants in them are defensively blinded from recognising the pains of racial trauma that are carried by both non-White and White members of them. This exemplifies the insidious power of systemic racism, which exemplifies the social unconscious as a property of the foundation matrix, and, thus, the ways in which it saturates the dynamic and personal matrices of organisations and groups within a particular society.

The fourth section of this volume addresses a selection of topics in the study of the social unconscious. The first topic concerns envy in the context of the intersectionality of class and gender. In Chapter 10, "'They Envy Us': Privilege and Power Relations in the Social Unconscious", Avi Berman focuses on envy in intergroup relations and considers several social defences against collective patterns and expressions of envy. This is particularly important in the study of the social unconscious, because envy is so often regarded by psychoanalysts as an expression of the death instinct rather than as a defence against helplessness (Hopper, 2003b).

In Chapter 11, "Bigenderality, Bisexuality, Foundation Matrix and the Social Unconscious", Gila Ofer explores gender and sex identity as rooted in the foundation matrix. She acknowledges the importance of unconscious aspects of bisexuality and bigenderality as well as fluidity. The distinction between sex and gender is at the very heart of the theory of the social unconscious, having been a particular interest in the work of early social psychoanalysts such as Karen Horney. One of the first references to the social unconscious in group analysis was that of Foulkes to the social nature of femininity.

In Chapter 12, "Fear of Envy and Dispossession: The Evil Eye", Leyla Navaro illustrates how women, especially in Turkey as a "traditional society", unconsciously avoid competition because "winning" is likely to lead to the experience of being envied, and, therefore, to various forms of "envy pre-emption" as socially patterned defences against this. She explores the dynamics of envy with particular reference to the "evil eye" as a talisman against malevolent envy and the destructive expressions of it. Navaro introduces the suggestive idea that envy can lead to the scapegoating of the "self" as well as of the "other".

The next topic is substance addiction and abuse. In Chapter 13, "Addiction in Egypt in the context of its Foundation Matrix", Mona Rakhawy and Nabil Elkot describe the history of addiction and substance abuse in Egypt, and the administration of the treatment of it. They recognise that at a particular time and in a particular society, it is not always clear whether addictive behaviours are regarded as pathological. They also recognise the political nature of the illegal use of substances and the social control of it.

In Chapter 14, "Dangerous Desire: Addiction, Consumption and Recovery", Martin Weegmann traces the etymology and imagery of addiction, mainly to alcohol and mainly in England. The use and abuse of alcohol is as ancient as our knowledge of how to manage the fermentation of various substances. It is socially and culturally patterned, as is the treatment of it.

The third topic concerns the inability to mourn the loss of various social, political, and economic arrangements, recognising that some sections of the population might welcome the loss of these arrangements, and even define this as a social gain. In Chapter 15, "The Brexit Referendum and the Inability to Mourn: Equivalence in a Large Group", Frances Griffiths considers some of the social dynamics that underpinned Brexit, of which people seem to be unconscious. This could be seen in a Large Group that was convened shortly after the Brexit referendum. She traces the dynamics of the inability to mourn in the foundation matrix of the contextual society, the dynamic matrices of the Group Analytic Society International and the Institute of Group Analysis (UK), and in the personal matrices of several participants in the group through their personification of roles that were unconsciously co-created in the group.

In Chapter 16, "The Inability to Mourn and the Manic Defense of Reconstruction in Post-World War Japan", Kai Ogimoto and Tomas Plaenkers describe the inability to mourn after World War II in Japan, and how the manic defences against the pain of mourning can be seen in the intensity of the subsequent investment in and the development of its economy. This socially unconscious defence is also traced to more traditional aspects of the society, such as various myths.

In Chapter 17, "Social Unconscious and Group Psychotherapy in Georgia", Rezo Korinteli describes the development and practice of group analysis and group psychotherapy more generally in post-Soviet Georgia, in which colleagues struggled with their confusions and conflicts concerning nostalgia and idealisation of Soviet rule, conflicts between biological and sociological world views, and the consequences of specific social traumas. The inability to mourn has influenced the development of treatment modalities.

This volume ends with Chapter 18, "The Trilogy Matrix Event (TME): A Setting for the Study of the System Dynamics of Large Group", in which Richard Morgan-Jones describes a new technique for the exploration of the dynamics of the tripartite matrix of larger groups. TME offers an exceedingly generative way for elucidating the various sub-matrices and their dimensions of the tripartite matrix of a particular organisation, and perhaps of a particular society more generally. This chapter, drawing on the study of constructed large groups as well as of social dreaming matrices, also functions as a kind of Epilogue. The continuing study of the social unconscious will always recognise that it is a dynamic function of the tripartite matrix as-a-whole.

Notes

1 This Introduction is based on an article in *Group* (2018a); an edited version was published in *Group Analysis* (2018b).
2 These confusions between homologies and analogies were hardly uncommon. For example, in the first edition of his *magnum opus*, Herbert Spencer referred to societies *as* organisms, but in the later editions of it said that they were *like* organisms. Of course, the basic conceptualisation of systems of social systems had not yet been developed.
3 This reminds me of Thornton Wilder's (1938) "Our Town", in which the problem of how to address letters is raised – in the US, as in the UK, the street address is given before the country, but in other countries, the street address is given after the country, which might well have unconscious implications for the balance between a local and a cosmopolitan identity.

References

Agazarian, Y. & Gantt, S. (2000). *Autobiography of a Theory: Developing a Theory of Living Human Systems and its Systems-Centered Practice.* London: Jessica Kingsley.

Bion, W.R. (1961). *Experiences in Groups.* London: Tavistock.

Bourdieu, P. (2000). *Pascalian Meditations.* Stanford, CA: Stanford University Press.

Dajani, K. (2017). The Ego's Habitus: An examination of the role culture plays in structuring the ego. *International Journal of Applied Psychoanalytic Studies*, 14: 273–281.

Dalal, F. (2022). Ethics and the bureaucratization of the psychotherapy professions. *Group Analysis*, 55 (3): 353–371.

Davies, J. (2018). *The Making of Psychotherapists: An Anthropological Analysis.* London: Routledge.

De Maré, P. (1972). *Perspectives in Group Psychotherapy.* London: Allen & Unwin.

Foulkes, S.H. (1948). *Introduction to Group Analytic Psychotherapy.* London: Karnac, 1983.

Foulkes, S.H. (Ed.) (1990). *S.H. Foulkes: Selected Papers.* London: Karnac.

Foulkes, S.H. & Anthony, E.J. (1957). *Group Psychotherapy: The Psychoanalytical Approach.* Second Edition. London: Karnac, 1984.

Frie, R. (2022). *Culture, Politics and Race in the Making of Interpersonal Psychoanalysis: Breaking Boundaries.* London: Routledge.

Fromm, E. (1970). *The Crisis of Psycho-Analysis.* Harmondsworth: Penguin.

Gonzales, F. (2020). First world problems and gated communities of the mind: Ethics of place in psychoanalysis. *The Psychoanalytic Quarterly* 89 (4): 741–770.

Hobson, R. (1974). *The Archetypes of the Collective Unconscious.* London: Routledge.

Hopper, E. (1975). A sociological view of large groups. In L. Kreeger (Ed.). *The Large Group: Dynamics and Therapy* (pp. 159–192). London: Constable. Reprinted in 2003 in *The Social Unconscious: Selected Papers.* London: Jessica Kingsley.

Hopper, E. (1981). *Social Mobility: A Study of Control and Insatiability.* Oxford: Blackwell.

Hopper, E. (2003a). *The Social Unconscious: Selected Papers.* London: Jessica Kingsley.

Hopper, E. (2003b). *Traumatic Experience in the Unconscious Life of Groups.* London: Jessica Kingsley.

Hopper, E. (2007). Theoretical and conceptual notes concerning transference and countertransference processes in groups and by groups, and the social unconscious: Part III. *Group Analysis*, 40 (2): 285–300.

Hopper, E. (Ed.) (2012). *Trauma and Organizations.* London: Karnac.

Hopper, E. (2018a). Notes on the concept of the social unconscious in Group Analysis. *Group*, 42 (2): 99–118.

Hopper, E. (2018b). The development of the concept of the Tripartite Matrix: A response to 'Four modalities of the experience of others in groups' by Victor Schermer. *Group Analysis*, 51 (2): 197–206.

Hopper, E. (2022a). Notes on the theory and concept of the fourth basic assumption in the unconscious life of groups and group-like social systems: Incohesion: Aggregation/Massification or (ba) I:A/M. In C. Penna (Ed.). *From Crowd Psychology to the Dynamics of Large Groups: Historical Theoretical and Practical Considerations* (pp. 176–208). London: Routledge.

Hopper, E. (2022b). From remorse to relational reparation: Mature hope, communication, and community in our responses to social conflict and to the virus as a persecuting object. *Contexts,* Issue 95, March.

Hopper, E. (2022c) (In Press). "Notes" on processes of fundamentalism in the context of the basic assumption of Incohesion: Aggregation/Massification or (ba) I:A/M. In G. Ofer. & A. Berman (Eds). *Tolerance – Coping with Painful Otherness: Psychoanalytic, Group Analytic and Organisational Perspectives.* London: Routledge.

Hopper, E., & Weinberg, H. (Eds.) (2011). *The Social Unconscious in Persons, Groups, and Societies: Volume 1: Mainly Theory.* London: Karnac.

Hopper, E., & Weinberg, H. (Eds.) (2016). *The Social Unconscious in Persons, Groups, and Societies: Volume 2: Mainly Foundation Matrices.* London: Karnac.

Hopper, E., & Weinberg, H. (Eds.) (2017). *The Social Unconscious in Persons, Groups, and Societies: Volume 3: The Foundation Matrix Extended and Re-configured.* London: Karnac.

Kaës, R. (2006). *Linking, Alliances, and Shared Space: Groups and the Psychoanalyst.* Andrew Weller (trans). London: Karnac.

King, P. & Steiner, R. (1991). *The Freud/Klein Controversies* 1941–45. London: Routledge, 2015.

Layton, L. (2020). *Toward a Social Psychoanalysis: Culture, Character and Normative Unconscious Processes.* London: Routledge.

Lewin, K. (1951). *Field Theory in the Social Sciences.* New York: Harper & Row.

Little, M. (1985). Winnicott working in areas where psychotic anxieties predominate: A personal record. *Free Associations*, 1: 9–42.

Loewald, H. (1978). *Psychoanalysis and the History of the Individual.* New Haven, CT & London: Yale University Press.

Long, S. (2013). The associative unconscious. In S. Long (Ed.). *Socio-Analytic Methods: Discovering the Hidden in Organisations and Social Systems.* London: Karnac. pp. 3–22.

Losso, R., de Setton, L. & Scharff. D. (2017). *The Linked Self in Psychoanalysis: The Pioneering Work of Enrique Pichon Riviere*. London: Karnac.

Mannheim, K. (1929). *Ideology and Utopia: An Introduction to the Sociology of Knowledge*. London: University of London.

Mies, T. (2022). Personal communication.

Mills, C.W. (1956). *The Power Elite*. Oxford: University Press.

Nitzgen, D. & Hopper, E. (2017). The concepts of the social unconscious and of the matrix in the work of S.H. Foulkes. In E. Hopper, & H. Weinberg (Eds). *The Social Unconscious in Persons, Groups, and Societies: Volume 3: The Foundation Matrix Extended and Re-Configured* (pp. 3–27). London: Karnac.

Ogden, T.H. (2005) *The Art of Psychoanalysis: Dreaming Undreamt Dreams and Interrupted Cries*. New York: Routledge.

Penna, C. (2015). Psychoanalytic investigations on collective grief. *Cadernos de psicanalise* (Rio de Janeiro) 37 (33): 9–30.

Penna, C. & Hopper, E. (2022). Commentary on the special edition on developments in the field theory of the European Journal of Psychotherapy & Counselling Fields, systems and silos: From Electromechanics to the matrix. *European Journal of Psychotherapy & Counselling*, 24 (1): 127–147.

Pertegato, E.G. & Pertegato, G.O. (Eds.) (2013). *From Psychoanalysis to Group Analysis: The Pioneering Work of Trigant Burrow*. London: Karnac.

Rao, J.M. (2022). The insistence on exclusion: The anti-integrative impulse and thwarted mourning in large groups. *International Journal of Applied Psychoanalytic Studies*, 19 (2): 217–229.

Scharff, D. & Scharff, J. (2011). *The Interpersonal Unconscious*. Northvale, NJ: Jason Aronson.

Scholz, R. (2022). 45th Foulkes Lecture "When foundation matrices move – challenges for a group analysis of our time". *Group Analysis*, 55 (4): 483–497.

Spector, E. (1992). Romantic love: At the intersection of the psyche and the cultural unconscious. In T. Shapiro and R. Emde (Eds). *Affect: Psychoanalytic Perspective* (pp. 383–411). New York: International Universities Press.

Wilder, T. (1938). *Our Town: A Play in Three Acts*. New York: Coward-McCann Inc. Reprinted in 2020 by Harper Perennial.

Part I

The tripartite matrix of social systems

1 The cornerstone, once more

Dieter Nitzgen

Ever since his first book, Foulkes pointed out the 'growing recognition of the basic importance of society' for psycho-analysis and group analysis alike (Foulkes, 1983, p. 11). In the 1960s, he refined this view when he said: 'In group analysis, and to growing extent in psychoanalysis, we realize that the social and cultural element is deeply ingrained in the individual and is, to a large extent, unconscious' (Foulkes, 1990, p. 163).

Introduction

For Foulkes, the notion of *interdisciplinarity* was a key feature of the group analysis. In my approach, he explained to the members of the British Psychoanalytical Society (BPS) in April 1946, 'the qualifying word "analysis" does not refer to psychoanalysis alone, but reflects at least, *three* different influences, all of which operate actively', namely 'psychological analysis' according to Kurt Goldstein and Adhémar Gelb (Foulkes, 1990, p. 129), 'psychoanalysis itself' (aao., p. 128)and 'sociological analysis' according to Karl Mannheim (aao., p. 131) and Norbert Elias (Foulkes, 1983, pp. 13–14). Favouring an interdisciplinary approach, Foulkes definitively differed from other contemporary psychoanalysts, like, for instance, John Rickmann who in his important paper on 'Numbers and the Human Sciences' privileged psychoanalysis as the *leading* science even beyond the classical setting (Rickmann, 1950; cf. Rickman, 1951). Following the scientific legacy of the *Frankfurt School* (Jay 1973; Rothe 1989), Foulkes was reluctant to consider group analysis as 'merely' an '*application*' of psychoanalytic principles (Foulkes, 1983, p. 154). As can be gathered from his papers, early and later ones, this legacy informed his whole work, and is perhaps most clearly spelt out in his reflections on social psychiatry (cf. Foulkes, 1969). Moreover, it also and crucially influenced the conceptualization of group-analytic *terms* which Foulkes insisted requires the elaboration of 'group' '*equivalents* of processes which are known to us from psychoanalysis' (Foulkes & Anthony, 1984, p. 263; italics i. orig.). A good example of this is the elaboration of the concept of the 'group-matrix'.

DOI: 10.4324/9781003425915-3

Theoretical foundations

The making of the matrix

The first time Foulkes referred to the 'group matrix' was in the very same paper in which he introduced the notion of the 'social unconscious' (Foulkes, 1950/1984, p. 52). Focusing on the group as a whole, he spoke of it as 'a common matrix inside which all other relationships develop' (Foulkes, 1984, p. 49). Building on this, he then described the group matrix as '*relatedness* seen as taking place within an all-embracing group matrix' (Foulkes & Anthony, 2014, p. 217; italics mine). Comparing it to the concept of repression which for Freud had been the 'cornerstone on which the whole structure of psychoanalysis rests' (Freud, 1915, p. 16), Foulkes considered the group matrix as 'the *cornerstone* of our working theory' (ibid.) this was, a stone on which he kept working and reworking. Although not always noted by his colleagues, the conceptualization of the matrix took time, basically from the 1950s to the 1970s. There are a number of milestones to map his progress.

The group as a model of the mental apparatus

The first milestone was to link the notion of the group matrix to mental representations. Elaborating what he called 'group equivalents of processes which are known to us from psycho-analysis' (Foulkes & Anthony, 2014, p. 249), Foulkes in the 1950s took an important step when he wrote: 'The group is *like* a model of the mental apparatus in which its / internal / dynamics are *personified* and *dramatized*' (Foulkes, 1984, p. 114). Due to this, he argued that in the group-analytic situation, the group members may represent the internal agencies of 'Freud's so called "structural model" of the psyche (Freud, 1923b), namely the ego, the superego and the id' (Foulkes, 1984, p. 112). However, and in addition to the *personification* of these intrapsychic agencies, Foulkes also forged a link between the notion of the group matrix and the psychoanalytic view of an inner world of conscious and unconscious self – and object *representations* (cf. Foulkes, 1984, pp. 113–115), namely the representations of family figures (mother, father, siblings) as well as 'parts of the *self*, the *body* (-*image*) and even "*collective* images"' (cf. Foulkes, 1984, p. 115; italics mine). Generalizing this, he concluded that due to their *personification,* 'unconscious processes can be *represented* by persons' (Foulkes, 1984, p. 289; italics mine). By considering the group situation as a locus of *mental* representations, he thus added clinical precision of what he had termed as a 'network of communication' (Foulkes, 1984, p. 66) in terms of a '*mental* field' or a '*mental* matrix' (Foulkes, 1984, p. 118). 'In the mental matrix', he wrote, 'individuals also emerge, but their boundaries do not run parallel of their physical person' (Foulkes, 1984, p. 118; italics mine). However, whilst in the 1950s the range of these mental representations was more or less limited to conscious and unconscious aspects of the self and the family, as in psychoanalysis, this view was extended in the 1960s.

Extending group representations beyond the family

From early on, Foulkes maintained that 'it is true that the family is a group but not that the group is family' (Foulkes, 1984, p. 60). In Northfield, he already realized that the group (as a whole) also 'symbolizes the community as a whole' (Foulkes, 1983, p. 168; cf. Foulkes, 1984, pp. 114–15). From this, he concluded that group members collectively '*constitute the very Norm from which individually the deviate*' (Foulkes, 1983, p. 29; italics mine). Due to this, socio-cultural values and norms always depend 'on the valuation of the particular community (tribe, nation, period)' to which its members '*implicitly* subscribe' (Foulkes, 1984, p. 92). Consequently, they are subject of and subjected to conscious and unconscious conflicts within themselves and within community that go beyond family matters. Hence, the vocation of group analysis already emphasized in its inaugural paper (Foulkes & Lewis, 1944) was to contribute to the group member's education as 'responsible citizens' (cf. Foulkes, 1984, p. 21; cf. 1984, pp. 64–65; de Maré et al., 1991, Hopper, 2003a). However, it was only in the 1960s, when Foulkes conceptualized this more systematically. In 1960, he wrote: 'The individual considered *in isolation* appears to be motivated by his *personal history* and the resources of his *body*' with psychoanalysis going 'farthest in this study' (Foulkes, 1984, p. 169; italics mine). However, he added, 'The individual in life is *equally* determined by the *various groups* of which he is a part, some more, some less fundamental: his *culture*, his *nation*, his *family*, his *clan*, his *time*' (Foulkes, 1984, p. 169; italics mine). Accordingly, individual group members not only represent themselves and/or their family of origin but also and always the various socio-cultural (sub-)groups they are part of. Putting this forward, Foulkes not only extended the range and scope of *conflicting* representations, conscious and unconscious ones in the group, but also that of analytic interventions to be applied in groups from the classical *interpretation* of (*repressed*) 'familio-centric' (de Maré et al., 1991, p. 8) meanings to the confrontation of *denied* social conflicts and social *trauma*. In a paper dedicated to clarify opposing views of 'social psychiatry', he neatly summarized the model of group analysis as it had emerged towards the end of the1960s. He wrote: 'Illness emerges as a social, interpersonal process' whose psycho-social analysis is of particular value in bringing to light the concealed meaning and significance (…) in which this illness appears by furnishing a key, in particular, to the approach to *unconscious processes* in three areas:

'the personal, repressed meaning based on the original family group, in psychoanalysis;
the unconscious, interpersonal interaction, the 'social unconscious' , in group analysis;
the society's ills, and the unconscious origins of much human behaviour' (Foulkes, 1990, p. 203; italics i. orig.).

It will be noticed though that at the end of the 1960s, Foulkes still opposed the range and scope of psychoanalysis and group analysis in terms of their scope, a view he then revised in the advanced model of the group matrix as the locus of socio-cultural inheritance and transmission.

The group matrix as the locus of cultural transmission

Towards the end of the 1950s, Foulkes turned from '*biological*' to '*cultural* inheritance' (cf. Foulkes, 1984, p. 155). Building on the evolutionary biology of Julian Huxley, he asserted that 'modern zoo-ology has arrived at the conclusion that cultural inheritance has superseded biological inheritance in its importance for the human species' (Foulkes, 1984, p. 142). Leaning on Huxley's conception of bio-psycho-social evolution, Foulkes envisaged an ongoing process of socio-cultural transmission 'from generation to generation from the earliest days onwards' (Foulkes, 1990, p. 252; italics ours), a process that he emphasized cannot be seen 'entirely or even predominantly as a genetic and biological one, but more as a cultural inheritance'.

Trying to meet the conceptual challenges of what Huxley dubbed as 'the modern synthesis' (Huxley, 1942), Foulkes in the 1960s called for more adequate concepts 'which from the beginning do justice to an integrated view' of biological and cultural evolution (Foulkes, 1984, preface). Due to this, he eventually revised some of the Freudian foundations of group analysis, for instance, Freud's view of the Oedipus-Complex as 'a precipitation of pre-history' (Foulkes, 1983, p. 14) and 'rooted in biology' (Foulkes, 1990, p. 235). He had already questioned this first book (Foulkes, 1983, pp. 14–15), but he now conceived it as 'a product of the whole family group' (Foulkes, 1990, p. 236). Moreover, he claimed that 'even the libidinal phases and bodily functions are *culturally* conditioned' (Foulkes, 1990, p. 275; italics mine) as is 'infantile sexuality' (Foulkes, 1990, p. 155). Finally, he also abandoned Freud's initial 'one-person concept' (Foulkes, 1984, p. 289) of free association as being based 'on traces in the brain' (Foulkes, 1990, p. 156) in favour its '*social equivalent*' (Foulkes, 1984, p. 289; italics mine), as 'a free association of ideas in the group' (ibid.). Positing that 'ideas and comments expressed by different members' have 'the *value* of unconscious interpretations' (Foulkes, 1990, p. 157. italics mine), he concluded that they are to be considered as 'quasi associations to a common /cultural / context' (Foulkes, 1990, p. 157) based on 'the common ground of members' 'unconscious *instinctive understanding* of each other' (ibid.). Regarding these revisions, Foulkes was well aware to have made 'a decisive step regarding method as well as theory' (Foulkes & Anthony, 1984, p. 29), a step whose importance at the time was neither fully realized by the members group-analytic community nor appropriately appreciated (cf. Brown & Zinkin, 1994, pp. 1–11, 232–253).

The individual as a representative of culture and society

The first time he publicly presented the revised foundations of group analysis was at the *Third International Congress of Group Psychotherapy* in Milan 1963 (cf. Foulkes, 1990, pp. 151–158; cf. Foulkes & Anthony, 1984, pp. 26–28). In Milan, he stated:

> The culture and values of the community to the growing infant by its individual father and mother as *determined* by the their particular nation, class, religion and region. They are transmitted *verbally* and *nonverbally, instinctively* and *emotionally* 24 hours a day.
>
> (Foulkes, 1990, p. 155; cf. Foulkes & Anthony, p. 1984, p. 29; i)

Moreover, he emphasized that 'even *movements, gestures* and *accents* are determined in this way by the *representatives* of the cultural group' (ibid.; italics mine). However, what applies to the individual parents also applies as we have already pointed out to each and every individual, namely that it represents not just itself, i.e. its self, but also the 'various groups of which he is a part' (Foulkes, 1984, p. 169). Compared to the initial definition of the individual as 'a nodal point' in a network given in his first book (Foulkes, 1983, p. 14), its revision as "a *representative* of its various socio-cultural 'groups of belonging'" (Rouchy, 1993, 1987; cf. Leroy, 1994) added considerable theoretical and clinical substance to its definition. Whilst the former was basically empty, the latter actually succeeded to link the psyche and the social world (and in so far it is closely related to what Elias (1939a, 1939b) and later Bourdieu (1982) described as '*habitus*'). Moreover, focusing on the process of transmission, Foulkes made it very clear in his description that as a process, transmission by far transcends the limits of *symbolic* language and speech. Proceeding *in* different *modes* or 'keys' (Foulkes, 1990, p. 181) and *on* different 'levels', 'conscious, preconscious and unconscious' (Foulkes, 1990, p. 213) as well as '*nonconscious*' ones (cf. Hopper & Weinberg; 2011). It includes 'acts, active messages, verbal behaviour, actions, movements, expressions of mood, various emotions, silent transmissions, eventually even "telepathic" ones (Foulkes, 1990, p. 213) and thus operates well beyond Freud's psychoanalytic notion of repression' (cf. Foulkes, 1984, pp. 260–262).[1]

The matrix as a tripartite structure

Viewed from the perspective of cultural inheritance and its transmission, the extension of the group matrix appears as a logical consequence. Confronted with the conceptual challenges involved in its conceptualization, Foulkes eventually realized that the concept of the matrix needed to be differentiated as this was the only way to conceptualize the two *dimensions* missing in his earlier model of group communication, namely that of *history* and of *evolution*. Neither of them could be elaborated in terms of a theory of communication confined to the here-and-now of the consulting room. Therefore, both could only be envisaged in the context of a theory of transmission from one generation to the other, i.e. over time and by integrating historical and evolutionary aspects. In other words, by a vision of the matrix as an ongoing process in which biological and cultural inheritance are completely intertwined. However, to develop such an integrated view depended on the possibility to distinguish different *domains* of the matrix, and thus to differentiate its *structure*. This is what Foulkes did in his opening address to the *First European Symposium of Group Analysis* in Estoril, 1970 where he first introduced such an advanced concept of the group matrix in terms of a '*dynamic*' and a '*foundational*' matrix, the latter to be understood as 'a pre-existing relatively stable part' of it (Foulkes, 1990, p. 215) and the former as a theatre of operation that develops 'under our eyes' (Foulkes, 1990, p. 213). However, it was only in his last book (Foulkes, 1975) where Foulkes supplemented the twofold structure of the matrix by the third element he termed as the 'personal matrix'. Thereby he finally established the 'tripartite matrix' (Burruth, 2008; Nitzgen & Hopper, 2017; Hopper, 2020, 2021) as the ultimate frame of reference for group-analytic theory and practice.

Notes on the 'personal matrix'

The concept of a 'personal matrix' came late in the work of Foulkes. There is only once reference to it in Foulkes last book on *Method and Principles* of group-analytic psychotherapy (Foulkes, 1986, p. 112). May be this is the reason why the last part of the group matrix remained an inchoate concept that never attracted much attention in the group-analytic community. However, conceptually, it is intriguing for various reasons. Representing an essential element of the matrix as a tripartite structure (Nitzgen & Hopper, 2017; Hopper, 2020), it functions as a key or capstone of the advanced model matrix. To remove it would render it as structurally incomplete, unmoored and loosing consistency. However, although it remained an unfinished project that Foulkes himself could not bring to fruition during his lifetime and thus left it a heritage and a legacy, the concept of the 'personal matrix' was Foulkes most advanced attempt to elaborate a group-analytic 'equivalent' of Freud's 'structural theory' of the mental apparatus (Freud, 1923b). To introduce it, Foulkes wrote: 'Just as the individual's *mind* is a complex of interacting processes (*personal* matrix), *mental* processes interact in the concert of the group' (Foulkes, 1986, p. 130; italics mine). This description relates to his earlier postulation of the existence of 'group mind' in addition to an 'individual mind' (Foulkes, 1984, p. 118) in the sense of a 'mental field' (ibid.). In the mental matrix, he wrote, 'individuals also emerge, but their boundaries 'do not run parallel of their physical person' (Foulkes, 1984, p. 118)'(...) However, although Foulkes since the 1950s had began to conceptualize the matrix as a locus of (internalized) mental representations, first 'familio-centric', later socio-centric ones, he was not yet able to theorize this in terms of the matrix itself as a *structure*. Accordingly, he did not yet think in terms of different 'parts' or 'domains' of it.

Therefore, although he already recognized the individual as being subjected to a *double* determination, namely to the constraints *and restraints* of the body and to those of his community and culture, Foulkes was also not yet prepared to understand this double determination and its dynamics as an expression of an ongoing *dialectic* between the family and its surrounding culture and society.

In the second issue of his book written by E.J. Anthony, he came closest to it when he wrote about this dialectic: 'The conflict at bottom is one between the individuals's instinctive impulses and his group's cultural taboos' (Foulkes & Anthony, 1994, p.26; cf. Nitzgen, 2015). Funnily enough, when he put this on paper, Foulkes had it already in mind that these 'impulses' themselves were as he would say 'culturally conditioned' (Foulkes, 1990, p. 275). To conceptualize this in terms of the matrix as a 'tripartite' structure would take the rest of life. However, by coining the concept of the 'personal matrix', he not only discovered the One in the Many but also the Many in One (Aristotle Metaphysics; cf. Tubert-Oaklander, 2014).

The dialectics of family and culture

For the later Foulkes, 'the family is deeply imbued and totally *conditioned* by the values of its surrounding culture and the reflection of this culture in the particular class to which it belongs' (Foulkes, 1990, p. 206) and whose cultural norms and values this transmits. Therefore, Foulkes posited a *dialectic* between the family and culture which he summarized in a pregnant formula. He wrote: 'In the group-analytic group, the original family is represented by *transference*, the cultural group by the *matrix* in so far as it is shared and has to be shared to start with the "foundation matrix"' (Foulkes, 1990, p. 277; italics mine), whilst the operative network is the 'treatment group itself' (Foulkes, 1990, p. 277). It is the ongoing conflict between both that is constantly played out in the arena of group and its driving force. This is why through the lens of 'tripartite matrix', the individual person appears as 'a *fragment* shaped dynamically by the group he first grew up' (Foulkes, 1990, p. 275; italics). More precisely, *fractal* simultaneously shaped by *transference* and by *tradition* jointly operated in the *dynamic* and the *personal* matrix. It is in this sense we should understand Foulkes' cryptic remark that '"the neurotic person is more *isolated* from society than is good for him", and more *fixated* upon his original group, namely the family group' (Foulkes & Anthony, 2014, p. 216; italics mine).

The social unconscious as part of the tripartite matrix

As we (Nitzgen & Hopper, 2017) have shown in a previous paper, Foulkes initially conceptualized the 'social unconscious' as a *supplement* to the unconscious 'in the Freudian sense', i.e. the *repressed* unconscious (Foulkes, 1984, p. 52; cf. Foulkes & Anthony, 2014, pp. 246–247). However, at some point during the 1960s, Foulkes abandoned this *psychoanalytically* informed understanding of the social unconscious as an 'agency' in its own right, *localized* in the 'mental apparatus' of the individual for a more group-analytic conceptualization of it, located in the group as a whole, namely in its *mental* matrix (Foulkes, 1984, p. 118). He did this by turning to Huxley's theory of socio-cultural inheritance and its transmission. In other words, he located the social unconscious in the ongoing process of transmission, and namely in its pre-conscious, unconscious and non-conscious aspects. However, by making the social unconscious a property of the group and its matrix, the 'old' juxtaposition between the *repressed* unconscious and the denied *social* unconscious becomes obsolete. This is because within the matrix as a tripartite structure, neither of its parts can be separated from other two: neither can the foundation matrix be separated from the dynamic matrix and both from the personal matrix, nor can the repressed unconscious (represented by transference) ever be separated from its socio-cultural foundations. Accordingly, Foulkes emphasized once more what he had claimed in the first book, namely that the 'old juxtaposition of an inside and outside world, constitution and environment, individual and society, phantasy and reality, body and mind, and so on, are *untenable*' (Foulkes, 1983, p. 10; italics), as they are *completely intertwined* within the group matrix.[2]

Clinical considerations

Communication under reduced censorship

Throughout his work, Foulkes insisted that to approach unconscious processes in groups, 'we want means of communication under reduced censorship' (Foulkes & Anthony, 1984, p. 56; italics ours). It is only by 'the relaxation of censorship' (Foulkes & Anthony, 1984, p. 42) that we can get access to repressed psychic facts and to denied social facts. Building on Freud's notion of free association in psychoanalysis, he termed this as a 'free-floating discussion' (Foulkes, 1983, p. 71) or 'free group association' (Foulkes, 1984, pp. 73, 117, 125) as '*the* method of choice' for investigating 'the unconscious mind' in individual and the group (Foulkes, 1983, p. 5). However, although for Foulkes there is but *one* group-analytic method, it is *not* immediately apparent *how* it can be applied to different clinical phenomena, for instance, to 'repressed' *psychic* facts according to Freud and/or to *unaware* social facts. To clarify this, we have to review the initial definition of the social unconscious (Foulkes, 1950). In it, Foulkes argued that 'the group analytic situation while dealing intensively with the unconscious in the Freudian sense brings into operation and perspective a totally different area of which the individual is equally unaware' (Foulkes, 1984, p. 52). Thereby he emphasized that the social unconscious can *only* be brought 'into operation and perspective' in the group while dealing intensively with the unconscious 'in the Freudian sense' (Foulkes, 1984, p. 52). Only *then* it will emerge as 'a totally different area of which the individual is equally unaware'. By using the word unaware (instead of unconscious), Foulkes highlighted the difference between unconscious psychic facts (due to repression) and unaware social facts (due to denial). Therefore, becoming *aware* of *denied* social facts cannot be separated from lifting the *unconscious* meaning psychic facts due to repression. However, although *clinically* both processes work hand in hand, *theoretically* they need to be differentiated from each other. Therefore, on close reading, we find that Foulkes made different *usage* of 'free floating group discussion, and thus opened up different avenues to ways of approaching both unconscious psychic and social facts in the group situation.

A first usage of free-floating discussion

Although he clearly distinguished between unconscious psychic facts and unaware social facts, Foulkes explained the application of 'free floating discussion' first of all with regard to unconscious symptoms (due to repression). Arguing as a Freudian psychoanalyst, in his first book he explained that *symptom*s 'in themselves autistic and unsuitable for sharing, exert for this very reason an increasing pressure upon the individual for expressing them' (Foulkes, 1983, p. 169). Therefore, 'as long as they cannot be expressed "in a better communicable way" the individual finds no real relief' (Foulkes, 1983, ibid.). Accordingly, he could rightfully claim that 'free group association' (Foulkes, 1984, S. 73) is the 'group equivalent' (Foulkes & Anthony, 1984, p. 263) of 'free association' in an individual analysis (Foulkes, 1983, p. 7) and thus the royal road of transforming the libidinal '*energies* invested into these symptoms can be retransformed into exchangeable value (cash, as it were)' (Foulkes, 1983, p. 169). Moreover, he also recognized that 'understanding *oneself*' is a social process involving 'at least two persons' as it 'goes hand in hand with understanding others and being understood by others' (ibid.; italics mine). Hence, the first usage to be made of 'free floating discussion' is the (re-)transformation of libidinal energies 'into ,socially acceptable, articulate language' (Foulkes, 1983, p. 169). However, there is a further use to be made of this discussion, a usage going beyond the interpretation of the repressed meaning of unconscious symptoms.

A further use of free-floating group discussion

One of the most important clinical observations Foulkes made at North-field was that groups and their members consciously and unconsciously talk about their social context. From this, he concluded that 'free association is in *no way independent* of the total situation' (Foulkes, 1983, p. 71), an insight he should elaborate in the course of his work. Building on this observation, Foulkes eventually widened the use and scope of 'free-floating discussion' *beyond* the interpretation of the unconscious meaning (cf. Foulkes & Anthony, 2014, p. 80). For instance, with regard to the understanding of *censorship*. He wrote: 'This reduced censorship must apply *also* to the patient's relationships to others, including the conductor' (Foulkes & Anthony, 2014, p. 80) and thus involves 'the frank disclosure of *personal* feelings and experiences and of feelings towards other members of the group' (Foulkes & Anthony, 2014, p. 82). It is a 'very important feature', he emphasized, that 'enables us to approach what might be called the *social* unconscious, i.e. such social relationships as are not *usually* revealed, or are not even conscious' (Foulkes & Anthony, 2014, p. 80; italics mine). Due to this 'additional advantage' of the group situation, 'each individual's feelings and reactions will reflect the influences exerted on him by other individuals in the group and by the group-as-a-whole' (Foulkes & Anthony, 2014, p. 63). However, there is still another factor inherent in the group situation which for Foulkes was of paramount importance in connection with the social unconscious, namely that 'the small therapeutic group also represents for its members other people or even the *whole community*' (Foulkes & Anthony, 2014, p. 62; italics mine). It is due to this last factor he claimed that the social unconscious is particularly open to 'exact investigation' (Foulkes & Anthony, 2014, p. 63).

The community in the treatment room

In Northfield, Foulkes made a number of observations he first presented in Amsterdam in 1947 and which he then kept reworking, refining and re-conceptualizing through his work. He noticed that:

the collective situation reduces the severity of censorship inside the individual and the Id becomes liberated (1984, p. 89; cf. Foulkes, 1983, p. 164);

at the same time, the group sets up its own boundaries and its own weighty authority 'which is a good match for the ancient superego' (ibid.), as a consequence of this;

the boundaries of the ego, both towards the Id and the superego, are under revision 'in favour of a freer stronger and Ego-structure' (1984, p. 89; cf. Foulkes, 1983, p. 164); and

'the working through of the transference situation in individual analysis has an *equivalent* in the group, namely the *observation* and *interpretation* of individual members' reactions towards the group as a whole towards its task, towards other groups, and of individual members towards each other, towards the group, as well as their reaction to the leader' (Foulkes, 1983, p. 164; italics mine).

A further insight which Foulkes considered as so important that he included it into the list of the four group 'specific therapeutic factors' found by himself and by Eve Lewis (Foulkes & Lewis, 1944; Foulkes, 1983, pp. 166–167) was 'the function of the group as a powerful forum' by symbolizing 'the community as a whole' (Foulkes, 1983, pp. 167–168). Due to this capacity, the group allows the individual to 'see himself in a new light by consent or disapproval' of his peers (Foulkes, 1983, p. 168), namely to compare the view of oneself with that of other group members. However, at this point, it is important to point out that with regard to peer-presence, Foulkes not only referred to the peers in flesh and blood, as persons, but also and especially to their *mental* presence and representation, conscious and unconscious, in *Gestalt* of the community as a whole. Building on this, he eventually came to claim that 'the community is *represented in* the treatment room' (Foulkes, 1990, p. 155; italics). This aspect is also highly relevant for the Foulkes' understanding of group dynamics. Due to the relaxation of censorship also, superegoic values and norms will come to the fore in the group situation and thus can become subject to *comparison* and *contrast* by the group members. Subsequently, it was the view of the group as an arena of conflicting valuations, values and norms which informed the conceptualization of group dynamics according to Foulkes.

A basic law of group dynamics

Foulkes summarized the nexus between the individual, the group and the community as a whole in terms of a structural formula he called '*A Basic Law of Group Dynamics*' (Foulkes, 1983, p. 29; italics i.orig.).

According to this law, 'the group members '*collectively they constitute the very norm from which, individual, they deviate*' (Foulkes, 1983, S. 29–30; italics i. Orig.). As it is too complex to be reviewed here in detail, we will focus on only *one* aspect of this law, namely that the individual is but 'a *variant* of the social norm'. To explain this, Foulkes argued that the community of which the group members are 'a miniature edition' 'itself *determines* what is normal, socially accepted behaviour' (Foulkes, 1983, pp. 29–30; italics mine). Therefore, although it is 'to a *large* extent part of the group to which it belongs', each individual 'to a *smaller* extent, deviates from the abstract model, the Standard, of this "Norm"' (Foulkes, 1983, p. 30; italics mine). Consequently, it is 'just this *deviation* /which / makes it an Individual, *unique*' (ibid.; italics mine). Therefore, structurally speaking for Foulkes, it would be pointless to speak of individual without referring to the social norm (and vice versa as Levi-Strauss has shown; cf. Descola, 2015, pp. 37–38). Moreover, as the individual is modelled on the values and norms of the particular community it is a part of, for instance, those of a military hospital, Foulkes assumed that the analytic group has an '*inherent* pull towards the socially and biologically established norm' (Foulkes, 1983, p. 166).[3]

Asking about the nature of this norm, Foulkes maintained that '*biologically* it is an abstract ideal (e.g. the anatomical norm); *culturally* it depends on the valuation of the particular community (tribe nation, period)' (Foulkes, 1984, p. 92; italics ours). Due to this, what the group members collectively reproduce (without being aware of it) are the valuations (ego, superego) of *their* particular community and/or society, to which they 'subscribe (…) and agree upon implicitly' (Foulkes, 1984, p. 92; italics mine). In this sense, he spoke of the neurotic as 'an exaggeration and caricature of the norm' (Foulkes, 1984, p. 88) and neuroses itself as 'an individual deviation / that / is in conflict with these values' and thus causes 'illness and inner conflict' (Foulkes, 1984, p. 92). However, as it is 're-established in our groups', this conflict becomes 'amenable to revision' (ibid.). Consequently, Foulkes insisted that 'neurosis is not a disease, but arises from problems which concern *everybody*' (Foulkes, 1984, p. 296; italics mine). For the same reason, he considered the group situation as 'an excellent forum for diagnosis and prognosis in a dynamic sense' (Foulkes, 1984, p. 90). However, from Northfield onwards Foulkes continued to emphasize that the 'working through' of conflicts in group-analytic therapy depends on the function of the group as a *forum* representing the community (Foulkes, 1983, p. 168), a function that is required to make a full use of 'free floating discussion'.

The group as a token community

Attempting to clarify some loose ends concerning the 'Basic Law of Group Dynamics' (cf. Foulkes, 1984, pp. 91–92; pp. 296–298), Foulkes remarked that 'the therapeutic analytic group is a *token* community with access to the social, interpersonal unconscious' (Foulkes, 1984, p. 296; italics mine). This is because the group situation itself provides 'the necessary *comparative* basis of observation' (Foulkes, 1984, p. 296; italics ours) to register 'a differential reaction to the same stimulus' (Foulkes, 1984, p. 297, italics i.orig.). Due to this, he argued that 'we can study the interactional processes *in between* persons as well as their *differential* reactions to the *same* current material' (Foulkes, 1984, p. 297; italics mine). Making this statement, he clarified why in his early work he had been shifting between speaking of a *social* and/or an *interpersonal* unconscious. The reason for this is a simple one because the *social* unconscious only emerges out of the group members' 'unconscious *interpersonal* interaction' (Foulkes, 1990, p. 203; italics ours). In other words, in contrast to the *repressed* unconscious, the social unconscious can only be observed and apprehended within the multipersonal group situation. Therefore, the royal road to it depends on a different usage of the group-analytic method of 'free floating group discussion, i.e. one that focuses on the registration and the subsequent analysis of social values and norms the group members *express* or *enact* without being *aware* of it. This is the reason why Foulkes many years later should say that in group-analytic psychotherapy, 'valuations and norms are *re-stated* and *modified* by *comparison, contrast* and *analysis*' (Foulkes & Anthony, 1984, p. 27; italics mine). Therefore, without really explaining, Foulkes since the 1950s made a double usage of 'free floating discussion' in groups, one in the service of uncovering the *meaning* of repressed psychic facts, and the other in the service of confronting *denied* social facts the group members are not consciously aware of. Although he continued to make this double usage of free-floating discussion in later work, Foulkes also continued to refine their theoretical foundations.

A comparative psychopathology

Apart from applying the principle of 'comparative observation' for exploring the social unconscious, Foulkes likewise applied it to psychopathology. 'All psychopathology', he claimed, 'is *essentially* comparative' (Foulkes, 1984, p. 297). Due to this, the group situation is 'an ideal setting' for studying such a 'comparative psychopathology in operation, i.e. in actual living reality' (Foulkes, 1984, p. 296).[4] To illustrate such 'comparative psychopathology', Foulkes referred to the case of the so-called 'murderous mothers' (Foulkes, 1984, p. 259; cf. Anthony, 1957, 2010). As this case has been discussed at some length in a previous paper (Nitzgen & Hopper, 2017, pp. 18–19), it should be enough here to report the gist of it by quoting from the account Foulkes gave on these mothers who harboured *conscious* death wishes towards their children. In his view, this wish was 'an expression of the progressive demoralization of the whole of our culture since the advent of Hitler and Stalin and under the impact of two World Wars and the murder of literary millions of innocent people' (Foulkes, 1984, p. 259). He also wrote that although 'a group of such mothers would show much of the psychopathology of this particular syndrome' (ibid.); the group conductor, E.J. Anthony, did not 'quite recognise this', but only arrived at a 'diagnostic differential classification of this types of mothers' (ibid.).

Notes on technique

As this chapter discusses the theoretical foundations of tripartite matrix, the group-analytic *technique* is not in the foreground.

However, this cannot be entirely ignored. This is why some notes on technique are offered here for reasons of clarification and further discussion. They will focus on two remarks that seem to be immediately relevant for working with the matrix as a tripartite structure. Referring to Fenichel's well-known recommendation to analyse 'from surface to depth' (Fenichel 1941), Foulkes offered an interesting, group-analytic reading of this principle. Making an interpretation, he wrote, 'we should start always from the surface of things, from what is manifestly present' (Foulkes, 1986, p. 115; cf. Foulkes, 1990, p. 182). In group analysis, he cautioned that 'what is surface *changes* as the group as the group progresses' (Foulkes, 1990, p. 181; italics mine). However, he argued that 'the key to what is the most relevant meaning at any time is provided by the group itself' (Foulkes, 1990, p. 181). Following this line of thought, Foulkes in his last book compared the meaning of the German word '*Deutung*' to of '*interpretation*' in English (Foulkes, 1986, p. 114), pointing out that the latter seems to have 'a more rational meaning' than the German original (ibid.). Therefore, '*Deutung*' in German has 'a more restricted field of application but goes *deeper*', whilst *interpretation* in English 'has a wider field of application but remains more on the *surface*' as it 'literary means to point to' (i.e. hin-deuten), namely 'to draw a person's attention to *another meaning* of the line of thought or action he is just pursuing' (Foulkes, 1986, p. 114; italics mine). From this, he concluded that 'to interpret, therefore, is to *transfer* or to translate something from *one context* to *another*' (Foulkes, 1986, 114; italics ours). Thereby he hinted a group-analytic 'equivalent' of interpretation in groups, particularly with regard to the tripartite matrix.

Notes

1 Current authors nowadays speak of 'a primary matrix of intersubjectivity' (cf. Ammaniti & Gallese, 2014, pp. 124–150; cf. Barwick & Weegmann, 2018, pp. 38–39). With the group-analytic model of transmission, Foulkes envisaged such 'primary' matrix, or *magma* (Castoriadis) which at bottom consists of '*objects, movements, gestures* and *accents*' (Foulkes & Anthony, 1984, p. 27) and thus a '*polyphony*' of voices (Bakhtin, 1929; cf Holquist, 1990) or a '*polylogue*'(Kristeva, 1977; cf. de Maré, 1991, p. 167).

2 However, and to avoid the danger of reification, it would perhaps be more appropriate to speak of social *unconsciousness* rather than of '*a* social unconscious' (cf. Weegmann, 2014, pp. 57–81).

3 Evidently, Foulkes modelled his '*Basic Law of Group Dynamics*' on Goldstein's '*Basic Law of Biology*' (Goldstein, 1934) built on 'the fact that the same external change, the *same stimulus* may result in *different reactions*'(Goldstein 2014, p. 100) and on the assumption of a 'relatively constant equilibrium' (Goldstein, 2014, p. 103), i.e. a middle state of tension that is 'specific' for each organism. (Goldstein, 2014, p. 102; cf. Foulkes, 1984, p. 58).

4 Saying this, he varied a principle of Kurt Goldstein who had shown that individual behaviour should not be (mis-) understood as a mere *reaction* to an external stimulus, but rather as a *response* of the organism towards its total situation. Therefore, even at the level of the 'reflex arc', such reactions and/or responses are not *uniform* but *vary* according to the organism's 'total situation' (cf. Goldstein, 2014, pp. 57–84; Foulkes, 1983, p. 1).

References

Ammaniti, M. & Gallese, V. (2014) *The Birth of Intersubjectivity. Psychodynamics, Neurobiology and the Self*, pp. 236. W. W. Norton & Company, New York.

Anthony, E.J. (1957) *A Group of Murderous Mothers. Protokolle of the Second International Congress on Group Psychotherapy (Zürich)*, pp. 137–142. S.Karger, Basle, 1959.

Anthony, E.J. (2010) My Psychoanalyic and Group-analytic Life with S.H. Foulkes. In: *Group Analysis*, 43(1), pp. 81–85.

Bakhtin, M. (1929) *Probleme des Schaffens von Dostojewskij. Dtsch: Probleme der Poetik Dostojewskijs.* Wien, Frankfurt, 1985.

Barwick, N. & Weegmann, M. (2018) *Group Therapy. A Group Analytic Approach.* Routledge, London.

Bourdieu, Pierre (1982) *Die feinen Unterschiede. Kritik der gesellschaftlichen Urteilskraft.* Suhrkamp, Frankfurt am Main.

Brown, D. & Zinkin, L. (Eds). (1994) *Developments in Group-Analytic Theory*, pp. 180–201. Routledge, London.

Burruth, M. (2008) Matriculating the Matrix. In: *Group Analysis*, 41(4), pp. 352–365. Sage, London.

De Maré et al. (1991) *Koinonia. From Hate through Dialogue to Culture in the Large Group.* Karnac, London.

Descola, Ph. (2015) Transformation Transformed. Keynote lecture for the Symposium "Living Structuralism/ Le structuralisme vif. Toronto 2016". *HAU: Journal of Ethnographic Theory* 6(3), 33–44.

Elias, N. (1939a) *Über den Prozeß der Zivilisation. Soziogenetische und psychogenetische Untersuchungen. Erster Band. Wandlungen des Verhaltens in den weltlichen Oberschichten des Abendlandes.* 20., neu durchges. und erw. Auflage, p. 76 u. 82. Suhrkamp, Frankfurt am Main. English: The Civilizing Process (re.edn) Oxford 2000 (Basil Blackwell).

Elias, N. (1939b) Die Gesellschaft der Individuen. In: Edited by Elias, N. *Die Gesellschaft der Individuen*, pp. 15–99. Suhrkamp, Frankfurt, 1988. *English:* The Society of Individuals. Oxford 1991 (Basil Blackwell).

Fenichel, O. (1941). *Problems of Psychoanalytic Technique.* [Trans. by D. Brunswick]. Psychoanalytic Quarterly, Inc., New York.

Foulkes, S.H. (1948) *Introduction to Group Analytic Psychotherapy.* Karnac, London, 1983.

Foulkes, S.H. (1950) Group Therapy. Survey, Orientation, Classification. In: *Therapeutic Group Analysis* Edited by Foulkes, S.H. 1984, pp. 47–53. Karnac, London.

Foulkes, S.H. (1963) Some Basic Concepts in Group Psychotherapy. In: Foulkes, S.H., 1990, Selected Papers: Psychoanalysis and Group Analysis. pp. 151–158.

Foulkes, S.H. (1964) *Therapeutic Group Analysis.* Karnac, London, 1984.

Foulkes, S.H. (1969) Two Opposed Views of Social Psychiatry: The Issue. In: Foulkes, S.H., 1990. Selected Papers. Psychoanalysis and Group Analysis, pp. 195–208.Karnac, London.

Foulkes, S.H. (1972) Oedipus Complex and Regression. In: Foulkes, S.H., 1990. Selected Papers. Psychoanalysis and Group Analysis, p. 135–248. Karnac, London.

Foulkes, S.H. (1975) *Group-Analytic Psychotherapy - Methods and Principles.* Interface, Gordon&Breach, London; repr. 1984 (Karnac).

Foulkes, S.H. (Ed.) (1990) Selected papers. *Psychoanalysis and Group Analysis.* London: Karnac.

Foulkes, S.H. & Anthony, E.J. (1957) *Group Psychotherapy. The Psychoanalytical Approach.* First Edition, repr. Karnac, London, 2014.

Foulkes, S.H. & Anthony, E. J. (1665) *Group Psychotherapy. The Psychoanalytical Approach*. Second Edition, repr. Karnac, London, 1984.

Foulkes, S.H. & Lewis, E. (1944) Group Analysis. A Study in the Treatment of Groups on Group Analytic Lines. In: Foulkes, 1984, pp. 20–37. Karnac, London.

Freud, S. (1915). Repression. *S.E. 14:*141 ff. Institute of Psychoanalysis. London: Hogarth.

Freud, S. (1923b) The Ego and the Id. *S.E.* 19: 1ff. *S.E.* Institute of Psychoanalysis. London: Hogarth.

Goldstein, K. (1934) Der Aufbau des Organismus. Einführung in die Biologie unter besonderer Berücksichtigung der Erfahrungen am kranken Menschen Hg. Thomas Hoffmann und Frank W. Stahnisch. Paderborn 2014 (Wilhelm Fink Verlag) English: Goldstein, K. (1939) *The Organism: A Holistic Approach to Biology Derived from Pathological Data in Man*. American Book Company, New York; New Edition with a foreword from Oliver Sacks. New York 1995 (Zone Books) In: Grossmark, R. & Pine, F. (Eds) *The One And The Many. Relational Approaches To Group Psychotherapy*. Routledge, New York, 2015.

Holquist, M. (1990) *Bakhtin and His World*. Routledge, London, 2002.

Hopper, E. (1985) The Problem of Context in Group Analytic Psychotherapy. A Clinical Illustration and a Brief Theoretical Discussion. In: Edited by M. Pines *W.R. Bion and Group Psychotherapy. A Critical Reappraisal*. Routledge & Kegan, London. Reprinted in Hopper (2003).

Hopper, E. (2003a) *The Social Unconscious: Selected Papers.*Jessica Kingsley, London.

Hopper, E. (2003b) *Traumatic Experiences in the Unconscious Liefe of Groups. The Fourth Basic Assumption: Incohesion: Aggregation/Massification or (ba)I:A/M.*Jessica Kingslesy, London.

Hopper, E. (2020). The tripartite matrix, the basic assumption of Incohesion, and Scapegoating in Foulkesian Group Analysis: Clinical and empirical illustrations, including terrorism and terrorists. *Forum*. Online

Hopper, E. & Weinberg, H. (Eds) (2011) *The Social Unconscious in Persons, Groups and Societies: Volume 1: Mainly Theory*. Karnac, London.

Huxley, J. (1942) *Evolution: The Modern Synthesis*. Allen & Unwin, London.

Jay, M. (1973) *The Dialectical Imagination. A History of the Frankfurt School and the Institute of Social Research 1923–1950*. Little Brown, Bosten Toronto.

Kristeva, J. (1977) *Polylogue*. Seuil, Paris.

LeRoy, J. (1994) Group Analysis and Culture. In: Edited by Brown, D. and Zinkin, L. *Developments in Group-Analytic Theory*, pp. 180–201. Routledge, London.

Nitzgen, D. (2015) Group Psychotherapy: The Psychoanalytical Approach by S.H. Foulkes and E.J. Anthony. From the First to the Second Edition. In: *Group Analysis*, 48(2), pp. 126–136. Sage, London.

Nitzgen, D. & Hopper, E. (2017) The Concepts of the Social Unconscious and the matrix in the work of S.H. Foulkes. In: Hopper. E. & Weinberg, H. (Eds) (2017 The Social Unconscious In Persons, Groups and Societies. Vol. 3 : The Foundation Matrix extended and Re-configured, pp. 3- 22 London 2017 (Karnac).

Rickmann, J. (1950) Number and the Human Sciences. A Short Communication. Based on a talk given to the BPAS in 1950. wellcomelibary.org/item/b20221101. Pp. 218-223.

Rickmann, J. (1951) Methodology and Research in Psychopathology. *Journal of Medical Pschology* 24, 1–7.

Rothe, S. (1989) The Frankfurt School: An Influence on S.H. Foulkes's Group Analysis? *Group Analysis* 22(4), 405–415.

Rouchy, J.-C. (1993) Identification and Groups of Belonging. In: *Group Analysis*, 28(2), pp. 129–140. Sage, London.

Tubert-Oklander, J. (2014) *The One and the Many. Relational Gsychoanalysis and Group Analysis*. Karnac, London.

Weegmann, M. (2014) *The World Within The Group*, pp. 57–81. Karnac, London.

2   The tripartite matrix in Foulkesian Group Analysis[1]

Earl Hopper

In this chapter, I will outline the theory and concept of the tripartite matrix, which I regard as the defining feature of Foulkesian Group Analysis, and as the insignia or hallmark of it. I will illustrate this concept with clinical data from two of my twice weekly groups, the details of which have been changed in order to protect the confidentiality of the members of the groups.

The tripartite matrix: realms and dimensions

In Group Analysis (in contradistinction to what is known in the United States as the "Tavi" orientation, with its emphasis on the work of Melanie Klein, Wilfred Bion, and Henry Ezriel, and on "the group as-a-whole" in the "Here and Now", and perhaps in contradistinction to what is known as "psychoanalytical group therapy", with reference to various psychoanalytical orientations and with less emphasis on the group-as-a-whole), the focus is on human beings/persons in the context of their groups as dynamic open social systems, and analysed in terms of their tripartite matrices. In Latin, "matrix" means fecund womb, and is a linguistic cognate of mater or mother. The word implies both conception and birth. In English, "matrix" means mould or die, the latter having somewhat oxymoronic implications.

As an essential characteristic of the social system of any human grouping, the concept of the tripartite matrix offers not only a way of perceiving society, community, organisations, family, and persons, but also a way of thinking about them. All groups are microcosms of their contextual society and its many organisations and institutions. To a degree, individual persons are also microcosms of their contextual entities, each of which is a kind of social-psychological-organismic fractal of the others (Hopper, 2003a,b, 2018a,b). Hence, the appreciation in Group Analysis of the "social unconscious", which pertains to the sociality of the human nature of persons as well as to the socio-culture of a group and/or of other socio-cultural entities of which their members are unconscious. However, it is important to take account of the fact that persons have bodies, that is, they have organismic materiality, which influences the structures of their social systems, which are rooted in the species but not exclusively so.

The intra-psychic life of persons must be described and understood in terms of the theory and concepts of various depth psychologies. Similarly, the organism of

DOI: 10.4324/9781003425915-4

each person must be described and understood in terms of the biology of it; the life of the group, in terms of group dynamics; and the life of a society, in terms of the social sciences. However, in order to have a more complete understanding of the processes of any one matrix, it is necessary to draw on the perspectives of each and all of the disciplines which specialise in the study of them. Group Analysis is, in effect, an interdisciplinary discipline (Foulkes, 1990, p. 127), or what today is often called a "transdisciplinary" discipline.

Many Jungian colleagues assume the existence of an omnipresent "cosmic matrix". Should this be a matrix in its own right, or a component of the organismic part of the personal matrix? Perhaps a cosmic matrix constitutes the environment of the social system in question. However, given the porous and intertwining nature of the realms of the tripartite matrix, in so far as one wishes to assume the existence of a cosmic matrix, it should be taken as transcending any notion of boundaries between the inside and the outside of any entity.

The equivalence of events among the realms or sub-matrices of the tripartite matrix

Events and processes in the foundation matrix of a contextual society tend to be recapitulated in the dynamic matrix of a group and in the personal matrices of the members of it, and to some degree vice versa. Group analysts refer to the "equivalence" of processes and events in one sub-matrix with those in the other sub-matrices.

The recognition of equivalence is a matter of the perceptions of a participant observer, based on an optimal degree of involvement and detachment (Elias, 1956). This is a matter of the gestalt of the perception of the object. An optician's box of lenses offers a useful metaphor in that any phenomenon can be viewed through the lenses of the foundation matrix, the lenses of the dynamic matrix, and/or the lenses of a personal matrix. This is not merely a matter of binocular vision. In this connection, Pines (1998) has discussed the perception of equivalent phenomena in terms of "frames of reference", which recognises the importance of fields of enquiry and schools of thought.

Equivalence is not only a matter of perception. Equivalence is not derived from the perceptual construct as much as the perceptual construct is derived from the reality of what is perceived.

The phenomenon of equivalence is driven by the need to defend against psychic pain. On the basis of the defences of repression and especially of the disassociative defences of denial and disavowal, what cannot be experienced and considered within a particular sub-matrix is likely to be enacted unconsciously within another sub-matrix in which it is thought that the narratives of these experiences are more likely to be heard and to be heard safely. For example, an angry feeling might be expressed in a person's borygmie, but not in verbal communications between one person and another; feelings and opinions might be expressed between two people, but not elaborated in the context of the group; and what might be elaborated in a group might not be communicated in another space within the contextual organisation and/or society. And vice versa.

Equivalence within the tripartite matrix is expressed through projective and introjective identification, mirroring, and resonance, the pathological and pathogenic forms of which are based on expulsion, sadism, control of the object, turning passive into active, and attempting to communicate that which cannot easily and readily be put into words. This is especially relevant for working with traumatic experience in which there is a desperate urge to communicate through the enactment of the stubbornly sub-symbolic elements of psychic life (Grossmark, 2017).

In the United States, colleagues refer to processes of equivalence in terms of "parallel processes", which implies that such processes are merely random. In systems-centred approaches to therapy and consultation, colleagues refer to processes/events in the group which are thought to be isomorphic with processes/events in a hierarchy of sub-systems (Gantt & Hopper, 2012). Modern Jungians regard equivalence in terms of "synchronicity", which is not a mystical process so much as it is one that is based on an almost infinite number of complex interactions.

The dimensions of the tripartite matrix

Each of the realms or sub-matrices of the tripartite matrix can be considered in terms of a number of dimensions: the patterns of interaction (interpersonal relations); the patterns of *normation* (values and norms); the patterns of communication (verbal and non-verbal); styles of thinking and feeling (for example, instrumental/expressive, local/cosmopolitan, concrete/abstract, visual/non-visual, and priorities of various senses); styles of leadership, followership, and bystandership, etc. The cohesion of the socio-cultural entities in which groups are embedded is based on the integration of their patterns of interaction and the solidarity of their patterns of normation. The dimension of communication is especially important in the dynamic matrix of a group because the cohesion of a group is based on the coherence of its patterns of communication (Hopper, 2003b; Pines, 1998).

Patterns of technology should also be specified (Hopper & Weinberg, 2011). For example, it is important to know how many people one can see and be seen by, and can hear and be heard by, whether or not what is said is commemorated for future generations, and so on. Information technology is virtually a sub-dimension of patterns of communication, especially in virtual groups (Hutchinson, 2017). However, this is alsoimportant more generally. For example, consider the implications of technology for sex and gender identity in connection with fertilisation, gestation, and birth. Does the scientist become father? Can a male be a mother? In the context of IVF, what is the meaning of "father" and "mother"? It may only be a matter of time before we have to redefine these words. Will it soon be easier to change through technology the basic parameters of the species than to change through political processes the basic parameters of our social institutions? After all, if T. S. Eliot could discuss the "linguistic imagination", then surely, we can discuss the "technological imagination". Clearly, patterns of technology shape interpersonal relations, influence values and norms, as well as patterns of communication. They also affect the curves of "effective intelligence" in the population as-a-whole.

Dimensions: Examples	Sub-matrices		
	Foundation Matrix	Dynamic Matrix 1. Organisations 2. Groups	Personal Matrix
Patterns of interpersonal relationships (the interaction system)			
Patterns of values, norms and beliefs (the normation system)			
Patterns of verbal and non-verbal communication			
Styles of thinking and feeling			
Styles of leadership followership and bystandersthip			
Patterns of technology.			

Figure 2.1 The Tripartite Matrix and a Selection of Dimensions of It.

This very condensed outline of the theory of the tripartite matrix is represented in Figure 2.1.

The Reader is invited to provide examples from clinical work in groups for each cell in this diagram of a tripartite matrix, perhaps using the clinical vignettes presented in the third section of this chapter.

Clinical illustrations of equivalence in the tripartite matrix

In clinical work, what is taken up for further exploration is always a matter of judgement. Such work is more of an art form than a matter of technique. Group analysts try to go where it is the "hottest", which is based on an appreciation of the need to work with transference and countertransference processes, especially with respect to all parts of the Oedipus complex and phases of the development of it. In the context of groups, such processes must be understood in both their vertical T and vertical CT-forms directed towards the conductor of the group, and in their horizontal t and horizontal ct-forms directed towards the members of the group (Hopper, 2006, 2007a,b). These processes are almost always interrelated, and define what we regard as a mental field. Moreover, we do not think about transference and countertransference processes only in terms of the repetition in the "Here and Now" of the "Here and Then", but also in terms of the repetition of the "There and Then" and the "There and Now". We are attentive to each cell in the time-space paradigm for each sub-matrix. This includes transgenerational and epigenetic processes within the foundation matrix of the contextual society.

Clinical Vignette 1

An example of equivalence in one of my twice weekly slow-open heterogenous groups can be seen in the symbolism of verbal communications, in a sub-symbolic personal encapsulation (Hopper, 2003b), and in the development of organisational and societal social psychic retreats (Mojovic, 2011):

> During a week in which there was an outbreak of anti-Semitic behaviour in many parts of London, as seen in graffiti and the defacement of tomb stones in two Jewish cemeteries, i.e., a feature of the foundation matrix of the society, a patient who was in training as a group analyst spoke about her anxieties concerning the development of an elitist and mostly Jewish sub-group within the training organisation, i.e. a feature of the dynamic matrix of an important contextual organisation. Another member of the group tearfully recalled traumatic experience that she had more or less encapsulated since she was a child, i.e. a feature of her personal matrix.
>
> At the next session a patient started the group by saying that she had discovered a lump in her breast, which she assumed was a cyst, i.e., a feature of her personal/organismic matrix, and that she had arranged to have this investigated by her surgeon whose name was Dr Greenbaum. The group discussed the likelihood that her surgeon was not only a Jew, but also that his last name sounded like "bomb". They then turned to their anxieties about meeting in an area of London which was regarded as "Jewish", which had become a de facto ghetto.
>
> By way of moving towards a more "complete interpretation" (Hopper, 2003a) of how these communications reflected the equivalence of the foundation, dynamic, and personal matrices of the group, I wondered aloud if there was a "connection" between the "green" of the Greenbaum, the green of so-called "leafy Hampstead", and the recent outbreak of anti-Semitic violence in this area of London. We discussed the symbolic meanings of "green", referring to the green of jealousy and envy, and to the green of hope.

I asked the woman who had begun to speak about her cyst if she felt that she had encapsulated the traumatic experience that was being discussed and experienced in the group, and if this encapsulated experience was also encysted in her breast. She began to cry, exclaiming that in this way she could at least be useful for other people. Another member of the group then replied that perhaps we could be useful to her in providing a space in which she could talk more about what she was locating in her breast. I asked if she regarded me as a kind of psychic surgeon or as a military specialist in defusing explosive devices, perhaps terrorist devices.

I would like to reassure the Reader that the cyst was benign. Dr Greenbaum dealt with it in a satisfactory way. The group continued to meet in leafy Hampstead.

Clinical Vignette 2

Equivalence can also be seen in the following vignette from another mature twice weekly slow-open heterogeneous group:

I brought a new patient into the group. She was the eighth member of the group, and filled a vacancy left by a man who had been in the group for five years. The new patient was thirty-five years of age, a psychiatrist, and a very dark-skinned Sri-Lankan who had come to London with her parents when she was about three years of age. Although she wore Western style clothes, she also wore a lot of jewellery, such as earrings and necklaces, made of chunky gold. She was treated somewhat contemptuously in the group, being teased as someone who could not quite make up her mind as to whether she wanted to be a modern Western woman or a traditional "Indian" woman. Two members of the group continued to use "Ceylon" rather than Sri Lanka. The women in the group expressed their envy of her "interesting" and "exotic" style. A man in the group welcomed her as "bringing something different to the party". Another man said that he was somewhat "frightened" by her "fully dressed" severity.

During the eighth session following her joining the group, a woman said that the group reminded her of what it was like in her own family after the birth of her younger brother. He was deemed to be a new Prince who could do no wrong and was regarded by their mother as having brought new gifts to the family. At the end of the session, the group left the room as usual, but the new patient remained in the foyer. She knocked on the door of my consulting room and reported that someone had "by mistake" taken her black rubber raincoat from the "coat peg", and that to her annoyance she would now be without protection from the rain on her way home.

At the next session, the woman who had taken the coat "in error" returned it to her and apologised for this. She acknowledged that within a few minutes of leaving the premises, she had become aware that she had taken the coat entirely by "accident". She had also become aware that the patient would be exposed to the rain, whereas she herself would be protected by the raincoat. This event was then discussed and explored at some length, often in a very heated way. The group focused on aspects of their personal matrices, such as their ambitions and their experiences as siblings, which involved their desires to have been the "favourite" and the "favoured" of their parents, desires which continued to have a hold on them.

Eventually I suggested that the new patient was experienced as a chosen little brother who was much loved by me. I stressed that not only was she the eighth member of the group, but also that the "accidental borrowing" of the raincoat took place on the eighth session after she was born into the group. I said that in the Jewish religion the eighth day was the day for the ritual circumcision of a boy. The raincoat was regarded unconsciously as foreskin. Obviously, "he" had to be circumcised.

A member of the group said that the new patient was arrogant, as many Jews are, implying that she seemed to think that she had no need for protection and safety as "ordinary" people did. She seemed to regard herself as special. The group discussed whether one had to be a Jew in order to be regarded as a Jew, and whether one had to be a male in order to be regarded as a male. The new patient said that in truth she was not afraid of a little moisture, and that in any case her life was always one of tears.

I said that gender identity was not only a matter of sexual identity, and being "Jewish" might not be merely a matter of ethnic or religious identity. For example, Jewish men were assumed to be more accepting of their "femininity". In an attempt to support me, a man exclaimed that the Ibo were the Jews of West-Africa.

Bringing a new member into the group provoked feelings of anxious resentment towards both the new member and the group analyst. It was necessary to understand the dynamics of sibling relations with regard to envy, competition, and rivalry, primarily in terms of the dynamic matrix of the group and the personal matrices of its members. However, it was also important to consider these issues in association with gender identity, ethnic group identity, and immigration in the context of the foundation matrix of the contextual society. For example, if this group had taken place in the United States, we would have explored feelings about President Trump and his policies concerning the Wall between Mexico and the United States, the relations between the people who support him and those who despise him, racism, social and political exclusion and inclusion, scapegoating, etc.; and if the group had taken place in Greece or Turkey, we would almost certainly have discussed the continuing crises in the Middle East, involving relations between Israel and Palestine, rivalry among ethnic groups, patterns of immigration, etc.

As the sessions continued, we explored many paths of enquiry, for example: the enactment of anti-social tendencies based on the fear of exploring in words and feelings the encapsulated experience of having been displaced by a younger brother; and the blackness of skin colour in "white" societies as a narcissistic injury.

We also explored our feelings about female genital mutilation (FGM) in various ethnic groups in England which were identified in terms of religion, skin colour, country of origin, etc. After all, some females are also circumcised!

Unfortunately, I will not be able to discuss my countertransference processes here, especially in terms of the socially unconscious aspects of them. However, I was undoubtedly challenged to work with many aspects of my social identity, such as my status as an American citizen but a British resident, my being a Jew, and my being the eldest of three sons. In reviewing this chapter, a colleague observed that perhaps I had overlooked the relevance of circumcision practices in the Muslim community. Another colleague observed that perhaps taking the black raincoat was an unconscious attempt to remove "blackness" from the group, and should have been understood as an enactment of reparation rather than as an envious attack. Yet, another colleague with whom I discussed my interpretation suggested that it was "imaginative", which in England means "far-fetched" even if "well meaning". In any case, I am sure that my interpretation reflected my conviction that socially unconscious processes are a function of the tripartite matrix as-a-whole, and that into every life a little rain must fall.

Note

1 This chapter is a revised version of parts of Hopper (2018a,b, 2020). For a more detailed discussion of the theory and concept of the tripartite matrix, see Nitzgen and Hopper (2017). The "tripartite matrix" was coined by Martin Bhurruth (2008). Especially incisive is Powell (1994) which builds on Hopper (2003a). For a general overview of the use of the concept of matrix in Group Analysis, see Ahlin (2019).

References

Ahlin. G. (2019). The group-analytic group matrix concept. *Group Analytic Society Contexts*, 84.

Bhurruth, M. (2008). Matriculating the matrix: A different understanding of psychic structure, resonance and repression. *Group Analysis*, 41, 4, 352–365.

Elias, N. (1956). Problems of involvement and detachment. *British Journal of Sociology*. 7,3, 226–252.

Foulkes, S.H. (1990). *Selected Papers of S.H. Foulkes: Psychoanalysis and Group Analysis*. London: Karnac.

Gantt, S. & Hopper, E. (2012). Two perspectives on a trauma in a training group: The systems-centred approach and the theory of incohesion. In Hopper, E. (Ed). *Trauma and Organisations* (pp. 233–254). London: Karnac.

Grossmark, R. (2017). Narrating the unsayable: Enactment, repair and creative multiplicity in group psychotherapy. *International Journal of Group Psychotherapy*. 67, 1, 27–46.

Hopper, E. (2003a). *The Social Unconscious: Selected Papers*. London: Jessica Kingsley Publishers.

Hopper, E. (2003b). *Traumatic Experience in the Unconscious Life of Groups: The Fourth Basic Assumption: Incohesion: Aggregation/Massification of (ba) I:A/M*. London: Jessica Kingsley Publishers.

Hopper, E. (2006). Theoretical and conceptual notes concerning transference and counter-transference processes in groups and by groups, and the social unconscious: Part I. *Group Analysis*, 39, 4, 549–559.

Hopper, E. (2007a). Theoretical and conceptual notes concerning transference and countertransference processes in groups and by groups, and the social unconscious: Part II. *Group Analysis*, 40, 1, 21–34.

Hopper, E. (2007b). Theoretical and conceptual notes concerning transference and countertransference processes in groups and by groups, and the social unconscious: Part III. *Group Analysis*, 40, 2, 285–300.

Hopper, E. (2018a). Notes on the concept of the social unconscious in Group Analysis. *Group,* 42, 2, 99–118.

Hopper, E. (2018b). The development of the concept of the tripartite matrix: A response to 'four modalities of the experience of others in groups' by Victor Schermer. *Group Analysis,* 51, 2, 197–206.

Hopper, E. (2020). The tripartite matrix, the basic assumption of Incohesion, and Scapegoating in Foulkesian Group Analysis: Clinical and empirical illustrations, including terrorism and terrorists. *Forum,* 8. Online.

Hutchinson, S. (2017). 41st Annual Foulkes Lecture "The Times They Are A-Changing: Evolving Group Analytic Identity". *Group Analysis*, 50, 4, 419–435.

Hopper, E. & Weinberg, H. (Eds). (2011).*The Social Unconscious in Persons, Groups, and Societies: Volume 1: Mainly Theory.* London: Karnac.

Mojovic, M. (2011). Manifestations of psychic retreats in social systems. In Hopper E. & Weinberg, H. (Eds). *The Social Unconscious in Persons, Groups and Societies: Volume I: Mainly Theory* (pp. 209–234). London: Karnac.

Nitzgen, D. & Hopper, E. (2017). The concepts of the social unconscious and of the matrix in the work of S.H. Foulkes. In Hopper, E. & Weinberg, H. (Eds). *The Social Unconscious in Persons, Groups and Societies: Volume 3: The Foundation Matrix Extended and Re-configured* (pp. 3–22). London: Karnac.

Pines, M. (1998). *Circular Reflections: Selected Papers on Group Analysis and Psychoanalysis.* London: Jessica Kingsley Publishers.

Powell, A. (1994). Towards a unifying concept of the group matrix. In Brown, D. & Zinkin, L. (Eds). *The Psyche and the Social World: Developments in Group Analytic Theory* (pp. 92–102). London: Routledge.

3 Improvised vocality of verbal communication in groups

A contribution to the conceptualization of the tripartite matrix in group analysis

Helga Felsberger

Introduction

The relevance of speech in clinical groups and groupings of marginalized peoples is a fascinating topic and an important field of research, as seen, for example, in the study of communicative intentions and the role of ostensive cueing (Csibra 2010, Sakkalou & Gattis 2012, Felsberger 2017). The voice and vocality with its vicissitudes of coherence and incoherence are crucial for fostering contact and the communication of affect. It is especially important in the development and maintenance of attachment and trust. Learning to communicate freely and courageously in a group is essential for the development of resilience, and for integrating into the wider community.

Although communication – verbal and non-verbal – undoubtedly connects us, it also divides us. Humans have developed a seemingly infinite number of systems of verbal communication, or in other words languages, with all their dialects, regiolects, sociolects and jargons. Languages allow for the construction and experience of personal and social identity, which involves both distinguishing one group from the other, and belonging to one or more of them. By speaking to one person but not to another, to one group or sub-group, but not to another, by recognizing some people but not others, by making some people feel heard and others unheard, we thereby include or exclude, prefer or ignore them. Languages get lost or even get wrested from a group as an expression of power in the context of power structures. In the context of communication between people and their groups, languages can either develop or deteriorate, or can become degraded or even extinct. Such processes are sometimes legalized through the exercise of political power.

Rarely are we fully aware of such dynamics, especially while they are occurring. This is an aspect of the social unconscious with particular reference to the power structures of any social system.

According to S.H. Foulkes, a foundation matrix of a society can be seen as the operational basis of all mental and bodily processes in the group with lines of forces passing through each and all of its individual members at all levels of communication, comparable to a magnetic field. "The individual is thought of as a nodal point of this network, suspended within it" (Foulkes & Anthony 1957, p. 259). In his later work, Foulkes puts more emphasis on the idea of "resonance"

DOI: 10.4324/9781003425915-5

in group processes (Foulkes 1974, p. 199). Foulkes had begun to distinguish the concept of the foundation matrix from the concept of the dynamic matrix of any particular group. Around the same time, the Portuguese group analyst Maria Rita Mendes Leal (1970, Manso Neto & França 2021) formulated a similar concept of the "internal interpersonal matrix" or "personal group matrix", holding that every individual has the whole object representations – so to speak, group representations – in his/her mind.

Hopper (1996) took up these ideas of the foundation matrix and defined the concept of the social unconscious in terms of

> … the existence and constraints of social, cultural and communicational arrangements of which people are unaware; unaware, in so far as these arrangements are not perceived (not known), and if perceived not acknowledged (denied), and if acknowledged, not taken as problematic ("given"), and if taken as problematic, not considered with an optimal degree of detachment and objectivity.
>
> (Hopper 2001, p. 10)

Based on his work with Dieter Nitzgen (Nitzgen & Hopper 2017), Hopper (2018) conceptualized the tripartite matrix, which consists of three overlapping and interpenetrating matrices, the "foundation matrix" of the wider contextual society, the "dynamic matrix" of a particular grouping and the "personal matrices" of the members of the particular social entity. Each of these three realms or sub-matrices can be understood along various dimensions:

> the patterns of *interaction* (interpersonal relations); the patterns of *normation* (values and norms); the patterns of *communication* (verbal and non-verbal); styles of thinking and feeling (for example, instrumental/expressive, local/cosmopolitan, concrete/abstract, visual/non-visual, priorities of various senses, etc.); styles of leadership, followership, and bystandership, etc.
>
> (Hopper 2018, p. 24)

The dimension of communication, especially in reference to speech and vocality, must be contextualized with respect to power structures. For example, we constantly engage in such communicative gestures that involve either listening to the other or sealing off our ears, in either hearing or ignoring him or her, and thereby depriving the "other" from relevance or even partaking in the annihilation of a people and their language. These processes are closely associated with normative secrecy and normative taciturnity, which can amount to a social trauma (Hopper 1981 [2003]). Doron (2017) describes "black holes", "material" that is denied and not available for narrative, as a collective defence against shared fears of annihilation. In the early 1900s, Georg Simmel (1908) defines the sociological aspects of secrecy and assumed that it is the capacity to speak, which conditions the human interaction and controls social relations by manipulating the ratio of "knowledge" to "ignorance".

Human speech is the infinite field in which social inclusion and exclusion, and also marginalization and expulsion, are executed. Being addressed and addressing an "other" is social participation. If I do not participate, I do not partake within *common sense* and on *common ground* as a lived body (Bizzari 2018). Consequently, I do not matter as a subject, but merely as the object of marginalization or expulsion. Facing this threat creates enormous fear of annihilation. "Sometimes I fear I am not even human", as one of my patients once said. It is also challenging to accept inevitable phases of incoherence. The suspension of coherence can then either feed the desire to dissolve the dissonance (like a leading-note in music) or result in petrifying the discord.

Incoherence can rigidify into communication blockages (Mies 1992), and finally lead to marginalization, exclusion, expulsion or annihilation processes in groupings and society at large. My assumption is underpinned by a recent "dialogical turn" (Marková 2016) in social sciences, which has led to conceiving the mind of the Self and the minds of the Others as interdependent. This interdependence constitutes an irreducible axiom. Multifaceted social realities, evolving in and through sense-making and sense-creating are situated in intrapersonal, interpersonal, intergroup, institutional, cultural and historical planes. A dialogical epistemology foregrounds interaction between the Self and the Others, places the focus on language as dialogue and not as a system of signs, on conversation and communication and not on the transmission of information, be it conscious or unconscious.

This perspective is also underpinned by an important axiom of dialogical epistemology: *epistemic trust/distrust* (Sperber & Wilson 1995, Fonagy et al. 2014, 2015). The ethical relation between the Self and the Other as rooted in daily life is an important element in the common ground of social reality, especially as seen in human intentions. Epistemic trust is the capacity and readiness to learn and accept knowledge and experience from one another, whereas epistemic distrust is a lack of the presupposition that temporarily we are living in a shared and co-created social world. When finally established, epistemic trust is implicitly taken for granted and ranges from micro-social to macro-social forms, and shows in communicative contracts of secrets and non-disclosure, or in other words the hermeneutics of trust and suspicion (Marková 2016). It is a challenge to navigate between epistemic trust and distrust; to endure the necessary vigilance and suspicion in the face of deceit, to allow for secrecy and non-disclosure. It is a challenge for human beings to rely on common sense and common ground, to shift flexibly between Self and Other while reaffirming the boundaries of their relations.

Vocality in the here-and-now in communication

When we discuss language, we usually think of verbal communication and refer to it as a system of signs. Nonetheless, "language" is an abstraction: it only becomes effective in the performance of spatio-temporally situated speech practices. The phonetic or vocal event in communication constitutes *the dimension of fundamental reference to the other*, in consenting/dissenting, attracting/rejecting. This occurs on the level of musical attributes such as synchronized or divergent speech rhythms. "In the voice a desire, a neediness, but also power and powerlessness over the Other articulate. Voice-based communication creates a situation of existential openness and exposure" (Krämer 2003, p. 11, transl. HF). Attraction, rejection, group formation and anti-group formation are all manifest and expressed in processes and patterns of speech, e.g. synchronized or divergent rhythms and accommodated or dissonant pitch. Convergence and divergence in speech patterns are person-based and group-based accommodative strategies depending on the motivation and interpersonal and/or intergroup needs of the participants (Gallois et al. 2005).[1]

"Affection of contact"[2] (Murakami 2008, 2013), which occurs in a body, and perhaps in particular in a glance or in a voice that addresses an "other", is where communication begins. Felsberger (2017) gives a detailed account of the necessary paradigm-shift when dealing with language and communication. The *phatic* (contact-holding) and the *pathic* (affect-contagious) functions of language are socially and biologically grounded and they form the embodied essence of a social feedback mechanism. As early as 1934, G.H. Mead (1934/1962) highlighted the process of speaking and listening as *the* social feedback mechanism for the way in which we experience ourselves and others in society. Hence, the pathic and phatic functions of spoken language decisively affect our experience in society in general and in groups in particular. These intercorporeal and inter-affective events contribute significantly to the development of secure attachment and of coherent communication in a group and in society, and ultimately to the promotion and facilitation of mentalizing and epistemic trust.

The acoustic event of an utterance involves more than one physical body with its respective anatomical, physiological and neurochemical structures. For example, the periaqueductal grey located in the midbrain is involved in the emotional colouring of the voice – more or less caring, friendly, curious, romantic, doubtful, ignorant or hostile – in the speakers and the listeners alike (Koelsch 2008). This simultaneous event most probably involves the mirror neuron system, which is actually not intersubjective (interpersonal) but rather inter-embodied. It is due to a resonance-based deictic (here-and-now) attunement of a quite particular sort (Stamenov & Gallese 2002): only in vocal interaction do all participants perceive the same emotional event at the same time, continuously in "now-moments" (Stern 1985). I hear my own voice speaking at the same moment that it is heard by the listener (Liberman 1996), which is different from my glance which I cannot see myself.[3] Speech as a bodily event and as a structure for inward and outward perceptions of emotional and social states is an expression of an important ego function. The human voice in speech is actually an extension of our bodies to the acoustic realm where this here-and-now attunement takes place. In fact, we can regard the experience of *presence* as essential for perceptual experience in the now-moment, which allows for remembering and imagining as distinct from perception in the moment (Ratcliffe 2015a). Without this capacity, it is easy to confuse the imaginary and the real as in hallucinatory processes.

Damasio (2010), like Freud (1923), suggests that the core of the self might be found in primordial feelings. He refers to Freud who suggested that we could know the mental life of another person by means of imitating the bodily state of another, as explored by Gaddini (1969) in his concept of imitative identification. However, understanding that speech is an aspect of the body/bodies allows us to avoid the conception of imitation, which nowadays is associated with a process of social learning involving higher, yet time-consuming, thought processes. If we accept Stamenov and Gallese's understanding of speech in language as inter-embodied due to a resonance-based deictic attunement, we come closer both to Freud's conception of the ego and to Merleau-Ponty's (1945) concept of "intercorporéité". Language is not only a symbolically mediated form of communication, but through its vocality language also functions as the deepest level of intercorporeal communication. This allows us to describe speech in terms that Flakne (2019) uses in order to describe dance – "Participatory Sense-making" and "Contact Improvisation" – as enabling intercorporeal sense-making. In other words, it takes two to tango. This constitutes the experience of perception – proprioception and alloception – the enactive bodily receptivity to sensory and kinesthetic processes of others, which are involved, e.g. in mind reading, perspective taking and mentalizing. In psychosis and states of social incohesion, these capacities are suspended.

Blockages in communication can eventually lead to symptoms at an individual level. The dual concept of primary "inner" psychodynamics and secondary "external" group dynamics becomes questionable and hence mental illness becomes a multipersonal phenomenon (Köhncke & Mies 2012). Accordingly, Robi Friedman (2004, 2019) conceptualizes "relation disorders" by locating dysfunctional behavioural patterns not within intrapsychic issues, but rather considering them as a function of the dynamics of group relations.

The vicissitudes in coherence/incoherence experienced in the vocality of communication in groups arouse trust or mistrust, safety or anxiety. The unconscious impact of divergence in vocality can even be considered as aggression in the context of power structures that can and often do perpetuate the marginalization of persons and sub-groupings. Withholding or depriving a person or a sub-group of the "affection of contact" (Murakami 2013) through speech and body contact is an anti-group process expressed in the incoherence of communication. The rhythms of the oscillation between coherence and incoherence can become rigid and inflexible, and conceptionally inelastic. Negative or no feedback is also an expression of language and speech as our main social feedback mechanism. In other words, the achievement of coherence is always a relational process.

Disturbance is no longer a matter of an isolated individual, but of a person in relationship to others from the very beginning of life. In this context, the concept of "location" (Foulkes, 1948) is especially useful. The disorder is not located inside the individual, but between individuals within their dynamic and foundational matrices. Foulkes had been very much inspired by Kurt Goldstein and his Gestalt psychological concepts. As early as 1948, Goldstein integrated contemporary developments in linguistics, psychology and neuropsychology, and formulated his principles of Gestalt together with his ideas on psychopathology. He studied the effects of brain damage (like with aphasia and schizophrenia) on abstraction abilities, the loss of which results in a "catastrophic situation". The loss of the *abstract attitude* – and being restricted to the *concrete attitude* – means a catastrophe for the organism, as it is the loss of integration of sensory experience, cognitive and emotional states, motivational drives and final motor actions especially with language and speech performances (Goldstein 1948).[4] Nowadays, we speak of mentalizing versus non-mentalizing capacity.

The stigmatization of psychosis causes incoherence in communication with others. Incoherence also shocks, shatters and eventually fragments the relational mind, leads to a breakdown of mentalizing, on both sides. As Chaika (1990) asks, "If the schizophrenic's meaning can be so very far removed from [that of] normals, how does anyone know what the schizophrenic means?" (ibid., p. 311). In other words, what comes first, the diagnosis or the clinical reality? The answer to this question is that both are always recursively relevant in the context of the dynamic matrix of the institution.

Studies suggest that in psychosis, the capacity to communicate, participate and partake in social relationships is in fact shattered. Epistemic biases often arise from severe childhood trauma and abuse (Ratcliffe 2015b). The capacity to recognize affective prosody (the emotions in the voice) and emotions in faces are crucial aspects of social cognition and social perception. Both are severely impaired in schizophrenia and severe forms of depression (Alba-Ferrara 2011, Rossell et al. 2013). This is not merely a symptom or a consequence of cognitive restraints and limitations. Sensory, intercorporeal and cognitive capacities that are acquired and sustained in social relationships are suspended. Social knowledge and the capacity spontaneously to attune oneself to the emotional lives and behaviours of others through the bodily process of spoken communication are inaccessible (Sass & Parnas 2003; Stanghellini 2004).

The relevance of hearing myself speaking to others

The significance of a group-therapeutic event arises from the fact that in the group the patients encourage each other to experience affect-contagious and contact-fostering moments. This important step in therapy with schizophrenic and other severely disordered patients can be challenging. After all, recent research identifies two sets of "negative" symptoms: reduced motivation as seen in avolition, anhedonia and asociality; and diminished expressiveness as seen in alogia, restricted affect (Blanchard & Cohen 2006). Schizophrenic patients often struggle to maintain a feeling of self-as-agent, including motivation and intention to reach out, to succeed in distinguishing self and other in the presence of the other, and to maintain an ability to take the perspective of another person. For example, Martin (29 years old) is a participant in my group of patients with psychotic disorders. In one session, he says:

> What I hear from you can bother me for a quite some time. Last week I felt awkward after the group session. Karin (48), you told us about your suicidal thoughts. I had this in my head and I didn't know what to make of it. These thoughts don't go away.

– "Does this mean, that I shouldn't tell you about my thoughts?" Karin wonders. "Well, I don't know". "But what happens to you? In what way are they there, my thoughts in your head?" "They make me sad. I imagine, that you kill yourself, and you won't be there anymore. This makes me very sad". "Ah, I understand...". Karin said rather thoughtfully.

Sharing one's feelings can be threatening, though. Hannah (51) is reluctant to speak openly in the group.

> When I tell my feelings in the group, someone can take them away and use them against me. There might be someone who uses what I have said to threaten me. Then I get paranoid and experience you and the other participants as being against me. This happened at work time and again. It always ended in the colleagues bullying me.

The co-conductor suggests, "You could give it a try and see what it does to you when you talk about feelings and memories here in our group". Hannah says, "You don't understand my paranoia. That's exactly the problem. I know what happens when I leave this room. My paranoid ideas will haunt me if I tell you too much". The co-conductor replies, "So what is it that you can talk about here?" Hannah answers:

> Well, certain topics, more superficial issues. I don't want to talk about very personal aspects and certain emotions and memories. That's too risky. ..... It is difficult and sometimes impossible to judge what is a real threat and what is only in my head.

Hannah struggles a lot with epistemic trust or distrust, as she can fully rely neither on the setting and confidentiality nor on her own perception and judgement. At the beginning of her group participation, she skipped every other group session because it burdened her, but now she can come and stay and talk about her difficulty. Her reluctance, her deliberate restraint gives her confidence as she is in control. We reflect on this progress as we all try to understand how Hannah feels.

The sense of security with regard to the source of information, be it the "other" or one's own bodily sensations, requires a kind of dialectical oscillation between trust and distrust, between the confidence in the validity of one's own perceptions and an openness to the others' perceptions – otherwise, one ends up in paranoia or fundamentalism. Building up the necessary flexibility in terms of epistemic trust with a sufficient degree of vigilance is a huge challenge. Schizophrenic patients often succumb to epistemic blurring in which boundaries are unclear and frightening and then their conclusions are drawn from little evidence. This is a deplorable state to be in. Losing the capacity for social participation has the severest consequences for a person's experience of self. "In the group, there is a me for the others and a me for me, which is hard to endure", a patient describes. Patients with a psychotic disorder often avoid close or even emotional contact because they are frightened by the possibility of psychic merger. However, at the same time, they long for social contact and to be included in social relationships. Therefore, in group-analytic psychotherapy with such patients, we try to encourage them to consider these obstacles in conversation together. The group conductors need to be very attentive regarding the boundaries of self-experience.

To seek or accept eye contact, to speak up in a group or be spoken to, and to hear oneself addressing others and sharing thoughts and feelings all require some security in distinguishing self from not-self (object). However, it is the only way to achieve some level of epistemic trust within a shared social space. It needs to be repeated within a meaningful group process in order to trust in the experience of being an individual (a sense of "me") and a group member (a sense of "me-as-part-of-the-group") at the same time. Our goal is to enable the participants to attune to each other and let themselves be touched and enlightened by each other's accounts and emotional expressions without getting lost. This involves participatory sense-making and contact improvisation (Flakne 2019). So, how can I tango and still be myself? Affective participation contributes to the construction of the shared and collective mental representations of the group.

Friedrich (45) suffers from paranoid schizophrenia and one day he comes to the group in an awful state and tells us of his frightening hallucinations. He saw snakes everywhere in his flat. Some of the other group members react with great empathy. Ignaz (52) tells him how he deals with such situations and others tell of their hallucinations. The following week, Friedrich reports back to the group that the previous group session had helped him a lot. He had noticed that the others stayed calm while he was telling about his weird hallucinations and were not terrified by his account. He understood that it "was only [his] hallucinations and nothing really frightening". He regularly stresses the benefit he gets from the group in this way. This is an example of the distinction between imagination and perception.

At the end of her group therapy experience, one of the patients said that for her the most significant experience was "hearing myself speaking to others". Another patient said that the group had helped him to communicate much more, saying, "I have so many new words now". Yet another said, "What I learned from the group is talking to people. Now I talk so much more. I didn't do this before".

The growing ability to raise and address their voices to the group, to listen to the others speaking to them, struggling but finally succeeding in making themselves understood.... all seem to have helped them negotiate their partly similar and partly differing understanding of another person's narrative and emotional reaction. Their increasingly free conversation facilitates the distinction between self and other, and, hence, the experience of themselves in shared group moments. Many of the participants say that they usually cannot interact like this in their social contexts. Friedrich (45), for example, appreciates the group as a space in which one can say anything. Outside the group, people would consider him mad and he would not dare to speak freely. In the group, he feels a normal human being, "it is like in the land of milk and honey".

Coherence/incoherence in marginalized groupings in society

The loss of attunement in the foundation matrix can be seen in the migration or flight (Van Os et al. 2010; Tost & Meyer-Lindenberg 2012) of minorities through which the death of entire language communities ("Sprachtod") results from the exercise of political power by the majority (Brizic 2006). In her sociolinguistic research from 1999 to 2003 in six Viennese elementary schools, Brizic showed that the children of Turkish migrants tend to find it much harder to learn German than the children from migrants coming from ex-Yugoslavia. When she considered the true linguistic background of their parents, she found out that a great percentage of the Turkish parents of her cohort were actually descendants of about 40 ethnic minority groups who had been deprived of their mother tongue by Atatürk's devastating language policy almost 100 years ago. Brizic states that this intergenerational transmission of language switching and death of language was not only a regrettable reduction of a former cultural plurality, but also a deprivation with severe and significant difficulties in language acquisition and learning in general for the following generations. Those who are dispossessed of their mother tongue and hence of their full competence to communicate and interact among themselves and across the generations suffer a kind of social trauma. They find themselves "disentitled" to share emotions, experiences and memories, to sing traditional and nursery songs, to recite rhymes and poems and, of course, to speak up publicly. The power aspect comes into play consciously and unconsciously in so far as a community is deprived of the connections between their language and a variety of their internalized objects, involving, for example, patterns of authority and gender roles. There are many more examples of such forms of annihilation, e.g. throughout Australia's colonial history, Indigenous people were completely stripped of their languages (Griffiths 2020). This instrument of power has often been used to rip out the tongues of helpless and dependent groups, which serves to make them even more helpless and dependent by limiting their ability to express their discontent. In fact, this is a form of socio-cultural disembodiment.

Such a process is an expression of "symbolic violence" (Bourdieu & Passeron 1973), which Regine Scholz (2011) sees as a dynamic within the "foundation matrix", like press censorship banning large bodies of emotional facts from public communication and prohibiting their surfacing in the conscious psychic life of individuals. As Doron (2017) has argued, this is a way of creating a "black hole" in the communication dimension of the contextual society. Similarly, a person's mental illness is not talked about by his family and his community. Might this be like the silent reverberations that followed the disappearance of people and their groupings during the Third Reich? Women who did not conform to the prevailing cultural norms were diagnosed as schizophrenic and disappeared forever in institutions, as a way of not listening and not hearing what they might have been trying to say. Our schizophrenic patients' frightening hallucinations and terrifying delusions together with their accounts of painful exclusion tell a story of another form of censorship.

In his linguistic research, Erez Levon (2010) detects

> a linguistic manifestation of an epistemology of sexuality that views lesbian or gay identity as separate from other aspects of social subjectivity. In other words, by altering mean pitch levels between gay and non-gay topics, ... (m)ainstream men and women ... construct distinct "gay" and "non-gay" voices with which to portray distinct "gay" and "non-gay" selves.
>
> (Levon 2010, 16)

For example, in Israel, gay and lesbian subjectivities are excluded from dominant narratives, which makes it difficult to identify as gay or lesbian and as Israeli at the same time. In an attempt to overcome and reconcile this inconsistency and potential conflict, people who identify as both gay or lesbian and as Israeli use characteristic language patterns with respect to mean pitch in order to construct identities which are acceptable to others (Levon 2010, 2012). Apart from the obvious "symbolic violence", the effect of the bodily disconnection, involving the exclusion from common speech practices and the affection of contact, may be even more devastating because it leads to petrified incoherence. It is likely that similar conflicts and patterns of resolution occur in other societies as well; this may be related to military activities and normative patterns of aggression and definitions of gender.

Conclusion

The communication process is a co-creation. As such, it allows the construction of meaning, to be in time and in tune with others, and the development of a shared sense of time passing, which is relevant to "now moments" (Stern 1985) and to "intersubjective time" (Wotton 2017). Intersubjective time is expressed through human relations and specific gestural narratives of voice and body – which we can also observe in psychotherapeutic interactions (Malloch 1999, 2015, Wotton 2017). "Communicative musicality" (Malloch & Trevarthen 2009) as an element in vocality reflects the influence of the body.[5] We gain presence through our voices immersed in the tonal ground of a speaking group. This experience of *presence* "means becoming physically and virtually a part of the experience itself" (Ermi & Mäyrä 2005).[6]

Through this special kind of listening and speaking, I, as a therapist, maintain the experience of self and social relatedness. This helps to develop the pathic and phatic functions of communication. Hence, a group-therapeutic process can become a we-formation, which then enables ego-formation. Hearing our voices embodied and embedded in our common speech is an act of shared consciousness and shared perception (Flakne 2005).[7] In the context of the vicissitudes of coherence and incoherence, the extinction of a language and/or the marginalization and even the exclusion of schizophrenic patients and other social groupings means that they are banned from communication as such.

> If schizophrenia can be conceived of as a loss of attunement to the social world through *sensus communis*, and if such a loss can be adequately understood in terms of social space, then its treatment should also primarily focus on the social space that *sensus communis* attunes – or fails to attune – us to.
>
> (Thoma & Fuchs 2018, p. 30)

Notes

1 Communication Accommodation Theory (CAT), e.g. Gallois et al. (2005), Giles and Ogay (2007), Soliz and Giles (2014).

2 "The eye contact of others precedes the perception of his body. In the natural situation of the non-autistic, the experience of others—before being perception of their body—is first of all experience of a glance, the call of a voice or body contact. This experience does not require knowledge of the other and the baby responds to the facial expression of his (her) mother. We call 'affection of contact' this primordial experience [...]. (which is an independent [and transcendental] 'category' irreducible to other moments of transcendental subjectivity)" (Murakami 2008, p. 17).

3 The listener and I hear my utterance simultaneously, but I cannot look into somebody's eyes and my own at the same time – not without temporal delay (not even if I use a mirror or during a video conference). Liberman (1996) recognizes a link between perception and production as necessary for successful verbal and non-verbal communication.

4 Goldstein (1948) first described his concept of the abstract versus concrete attitude in his work on "Languages and language disturbances" studying patients with aphasia and schizophrenia. According to his findings, a person can assume the abstract attitude deliberately unless he suffers from severe neuronal or psychiatric disorders. "The abstract attitude is basic for the following potentialities:

1 Assuming a mental set voluntarily, taking initiative, even beginning a performance on demand.

2 Shifting voluntarily from one aspect of a situation to another, making a choice.

3 Keeping in mind simultaneously various aspects of a situation; reacting to two stimuli which do not belong intrinsically together.

4 Grasping the essentials of a given whole, breaking up a given whole into parts, isolating them voluntarily, and combining them to wholes.

5 Abstract and common properties, planning ahead ideationally, assuming an attitude toward the 'merely possible', and thinking or performing symbolically.

6 Detaching the ego from the outer world" (Goldstein 1948, p. 6).

5 Foulkes did not elaborate this idea very precisely although he based his group-analytic approach on it drawing a lot on musical metaphors. In an effort to pursue the location of the disturbance, the group conductor's task is to "divine" the key and then talk back to the group in the same key (Burman 2017).

6 "Presence derives mainly from the perception of sound [...] Our locating of sound into the environment is 'a means of reaching out into the world', distinguishing self from nonself and thus achieving presence, and the ability to act in that space" (Grimshaw 2017, p. 294). According to music psychologist Luke Windsor (2017), sound is placed in the environment where it makes cognitive sense to locate it – and therewith creates environmental affordances, for those perceiving. According to Wotton (2015), innate musicality enables the shared meaning of experience.

7 For if it is possible to live with and share the perceptions [*sunaisthanesthai*] of many at once, it is most desirable for them to be the largest possible number; but as that is very difficult, active community of perception [*sunaistheeseoos*] must of necessity be in a smaller circle" (EE1245b22–24). This refers to Aristotle's idea of embodiment and embeddedness in his concept of Sunaisthesis (friendship) in the course of which he already identified the immense importance of joint attention and shared perception for the experience of Self (Flakne 2005, pp. 57–58).

References

Alba-Ferrara, L. M. (2011). Emotional Prosody Processing in the Schizophrenia Spectrum. Durham thesis, Durham University. Available at Durham E-Theses Online: http://etheses.dur.ac.uk/3185/

Aristotle. Eudemian Ethics (EE1245b22–24).

Bizzari, V. (2018). Schizophrenia and Common Sense: A Phenomenological Perspective. In: Hipólito, I., Gonçalves, J. G. & Pereira, J. (Eds.). *Schizophrenia and Common Sense. Explaining the Relation between Madness and Social Values. Series: Studies in Brain and Mind 12* (pp. 39–54). Cham: Springer International Publishing.

Blanchard, J. J. & Cohen, A. S. (2006). The Structure of Negative Symptoms within Schizophrenia: Implications for Assessment. *Schizophrenia Bulletin* Apr; 32(2): 238–245. http://dx.doi.org/10.1093/schbul/sbj013. Epub 2005 Oct 27. PMID: 16254064; PMCID: PMC2632211.

Bourdieu, P. & Passeron, J.-C. (1973). *Grundlagen einer Theorie der symbolischen Gewalt. Kulturelle Reproduktion und soziale Reproduktion.* Frankfurt am Main: Suhrkamp [French: *La Reproduction: Éléments* pour une théorie du système d'enseignement. Paris: Minuit, 1970].

Brizic, K. (2006). The Secret Life of Languages. Origin-Specific Differences in L1/L2 Acquisition by Immigrant Children. *International Journal of Applied Linguistics (INJAL),* 16(3): 339–362.

Burman, E. (2017). The Location of Disturbance: Situating Group Analytic Practice. *CUSP: Critical Cultures and Cultural Critiques in Psychology,* 1(2). http://www.cuspthejournal. com/issue2/erica1.html

Chaika, E. (1990) *Understanding Psychotic Speech: Beyond Freud and Chomsky.* Faculty Books. Book 1. http://digitalcommons.providence.edu/faculty_books/1

Csibra, G. (2010). *Recognizing Communicative Intentions in Infancy.* Whiley Online Library. First published: 15 March 2010

Damasio, A. R. (2010). *Self Comes to Mind: Constructing the Conscious Brain.* London: Heinemann.

Doron, Y. (2017). "Black Holes" as a Collective Defence against Shared Fears of Annihilation in a Small Therapy Group and in Its Contextual Society. In: Hopper, E. & Weinberg, H. *The Social Unconscious in Persons, Groups, and Societies. The Foundation Matrix Extended and Re-configured* (pp. 107–126). London: Karnac.

Ermi, L. & Mäyrä, F. (2005). Fundamental Components of the Gameplay Experience: Analysing Immersion. Presented at *Changing Views Worlds in Play,* 16–20 June, Toronto.

Felsberger, H. (2017). Vokale Matrix und Gruppenbindung – wie Hören und Sprechen in der Gruppe mentalisierte Affektivität und epistemisches Vertrauen ermöglichen. Gruppenpsychotherapie und Gruppendynamik. *Vandenhoeck & Ruprecht. Göttingen,* 53/3: 188–225.

Flakne, A. (2005). Embodied and Embedded: Friendship and the Sunaisthetic Self. *Epoché,* 10(1): 37–63.

Flakne, A. (2019). Contact Improvisation and Embodied Social Cognition. In: *The Oxford Handbook of Improvisational Dance,* edited by V. Midgelow, 528–44. Oxford: Oxford University Press.

Fonagy, P. & Allison, E. (2014). The Role of Mentalizing and Epistemic Trust in the Therapeutic Relationship. *Psychotherapy,* 51/3: 372–380.

Fonagy, P., Luyten, P. & Allison, E. (2015). Epistemic Petrification and the Restoration of Epistemic Trust: A New Conceptualization of Borderline Personality Disorder and Its Psychosocial Treatment. *Journal of Personality Disorders,* 29(5): 575–609.

Foulkes, S. H. (1948) *Introduction to Group Analytic Psychotherapy.* London: Karnac.

Foulkes, S. H. (1974). *Therapeutische Gruppenanalyse.* München: Kindler.

Foulkes, S. H. & Anthony, E. J. (1957). *Group Psychotherapy: The Psychoanalytic Approach.* Harmondsworth: Penguin Books.

Freud, S. (1923). The Ego and the Id. In: *The Standard Edition of the Complete Psychological Works of Sigmund Freud*, Volume XIX (pp. 1923–1925). The Ego and the Id and Other Works, 1–66. London: Hogarth Press.

Friedman, R. (2004). Safe Space and Relational Pathology. *International Journal of Counseling and Psychotherapy*, 2: 108–114.

Friedman, R. (2019). *Dreamtelling, Relations, and Large Groups: New Developments in Group Analysis*. London: Routledge.

Gaddini, E. (1969). On Imitation. *International Journal of Psychoanalysis*, 50: 475–484.

Gallois, C., Ogay, T. & Giles, H. (2005). Communication Accommodation Theory: A Look Back and a Look Ahead. In: Gudykunst, William B. (Ed.). Theorizing About Intercultural Communication (pp. 121–148). Thousand Oaks, CA: Sage. ISBN 978-0-7619-2749-5

Giles, H. & Ogay, T. (2007). Communication Accommodation Theory. In: Whaley, B. B. & Samter, W. (Eds.). *Explaining Communication: Contemporary Theories and Exemplars* (pp. 293–310). Mahwah, NJ: Lawrence Erlbaum Associates Publishers.

Goldstein, K. (1948). *Language and Language Disturbances: Aphasic Symptom Complexes and Their Significance for Medicine and Theory of Language*. New York: Grune & Stratton.

Griffiths, J. (2020). Indigenous Australians had their languages taken from them, and it's still causing issues today. CNN. https://www.cnn.com/2020/07/20/australia/australia-indigenous-language-rights-intl-hnk/index.html

Grimshaw, M. (2017). Presence Through Sound. In: Wöllner, C. (Ed.). Body, Sound, and Space in Music and Beyond. Multimodal Explorations (pp. 279–297). Abingdon, New York: Routledge.

Hopper, E. (1981) [2003]. *Social Mobility: A Study of Social Control and Insatiability*. Oxford: Blackwell. Excerpts reprinted in Hopper, E. (2003) *The Social Unconscious: Selected Papers*. London: Jessica Kingsley Publishers.

Hopper, E. (1996). The Social Unconscious in Clinical Work. *Group*, 20(1): 7–42.

Hopper, E. (2001). The Social Unconscious: Theoretical Considerations. *Group Analysis*, 34: 9–27.

Hopper, E. (2018). Notes on the Concept of the Social Unconscious in Group Analysis. *Group*, 42(2): 99–118.

Koelsch, S. (2008). Die emotionale Stimme. *Musiktherapeutische Umschau*, 29: 201–208.

Köhncke, D. & Mies, T. (2012). Der Matrixbegriff und die intersubjektive Wende – Der gruppenanalytische Blick auf das Unbewusste. *Gruppenpsychotherapie und Gruppendynamik*, 48: 26–52.

Krämer, S. (2003). Negative Semiologie der Stimme. Reflexionen über die Stimme als Medium der Sprache. https://www.geisteswissenschaften.fu-berlin.de/we01/institut/mitarbeiter/emeriti/kraemer/PDFs/Negative_Semiologie_der_Stimme.pdf

Leal, M. R. (1970). Le Transfert analytic dans l'analyse de groupe. *Bulletin de Psychologie de l'Université de Paris*, 285(XXIII): 13–16, 760–764.

Levon, E. (2010). *The Politics of Prosody: Language, Sexuality and National Belonging in Israel*. Queen Mary University of London. October 2010. www.qmul.ac.uk › sllf › 16-QMOPAL-Levon-Prosody

Levon, E. (2012). The Voice of Others: Identity, Alterity and Gender Normativity among Gay Men in Israel. *Language in Society*, 41: 187–211.

Liberman, A. M. (1996). *Speech: A Special Code*. Cambridge: MIT Press.

Malloch, S. (1999). Mothers and Infants and Communicative Musicality. Special Issue of *Musicae Scientiae: Rhythm, Musical Narrative and Origins of Human Communication*, 3 (1 suppl): 29–57. https://doi.org/10.1177/10298649000030S104

Malloch, S. (2015). http://www.psychevisual.com/Video_by_Stephen_Malloch_on_The_ Musicality_of_Therapeutic_Conversations.html

Malloch, S. & Trevarthen, C. (Eds.) (2009). *Communicative Musicality: Exploring the Basis of Human Companionship*. Oxford: Oxford University Press.

Manso Neto, I. & França, M. (Eds.) (2021).*The Portuguese School of Group Analysis. Towards a Unified and Integrated Approach to Theory Research and Clinical Work*. London: Routledge.

Marková, I. (2016). *The Dialogical Mind: Common Sense and Ethics*. Cambridge: Cambridge University Press.

Mead, G. H. (1934/1962). *Mind, Self and Society*. Chicago, IL: The University of Chicago Press.

Merleau-Ponty, M. (1945). *Phénoménologie de la perception*. Paris: Gallimard.

Mies, T. (1992). Thesen zum Matrixbegriff von Foulkes. Individuelles und gemeinsames Unbewusstes in der Gruppe. *Arbeitshefte Gruppenanalyse*, 1992, 1–8.

Murakami, Y. (2008). *Hyperbole – pour une psychopathologie lévinassienne* (pp. 1–110). Amiens: Association pour la promotion de la phénoménologie.

Murakami, Y. (2013). Affection of Contact and Transcendental Telepathy in Schizophrenia and Autism. *Phenomenology and the Cognitive Sciences*, 12(1): 179–194.

Nitzgen, D. & Hopper, E. (2017). The Concepts of the Social Unconscious and of the Matrix in the Work of S.H. Foulkes. In: Hopper, E. & Weinberg H. (Eds.). *The Social Unconscious in Persons, Groups, and Societies. The Foundation Matrix Extended and Re-configured* (pp. 3–25). London: Karnac.

Ratcliffe, M. J. (2015a). How is Perceptual Experience Possible? The Phenomenology of Presence and the Nature of Hallucination. In: Breyer, T. & Doyon, M. (Eds.). *Normativity in Perception* (pp. 91–113). Basingstoke: Palgrave Macmillan.

Ratcliffe, M. J. (2015b). The Interpersonal World of Psychosis. *World Psychiatry*, 14(2): 176–178.

Rossell, S. L., Van Rheenen, T. E., Groot, C., Gogos, A., O'Regan, A. & Joshua, N. R. (2013). Investigating Affective Prosody in Psychosis: A Study using the Comprehensive Affective Testing System. *Psychiatry Research*. http://dx.doi.org/10.1016/j.psychres.2013.07.037

Sakkalou, E. & Gattis, M. (2012). Infants Infer Intentions from Prosody. *Cognitive Development*, 27(1): 1–16.

Sass, L. A. & Parnas, J. (2003). Schizophrenia, Consciousness, and the Self. *Schizophrenia Bulletin*, 29(3): 427–444.

Scholz, R. (2011). The Foundation Matrix and the Social Unconscious. In: Hopper, E. & Weinberg H. (Eds.). *The Social Unconscious in Persons, Groups, and Societies: Mainly Theory* (pp. 265–285). London: Karnac.

Simmel, G. (1908). *Soziologie. Untersuchungen über die Formen der Vergesellschaftung*. Leipzig: Duncker und Humblot.

Soliz, J. & Giles, H. (2014). Relational and Identity Processes in Communication: A Contextual and Meta-Analytical Review of Communication Accommodation Theory. In: Cohen, E. (Ed.). *Communication Yearbook* 38 (pp. 106–143). Thousand Oaks, CA: Sage.

Sperber, D. & Wilson, D. (1995). *Relevance. Communication and Cognition*. Oxford, Cambridge, MA: Blackwell Publisher Ltd.

Stamenov, M. I. & Gallese, V. (Eds.) (2002). *Advances in Consciousness Research, Vol. 42. Mirror Neurons and the Evolution of Brain and Language*. John Benjamins Publishing Company. https://doi.org/10.1075/aicr.42

Stanghellini, G. (2004). *Disembodied Spirits and Deanimated Bodies. The Psychopathology of Common Sense*. Oxford: Oxford University Press.

Stern, D. (1985). *The Interpersonal World of the Infant: A View from Psychoanalysis and Developmental Psychology*. New York: Basic Books.

Thoma, S. & Fuchs, T. (2018). Inhabiting the Shared World: Phenomenological Considerations on *Sensus Communis*, Social Space and Schizophrenia. In: Hipólito, I., Gonçalves, J. G. & Pereira, J. (Eds.). *Schizophrenia and Common Sense. Explaining the Relation between Madness and Social Values. Series: Studies in Brain and Mind 12* (pp. 39–54). Cham: Springer International Publishing.

Tost, H. & Meyer-Lindenberg, A. (2012). Puzzling Over Schizophrenia: Schizophrenia, Social Environment and the Brain. *Nature Medicine*, 18: 211–213.

Van Os, J., Kenis, G. & Rutten, B. P. F. (2010). The Environment and Schizophrenia. *Nature*, 468: 203–212.

Windsor, L. (2017). Instruments, Voices, Bodies and Spaces: Towards an Ecology of Performance. In: Wöllner, C. (Ed.). *Body, Sound, and Space in Music and Beyond. Multimodal Explorations* (pp. 129–128). Abingdon, New York: Routledge.

Wotton, L. (2015). Improvising a Home among Strangers. *Group Analysis*, 48(4): 447–454.

Wotton, L. (2017). The Musical Foundation Matrix: Communicative Musicality as a Mechanism for the Transmission and Elaboration of Co-Created Unconscious Social Processes. In: Hopper, E. & Weinberg H. *The Social Unconscious in Persons, Groups, and Societies. The Foundation Matrix Extended and Re-Configured* (pp. 107–126). London: Routledge.

Part II

Personifications and the interpersonal matrix

4 Personification and polarization within the foundation matrix of Israel

A case example[1]

Joseph (Yossi) Triest

> To a degree, individual persons are also microcosms of their contextual entities, each of which is a kind of social-psychological-organismic fractal of the others.
>
> (Hopper & Weinberg, 2011)

The mutual links and inter-relations between the individual and society have usually been reviewed from the perspective of the psychology of groups, starting with Freud's (1921) keystone article on 'Group Psychology', and continuing with Bion's 'Experiences in Groups' (1961) and with the works of Foulkes's (1964, 1975). These seminal contributions have generated an extensive literature concerning the study of the social unconscious and the tripartite matrix of which this book and its immediate predecessors (Hopper, 2003a, 2003b, 2018a, 2018b; Hopper & Weinberg, 2011, 2016, 2017) are an important part.

This chapter moves from the particular to the general and analyses a traumatic moment of collapse in the life of an **individual** who was in some (unconscious) ways a 'representative of the people', were it only from the way the media and press 'marked' and reflected his personal style of 'carrying' the symbols of his social-political status. My aim is to explore how the personal intrapsychic process reflects the tectonic movements in the foundation matrix, as well as the interpersonal and transpersonal 'blast waves' that occur in society when a whirl is created around such crisis events.

It must be noted that the reason for writing was not the case itself – as harsh as it may be – but, rather, the result of a larger attempt to track the virtual biography of the analytic subject in its relation to 'The Place Where We Live' (Winnicott, 1971a) and 'The Location of the Cultural Experience' (Winnicott, 1971b):

> "I am thinking of something that is in the common pool of humanity, into which individuals and groups of people may contribute, and from which we may all draw if we have somewhere to put what we find" (Winnicott, 1971b, P. 99) ... Can we gain some advantage from an examination of... the possible existence of a place for living that is not properly described by either of the terms 'inner' and 'outer'?
>
> (Winnicott, 1971a, p. 106)

DOI: 10.4324/9781003425915-7

Armed with Bion's binocular vision[2] (1961), I tried to explore this 'place for living' in order to follow the process of the historical-conceptual formation of the notion of 'subject' in psychoanalysis – a subject who was born (long before Winnicott's above citation) on the couch of Freud's analysis and continued Its crystallization in the various models created under the roof of the theory. Evolving from the conceptual 'stem cells' of the Freudian drive model, he made his way through the American ego-psychology, the revolutionary interpretations of French psychoanalysis to Freud's work (Lacan, Laplanche, Pontalis, Green, etc.), Klein's Object Relations model, Winnicott's theory of the Self and, in contrast, Kohut's approach – until he reached finally (so far) the Relational approach which offered 'intersubjectivity' as a meeting-point where subjects are supposed to co-create each other. All these may be seen as short-term inns where the subject stayed and was fed over his peregrination. Obviously, he changed during those years and shifted shapes in each stop along his journey, while his identity becomes gradually more and more complex and multi-dimensional.

A thorough exploration of these statements is naturally beyond the scope of this chapter but suffice it to say that mapping the subject's dialectical conceptualization process, at a theoretical level and in the history of psychoanalytic ideas, may prove highly relevant also to our understanding of the process of identity constitution at both the developmental and clinical levels (Triest, 2014). It had though to prevail the tendency to isolate 'the subject' in the role of 'patient' – a well-distinct entity kept under strict sterilized laboratory settings that should prevent 'infection' and ensure the continuity of the 'psychic skin' tissue as a defence against a trauma caused by impingement of an oversaturated reality.

It turned out that the understanding of the subject in the way I see it, namely as the outcome of his own dialectical attempts to both differentiate himself from *and* merge with his surroundings, has already been decided in advance by Freud's (implicit) basic definition, at the very beginning of the journey (Breuer & Freud, 1895), which *essentially* boils down to the following: ***The analytic subject is he whose identity is founded by an unconscious component – his sexuality.***

In a broad, overall perspective, this fundamental description has far-reaching repercussions in the way we understand the mutual relationship between the subject and the world of objects with its social, cultural and historic dimensions:

Since the subject's identity is constituted and driven by unconscious forces,[3] he is inherently dependent upon the object to know himself.[4] But there's a catch: being a subject also means defining one's own identity solely from *within*. The search for the object's definitions of his own identity therefore unfolds as a dialectical, never-ending, pendulum-like movement aimed to recognize, know and negate (sooner or later, one way or another) whatever the object's responses to the Shakespearian (eternal) question of 'Who's there?'[5])and who am I? (might have been (Ogden, 1994). This back-and-forth movement between the pole of the subject and the pole of the object can be seen as the substrate on which the representations of both 'self' and 'other' are **created, negated, re-created and even co-created** (Triest, 2014).

Whether that (negated) object by which identity is defined in countless ways is **one person** (even if experienced as an undifferentiated 'me-extension'), **two**

persons (a dyad; mother-child), **three persons** (the Oedipal triangulation), **a small group** (Bion, 1961; Foulkes & Anthony, 1975), **a very large group** (the mass – Freud's 'Group Psychology'; 1921) or a **meta-group** (the Foulkesian Matrix – abstraction of the group as a communication network), the **dialectic** way in which they co-create and negate one another puts them on a kind of Möbius strip running from the individual to the Matrix and back again to the individual, who is now enriched (or poisoned; and usually a little of both) with the capacity to co-create and take part in a network of unconscious communication between minds.

Thus, as I was trying to track down the development of the contemporary subject's unique portrait into a human-tech hybrid, a centaur, if you would, whose body is individual but whose head is that of a group, whose smartphone – that ultimate epitome of the quantum leap in the evolution of our generation's cyberspace and social networking technologies – is rooted as an extension of his palm and serves as a bidirectional umbilical cord through which materials from the interpersonal and intrapersonal spaces become mixed – came the COVID outbreak, which definitively shattered the illusion of the subject's separateness and distinctness (Triest, 2017).

At the level of unconscious anxieties, the virus's ultimate *otherness* challenged, in one fell swoop, both the politically correct tolerance towards otherness praised by enlightened society, and the usually quite efficient denial of awareness to death. Moreover, the fact that a single breath of toxic oxygen (COVID-19 in the order of the Real, or the terrifying virus of uncanny dread in the Imaginary) suffices to turn one into the bad object's victim, and that the next exhaled breath will transform that victim into the same bad object, is more than enough to shatter the individual (and collective) mental immune system, including the split mechanisms it uses as emergency safeguards, and bring about a kind of chaos whose psychological qualities may be even more catastrophic than the physical ones (Triest, 2021).

Adding insult to injury, note that in Israel (very similarly to what happened in the US under Trump's administration), the pandemic's inherent onslaught on the consciousness of the very concept of boundary was used by Benjamin Netanyahu, the state's leader accused of criminal charges, to wage psychological warfare designed to save him from the dread of the legal proceedings against him. He did that by systematically crushing the judicial authorities, defaming position holders (magistrates, senior police officials) and paralysing crucial state institutions (the parliament, the State Comptroller; even the fight against COVID was life-threateningly subjected to narrow political interests) by employing unbridled intentional incitement, by spreading hate (as a political strategy) and by systematically promoting a culture of Orwellian fake discourse. The goal seemed far-reaching: to shatter the very capacity to distinguish good from evil, truth from lie, universal law from private interest, etc. This betrayal of the collective and universal appeal of any post-traumatic group of people in distress to seek refuge in a protective mother's figure bosom or to find shelter under the wings of a strong father figure who can ensure survival illustrates how close the Israeli society was to break down – and the extent to which MZ, an individual who stood on the narrow bridge that connects between Israel's life culture and death culture, was prone to fall into the abyss when bridges and boundaries started to collapse. I maintain that his personal story reveals not only the broken and torn fabric of relations between religious and non-religious people in Israel, but also the very heart of the nightmarish conflict of life and death, as it is represented (repressed, denied, projected and split) in the unconscious foundation matrix of Israel.

The case of MZ

During the COVID crisis, a scandal of 'sex and death' exploded in the media: MZ, one of the distinguished nominees of the 'Israel Prize' (the highest distinction awarded by the State to private individuals), was publicly suspected of prolonged serial sexual assaults against men and women, some of them minors, who over the years came to him for help and advice. The scandal broke out – the timing, I believe, betrays an eruption of the collective unconscious – when some of the victims decided to come out and described their experiences in an open account in a press interview. One day before the interview was supposed to be aired on one of the main TV channels in Israel, MZ committed a suicide attempt, following which he was hospitalized in a nursing hospital, reportedly due to irreversible damage (specific details were not made public). He died a year later, in 2022.

MZ was a public activist, founder and chairman of a voluntary NGO dedicated to the identification of disaster victims. Specifically, the organization took upon itself the task of locating, collecting and identifying victims' bodies, which often meant – in cases of terror acts, suicide bombers or military operations – finding and collecting victims' remains and body parts (one of the most shocking iconic war photographs in the gallery of the Israeli social unconscious shows rows of soldiers endangering their lives while sifting through sand in order to find body parts of soldiers killed in an explosion in Gaza). This task is considered not only as a humanitarian deed but is also a religious commandment in the Jewish tradition and is highly respected by both religious and non-religious Israelis.

Interestingly, MZ was embraced not only by official authorities (police, army, religious authorities) but also by the Israeli public. His life-story reveals highly contradictory stages he went through: from a provocative, virulent, insidious and controversial representative of extremist Jewish ultra-Orthodoxy (a community harshly criticized by the mainstream for their anti-Zionist views), he turned into a bridgehead linking ultra-Orthodox factions, Israeli government officials and the whole non-religious part of Israeli society. Over years of activity, he became a well-known figure who was generally appreciated for his courage to cross some of the most rigid boundaries (seemingly) without burning any bridges – and for his astonishing ability to remain, quite literally, on everyone's side.

Blessed with great personal charm and eloquence, he was unsurprisingly embraced by the media, too, but when the fact was made public that he was an Israel Prize nominee, testimonies about his conduct started to surface. It turned out that his deeds were actually known to many who had until that moment chosen to remain silent. One of many testimonials that was made public caught my attention, that of a woman who described his response when she tried to turn down his advances by claiming that she was menstruating (which, in Judaism, is a period when sexual intercourse is prohibited; see below): 'Surely you must know', he reportedly said, 'that blood doesn't frighten me'. As morbid as this may sound, it also offers a link to the (social) unconscious, where Eros and Thanatos are supposed to be interwoven (Freud, 1920) as indeed implied by MZ's cynical comment.

Discussion

Earl Hopper writes:

> …to understand human beings/persons we have to see them… in the context of their groups, which are regarded as dynamic open social systems, and analyzed in terms of their tripartite matrices, consisting of the foundation matrix of the contextual society, the dynamic matrix of the particular group, and possibly of the larger organization which sustains and sponsors it, and the personal matrices of the participants in it. In effect, the tripartite matrix refers to the socio-cultural structure of the social system of any human grouping.
>
> (Hopper, The Tripartite Model, 2003, 2018a,b)

MZ placed himself at one of the most vulnerable and explosive junctions of the Israeli matrix. In a way, we can regard him as having been 'sent' out (by social unconscious forces) on a mission to the 'desert of the real')Žižek, 2002) – to barehandedly touch Israeli society's bloodiest wound – it's daily Isaac's sacrifice of all those who, unlike the biblical Isaac, were not saved in the last minute. The other side of his Janus face, the uproar about the sexual behaviour which was attributed to him, may be seen as a failed attempt to lay down yet another bridge – perhaps one too far – in his efforts to survive the horrible world in which he lived – a bridge between the death culture and a twisted version of life culture – 'Eros and Thanatos' as Freud (1920) conceptualized these basic drive-forces.

The ghoulish link between 'blood' and 'blood' – the lifeblood of menstruation and the death-blood of the victims – is perhaps the lead into one of the darkest corners of the unconscious matrices, of which MZ is a kind of fractal. Indeed, at the time of writing, a truly bizarre campaign is being conducted in Israel, like a geyser suddenly gushing from underneath a rock due to some invisible turbulence, in which non-religious female 'influencers' and celebrities are recruited and handsomely paid to convince 'the daughters of Israel' to observe the religious commandment of 'Niddah'[6] and maintain what is referred to as 'family purity'. The laws of 'tummah' and 'tahara' (ritual purity and impurity) in Jewish law are among the most mystical, arcane and psychologically fascinating injunctions. Menstruation blood, similarly to touching the body of a dead person, involves impurity. The 'impurity' of *menstruation* may be resolved through the ritual immersion in a 'Mikveh', a ritual bath, which is usually managed by the religious establishment. But in order to purify oneself from the impurity of the *dead,* the religious injunction is to be immersed in water mixed with the ashes of a 'red cow'; the problem is that, except for some messianic circles who are actually aspiring to raise one, no one knows what a red cow is or where it may be found. In the Israeli reality, the fact is therefore that it is actually impossible to be purified from the impurity of the dead (that is why most orthodox Jews are prohibited from going to pray on Temple Mount – an act which would probably generate, if it happened, an all-out war with the Muslim world). Be it as it may, we can see how death and sexuality are closely interconnected in the social unconscious, even if the guilt involved in each of them has entirely different destinies.

No wonder that the culture of death in Israel is an idealized area – usually respected by many as a holy place where one tiptoes quietly and in perfect order. While in the Palestinian society (which, of course, I see as part of the relevant social matrix) scarifying oneself – even in murderous terror acts – is at least publicly celebrated as a transformation of the dead into a 'Shahid' (martyr) on his way to Paradise, for the Israeli side, dying or killing in war is perceived as an heroic act of resurrection, which breathes life into the huge historical graveyard where time froze over the six million victims of the Holocaust, as well as all other victims of all the bloody struggles the Jewish people and Israel were involved in.

No cultural phenomenon is so typically Israeli as the wail of sirens heard throughout the country on two official anniversaries (but in no other official event) – Memorial Day and Holocaust Day. It is a shrill sound announcing a moment of silence, in which traffic stops even in the busiest arteries and highways and *most* Jewish Israeli citizens stand still regardless of whether they are out on the streets or by themselves in the innermost rooms of shops or homes. *Most* Israeli citizens, I said, the exception being Arab citizens and the ultra-Orthodox, of which MZ is part.

Life in Israel is a noisy, bustling market of impressive activities and exceptional creative development capacities in many areas – science, medicine, agriculture, business entrepreneurship… But it is also a battlefield where wars are being waged against enemies – from without, but to no lesser extent also from within. It is a space where all the tribes that constitute the colourful mosaic of Israeli immigration society vie with each other for supremacy. Even before the COVID outbreak, Israel became (especially under the leadership of PM Netanyahu) a torn-apart tribal society, a confederation of cultural, ethnic and religious communities bound together by their history as well as by links of competition, hatred, envy and fear – each community fighting for its rights in what seems like an increasing willingness to sacrifice the greater good for the benefit of that community's good. So here's the paradox; while death is seen as a unifying force, life is perceived as a divisive one. And MZ was moving in and out between the two.

'Can these bones live…' (Ezekiel, 37, 3) if not charged with libido? And can sexuality (representing a 'life giving' activity) survive in such a morbid field of part-objects (quite literally) unless it is distorted and perverted to such a degree that it turns even human subjects into partial objects?

The (religious) vision of the Dry Bones (book of Ezekiel) and the (non-religious) vision of the resurrection of Israel (a phoenix-like nation reborn out of the ashes of the victims of the Holocaust, thanks to the steadfast hold onto its lands by early Zionist settlers) both seem to be a distorted and twisted reflection that MZ may have represented unconsciously to Israeli society.

One can only imagine what was standing before someone like MZ, a public envoy whose job was to collect real body parts of real victims of real terrorist acts for burial; and we can only speculate how the pandemic contributed to the thrusting of death consciousness in humanity's face, and to the ensuant further destabilization of the local status-quo which, until that point, allowed MZ to keep operating in 'split-screen' mode – probably torn between his respectful appearance in the public area and apparently hiding his private (drive-driven) life in the darkness of guilt and shame.

When the boundaries of MZ's inner world collapsed – rigid boundaries, I assume, which had to be erected in order to keep his (too many) multiple selves apart (Bromberg, 1996), death must have seemed the only place where these opposites could finally rest together.

MZ's story can be seen as representing a dark version of the curse of the 'decentered subject' (Ogden, 1992a,b) – a generic figure who experienced the many escape routes offered by the cyberworld in manic amplification, and whose life's structures collapsed into chaos when his boundaries were penetrated by the 'bad object-virus' of deadly otherness.

This may also shed some light on the private AND collective psychic context in which a system of social defences evolved, which brought about a socio-political reality that mobilized a process of splitting of the Israeli society – probably as a defence against total chaos, when the perception of reality threatens to collapse into Beta Elements (Bion, 1962). One way or another, it created two camps united mainly by their mutual hatred. The tension between the camps is ostensibly attributable to the disagreement between 'right wing' and 'left wing' on Israel's right to colonize the territories conquered from the Palestinians during the Six Days War. It is manifested as a bitter conflict between those who see the 'liberated' lands as a historic heirloom, the colonization of which is perceived as no less than redemption, salvation and therefore keeping Zionism alive – and those who see the act of settlement as a forceful occupation leading to an 'apartheid nation' and therefore as the rule of a regime of death (the death of Zionism).

It is interesting to notice that, in Hebrew, the words for ownership and sexual penetration are variations of the same root ('BAAL'); according to the latter group, forceful intercourse and forceful ownership of lands as part of a land-redemption campaign may be much closer together, psychologically, than we may care to admit.

I maintain that this **dynamic of splitting and objectification,** as demonstrated by this case, is primarily designed to rid the individual, rooted in the Israeli-Palestinian matrix, of the horrifying recognition (whenever looking at the mirror during morning tooth-brushing) of his direct responsibility and accountability (through his actions and inactions) for both Isaac's sacrifice and the expulsion of Ishmael, acts blown up by a bloody conflict in a way that seems to be without hope or way out. In blunter terms: the recognition by the parents' generation of their sacrifice of their sons, the fact that as a society (Palestinian and Israeli alike) we sacrifice our sons on the altar of an ideology (some would call it messianic-utopian), which precludes any possible compromise that could make living together possible.

A way out?

Is there any real practical value in investigating the conscious and mainly unconscious mutual relationships between the individual and his group of belonging, between the subject and the matrix of which he is not only a member but also a co-founder?

I would like to believe that the very possibility of adopting a view-point that allows – indeed, demands – for a self-conscious examination of the mutuality of relationships between individuals and society (without cancelling out the individual's full moral responsibility for his own actions – but, however, without denying the fact that anyone standing on a cliff is in danger to be pushed into the abyss by a blind and 'innocent' crowd of people who only push the back of a person standing in their way, without wanting to know anything about those who are pushed by this move over the edge), may contribute to the establishment of a civil code of ethics – one that would be based on more awareness of the power and dangers embodied in our unconscious group-life and the way present-day technology (Triest, 2013) shapes the 'place in which we live'. My hope is that it may facilitate a higher sensitivity to the potential danger of destructiveness (mental lynching, shaming, etc.) the technological breakthroughs to which our generation is exposed, put in the hands of the Social Networks (a phenomenon which is no less momentous than the discovery of nuclear fission), a power that is both a blessing and a curse (Weinberg, 2014), a prize gained by our generation without adequate preparation and in a human society that is sorely lacking in psychic maturity, and still needs time to develop and digest the technological quantum leap which in a way caught us by surprise.

Notes

1 The information related to MZ's case is based on the media and press publications. Although this state of affairs suits our purpose perfectly – since the topic at hand is not the 'real' facts but the public record of the story – it also calls for an important caveat: all that is mentioned in these pages about MZ does not purport to be an accurate or comprehensive representation of any facts and does not presume to provide any description of what MZ did or did not do.

2 I am impressed, as a practising psycho-analyst, by the fact that the psychoanalytic approaches, through the individual, and through the group, are dealing with different facets of the same phenomena. The two methods provide the practitioner with a rudimentary **binocular vision**. The observations tend to fall into two categories, whose affinity is shown by phenomena which, when examined by one method, centre on the Oedipal situation, related to the pairing group, and, when examined by the other, centre on the sphinx, related to problems of knowledge and scientific method (Bion, 1961. Introduction, p. 8).

3 Sexuality, and in Freud's terms from 1920: Eros-Thanatos interwoven (Freud, 1920).

4 In Hebrew – 'knowing' has a double meaning – search for knowledge (also close to consciousness) but also intercourse (…and Adam knew Eve his wife…).

5 The guard's question in Hamlet – also quoted by Ogden (1994).

6 This commandment prohibits women who are menstruating from having sexual intercourse or almost any other direct interaction (including any physical contact, sleeping in the same bed or even passing objects) with any male for a predefined duration, essentially because menstruating women are deemed 'impure'.

References

Bion, W. R. (1961). *Experiences in Groups and Other Papers.* London: Tavistock.

Bion, W. R. (1962). *Learning from Experience* (Vol. 3, pp. 24–27). Routledge, London and New York: Maresfield Library.

Breuer, J. & Freud, S. (1895). Studies on Hysteria. *S.E.* II, 1–323.

Bromberg, P. M. (1996). Standing in the Spaces: The Multiplicity of Self and the Psychoanalytic Relationship. *Contemporary Psychoanalysis, 32,* 509–535.

Foulkes, S. H. (1964). *Therapeutic Group Analysis.* London: George Allen & Unwin.

Foulkes, S. H. & Anthony, E. T. (1975). *Group Psychotherapy: The Psychoanalytic Approach.* London: Penguin.

Freud, S. (1920). Beyond the Pleasure Principle. *S.E.* XVIII, 1–64.

Freud, S. (1921). Group Psychology and the Analysis of the Ego. *S.E.* XVIII, *65–143.*

Hopper, E. (2003a). *The Social Unconscious Selected Papers.* London: Jessica Kingsley Publishers.

Hopper, E. (2003b) *Traumatic Experience in the Unconscious Life of Groups.* London: Jessica Kingsley Publishers.

Hopper, E. (2018a). Notes on the Concept of the Social Unconscious in Group Analysis. *Group,* 42, 2.

Hopper, E. (2018b). The Development of the Concept of the Tripartite Matrix: A Response to 'Four Modalities of the Experience of Others in Groups' by Victor Schermer. *Group Analysis,* 51, 2, 197–206.

Hopper, E. & Weinberg, H. (Eds) (2011). *The Social Unconscious in Persons, Groups, and Societies: Volume 1: Mainly Theory.* London: Karnac.

Hopper, E. & Weinberg, H. (Eds) (2016). *The Social Unconscious in Persons, Groups, and Societies: Volume 2: Mainly Foundation Matrices.* London: Karnac.

Hopper, E. & Weinberg, H. (Eds) (2017). *The Social Unconscious in Persons, Groups, and Societies: Volume 3: The Foundation Matrix Extended and Re-configured.* London: Karnac.

Ogden, T. H. (1992a). The Dialectically Constituted/Decentred Subject of Psychoanalysis. I. the Freudian Subject. *International Journal of Psychoanalysis,* 73, 517–526.

Ogden, T. H. (1992b). The Dialectically Constituted/Decentred Subject of Psychoanalysis. II. The Contributions of Klein and Winnicott. *International Journal of Psychoanalysis,* 73, 613–626.

Ogden, T. H. (1994). *Subjects of Analysis.* Northvale, NJ: Jason Aronson.

Triest, J. (2013). The "Faceless Mother": Facebook and the Unconscious Perception of Leadership. *Socioanalysis,* 15, November, 72–83.

Triest, J. (2014). "The Witch and the Child" – Reflections about the Changing Notions and Theoretical Development of Subject and Object in Psychoanalysis. *Sihot,* 1–14. XXIX, 1, December.

Triest, J. (2017). Thoughts About a New Subject of Psychoanalysis: The iGroup. In: *Not Knowing, Knowing, not Knowing – Festschrift Celebrating the Life and Work of Shmuel Erlich* (pp. 129–115). Ed. Mira Erlich- Ginor. Astoria, NY: IPbooks – International Psychoanalytic Books.

Triest, J. (2021). Das Virus des Schreckens. Notizenzur Coronazeit. *Psyche,* 2, 165–171.

Weinberg, H. (2014). *The Paradox of Internet Groups: Alone in the Presence of Virtual Others.* London: Karnac.

Winnicott, D. W. (1971a). The Place Where We Live. In: *Playing and Reality* (pp. 17:-104–110). Ed. W. D. Winnicott. London: Tavistok [1971].

Winnicott, W. D. (1971b). The Location of Cultural Experience. In: *Playing and Reality* (pp. 17:95–103). Ed. W. D. Winnicott. London: Tavistok [1971].

Žižek, S. (2002). *Welcome to the Desert of the Real.* London and New York: Verso, October.

5 Nikola Tesla and the social unconscious of Serbs

The dance of science with poetry, and of the earthly with the heavenly

Marina Mojović and Jelica Satarić

From time to time, in rare intervals, the Great Spirit of Invention descends to Earth, to tell a secret which is to advance humanity. He selects the best fitted, the most deserving, and whispers the secret in his ear. Like a flash of light the precious knowledge comes. As he grasps the hidden meaning the fortunate sees a magic change...He knows there is not a shadow of a doubt in his mind, in every fiber of his body he feels: It is Great Idea!

Tesla (1904)

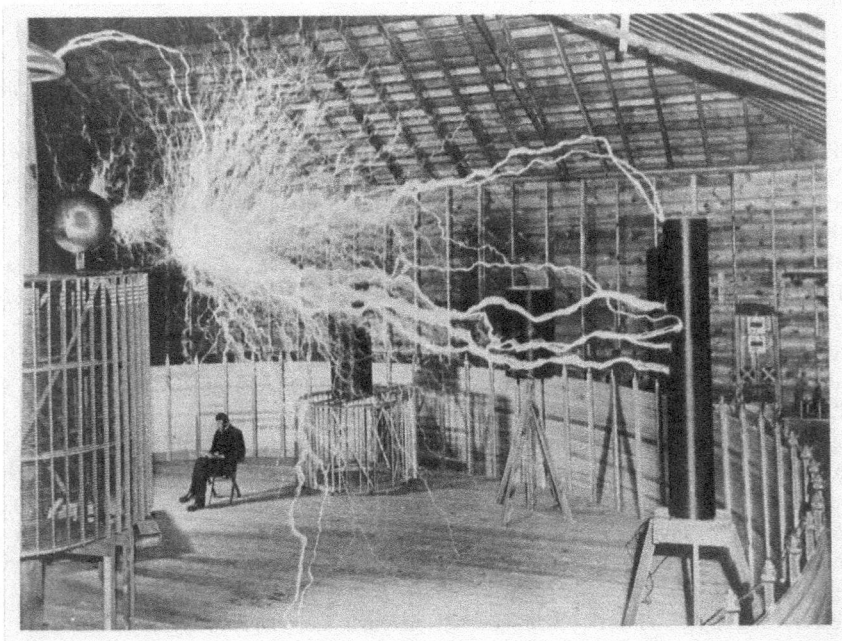

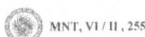 MNT, VI / II , 255

Figure 5.1 Tesla is his Colorado Springs laboratory in experiments with oscillating transformer with a 12-million volt. Photograph by Dickson Alley in Colorado Springs, 1899. Permission for using the image by Tesla Museum Belgrade.

DOI: 10.4324/9781003425915-8

Introduction

In this chapter, we consider aspects of the social unconscious of Serbs through the study of the Serb-American scientist Nikola Tesla. The concept of the social unconscious refers to the existence and constraints of social, cultural and communicational arrangements of which people are unaware (Hopper, 2003), especially within the context of a particular social system (Hopper & Weinberg, 2011). We will focus on the arrangements/interplay of the earthly and heavenly dimensions of life, the "dance of science with poetry" or on the ways of perceiving what Tesla has called the *Great Spirit*. Actually, we ourselves experience the social unconscious of Serbs as one of the manifestations of the Great Spirit (Logos), perhaps due to our Serbian roots, which has undoubtedly influenced our writing this chapter, especially in our own way and style.

The writing process, which included discussions with our editors, challenged our identification with Tesla's destiny, especially linked to issues of the worldview discrimination – particularly the Western denigration and persecution of the Serbian identity. The lack of recognition of Serbs' creativity as well as of their significance in the European history related to their/our anti-imperialistic and anti-fascistic fighting for freedom, justice and equality with readiness to sacrifice for those values is deeply embedded in the social unconscious of Serbs – an aspect of character.

Long-term bitterness due to the unfairness of the West is well portrayed in the way that Serbs perceive Tesla's fate: in spite of his extraordinary scientific gifts to the world, as are alternating current, radio and endeavoring to enable free electricity for all people, he stayed unrecognized and died in poverty. However, might certain constraints in the pragmatic and materialistic dimensions collude with the unfairness?

Leaving our hometowns and country in search for actualizing our talents and visions in the West certainly brings appreciation of the new life/work systems. However, it is always mixed with the pain of being *the other*, which can at times be unbearable. Endeavors to resist defensive escapes from such difficult feelings activate complex integration work, which involves social unconscious fields. Balancing between manic-narcissistic reactions to traumatic losses in the material/ *earthly* reality with retreating into the *heavenly* (which we tend to keep an eye on throughout the chapter) and the mourning processes, eventually with reaching authentic hope, faith and integrated knowledge, are ongoing life challenges – Tesla as an internal figure keeps helping us. How might this be linked to the socially unconscious character of Serbs?

The psycho-analytic understanding of the character formation has been modified since the classical Freudian model was developed, as outlined by Fenichel (1945). Social-psychological perspectives have become much more important. For example, Fromm's early descriptions of the "authoritarian" and "revolutionary character" were influential, as was Erikson's later psycho-social- biographical studies, e.g. Gorki, Hitler, Luther and Ghandi. American sociologist Gerth and Mills have in their "Character and Social Structure" (1953) built a model, which included the concept of the social role as a linkage between the character and the social structure. Hopper (2003) cites "A memoir of my father", by Bendix (1966), who was a German/American sociologist, as an elucidation of the personification of social forces. This resonates with the description of Tesla by Jovan Cvijić, Serbian social-geographer and ethnologist, contemporary of Tesla (at the time, president of the Serbian Royal Academy of Sciences, rector of the Belgrade University). The character/mentality type of Serbs as *Dinaric type* linked to Dinar Mountains: lively rich spirit, driven by imagination and poetry, sophisticated intelligence, high emotionality and faith, "usually inspired by moral and spiritual drives, whereas the material interests are of lower role...Ideals of justice and freedom move them much more than selfishness/self-centeredness" (Cvijić, [1922] 2011, p. 367). Many, who like Tesla immigrated to America, were able to advance the earthly/heavenly balance for themselves and societies. Tesla as a spokesperson for the wider society brings us closer to these aspects of the socially unconscious character of our fellow people, historical and cultural individuals, our ancestors and clients – whispers the precious secrets if we attune the "ears" (Tesla-receivers).

Entering with "zvezdobrojac"

Like the countless stars in the sky, the possible entries into the subject of this chapter seem endless, as often occurs with any topic in the field of the social unconscious. In line with this imagery: if we focus our vision only toward one of the stars (in Serbian "zvezda"), how can we then embrace a broader figure-ground mobility – expected from explorers in this field? How are we to know what is really the "Great Idea"? To mention the recent controversy around the winner of the 2019 Nobel Prize for literature, Austrian author Peter Handke: linked to his decades-long research into the Serbian perspective of life and history, he was boycotted by several countries, accused of racism and of denying the guilt of Serbs in Srebrenica massacres. His response to the media's simplified questioning was: "I prefer toilet paper to your empty and ignorant questions".

Is there a parallel here with the Serbian/American visionary, Tesla, one of the greatest scientists in the history of the mankind (in Serbian eyes for decades and now for many Americans as well)? For long, he was kept away from the Western mainstream, and only recently his popularity resurfaced. The theme, suggested by our editors, which links Tesla and his destiny with the social unconscious and the character of Serbs, is vast in its own right. Perhaps we should take a chance with the concept of "zvezdobrojac" so as to start clearing the way – as a vehicle or a lighthouse for traveling through the chapter. Zvezdobrojac (in direct translation: counter/mathematician of the stars) means a person attached to the stars and the cosmos in a broader sense. For Serbs, Tesla is a zvezdobrojac. We hope that mutual mirroring between zvezdobrojac and the theme, in a commensally containing relationship (Bion, 1970), will help us in unpacking the layers of complexity.

Tesla was born in the Serbian Lika village of Smiljan in 1856 during an extremely stormy night of the 10th July (28th June in the Julian calendar). This was in the white parochial house of the small Christian Orthodox Church, in which Tesla's father, Milutin, served as a priest, expecting his son to continue the same devotion, as did many distinguished members from both family sides. The house was miles away from any inhabited area, the sky shining with thunders, when the scared mid-wife said: "This will be a **Child of the Storm**", but Nikola's mother Đuka replied: "No, it will be a **Child of the Light!**" (Carlson, 2013, p. 24). Đuka's visions, included that her son becoming an inventor (as she and many of her ancestors had been), and Nikola's confidence that he was always in his mother's thoughts, never left him throughout his turbulent life.

In his personality, this "child of the light" (zvezdobrojac) was gifted with a poetic freedom to keep playfulness alive with thundering and lightning. It enabled him to *grasp the hidden meanings,* even from the repetitive flashes of light in his eyes (Tesla, [1919]2016), *revealing secrets* from the universe, which became *great ideas* for the advancement of science.

Promethean perspective on Tesla as zvezdobrojac

Tesla's story is often seen as a Promethean tale: like the culture-hero from Mythology – the creator of science and art and a trickster figure, who defies the gods by stealing fire and giving it to humanity, with the risk of overreaching, embodying the lone genius ultimately punished – so was Tesla: always looking into the future, sought to wrench lightening from the heavens and harness it to man's will, but spent his last years alone, tormented by poverty (Gunderman, 2020).

The ethereal dance between science and poetry, between the earthly and the heavenly, was successful in Tesla's creative work, but he would at times lose the fortunate-enough balance and collapse into life's voids/despairs – particularly financially. Identification of the Serbs with their *heavenly people* myth, as one of the essentials of their social unconscious, comes to mind. The strong idea among Serbs about historically making sacrifices for Europe – over centuries defending it from the Ottoman invasion, initially admired, but later unrecognized and seriously punished – is linked to this myth. In the tradition of Saint Sava (the patron saint of Serbs, who was a prince by birth, then a monk, and the first Serbian archbishop in the 13th century, the founder of autocephaly of Serbian Orthodox Church, ecclesiastical law, medicine, national literature, schooling – his fresco-image is in every Serbian classroom), the zvezdobrojac aspect means to look into the stars but to keep contact with the earthly needs of fellow people and oneself – in steady devotion to humbleness, mercy and forgiveness. We will follow this thread with the attempt to discern the deeper shades, both in Tesla's own life and in the meaning it plays in the social unconscious of Serbs in connection to Tesla.

*

Nikola Tesla (1856–1943) became an inventor, scientist and visionary, among the greatest geniuses of the modern civilization. His innovations led to the Second Industrial Revolution – the Electric Age, as well as to the Third – the Digital Age (Rifkin, 2017). Through his relentless work, sleeping usually just three hours, Tesla was devoted to helping people reach more joyful and peaceful life – decrease inequality. This included the care for the environment. He denounced the acquisition of energy through splitting atoms as unnatural, envisioning enormous dangers for the future of the world; advocated instead for costless energy directly from nature.

His successes were based on his exceptional talents, high education and extremely disciplined lifestyle. However, they were also deeply rooted in altruism and an attachment to poetry with spirituality, perhaps linked to the love legend of his parents: Milutin, publishing articles promoting equality in education for all children, thrilled/elated Đuka, from the prominent priest's family. Tesla "lit the light for mankind, enabled human voice and music to be transmitted around the planet, and wanted to bring free electric energy to all the people around the world" (Carlson, 2013, p. 53) – all linked with his intensive altruistic urges.

With his discoveries of the alternate current (AC) and high-frequency currents, which became the dominant, long-distance transmittable power-system of the 20th century, then of radio, Tesla-transformers, wireless transmission, remote-control, robotics and many other of his 700 inventions, he made significant quantum leaps possible in science and in the way we live. He laid the foundation for numerous scientific fields ranging from the lighting-engineering, radio-technology and medicine, to many original inventions in mechanical and aircraft engineering. To no surprise, Tesla's nicknames continue to proliferate: *The Man who Invented the 20th Century* (Lomas, 1999), *Prometheus of our Times, Father of the Radio, Inventor of the Modern* (Munson, 2018), *Wizard of Electrics,* and in Serbia, among others, *zvezdobrojac* – meaning a scientists' attachment to the stars and heaven, to altruism and poetry.

Interestingly, in spite of all that, in the West, Tesla was forgotten by educators and in the public life. Still, in random conversation, even with educated people, we can hear even nowadays: "Which Tesla? You mean Tesla, the car?" We may ask ourselves a question: how is this possible? Only in the last years has his legacy been reemerging in the wider world (through a proliferation of research projects, institutes, publications, films).

Take a look at the dates of Tesla's birth and death. Interestingly enough, both have a special meaning for Serbs. The 28th of June always evokes the strongest psychosocial reactions: as it is the Serbian patron-saint-day Vidovdan, the celebration of Saint Vid. "Vid" means sight, vision and visionaries and stems from the old pagan Slavic Mythology – of God Vid or Svetovid, who represents the supreme solar Ancient Serbian celestial being, deity of the Light. On this day, in 1389, the Kosovo Battle between the Ottomans and the Serbian King's Army took place and it is then that the myth of *heavenly people* re-emerged. Many other significant historical events took place on the same day. Just to mention a few: in 1876, Serbs declared the final war on the Ottomans; in 1914, the Austro-Hungarian Prince Ferdinand was assassinated in Sarajevo, followed by the Ultimatum for Serbia in such a way that Serbia had to enter the war, although fully aware of the David and Goliath kind of relationship. WWI began, in which Serbia suffered the greatest losses of all the world nations (half of all its men, and a third of the population). In 1989, for the 600th centenary of the Kosovo Battle, the president of Serbia, Milošević, gave his influential speech at the Kosovo Field; in 2001, he was extradited to Hague on Vidovdan; every year, many memorials and new social turbulences continue to emerge on Vidovdan.

Tesla passed away as an American citizen, alone in his New Yorker Hotel room. It was on the Orthodox Christmas Day, 7th January 1943. At his funeral, the representatives of the US president Roosevelt delivered speeches; the mayor of New York said: "Tesla died in poverty, but he was one of the most useful and most successful men who ever lived. His achievement was great, becoming greater as time goes on" (Matić, 2015, p. 147). After the Orthodox Christian rituals, the poem "There, faraway" (*far from the sea, there is a village of mine*) was played commemorating the greatest Serbian tragedy in WWI. Tesla's ashes along with his belongings and many documents were brought to the Tesla Museum in Belgrade – among them, his knitted bag from Smiljan, his faraway village.

Balancing between the East and the West by Serbian zvezdobrojci

Nikola Tesla had to balance in himself different aspects of the social unconscious: those from the Eastern and the Western Worlds – as Serbs, by geographical and cultural destiny, happened to live in a transitory zone. It is emphasized in his biographies that even in his last years, when the war in Yugoslavia was raging, "his destiny was that he became a pawn between the East and the West" (Chany, 1981, p. 349). The words of Saint Sava in 1221 are often mentioned:

At first we were confused. The East thought that we were West, while the West considered us to be East. Some of us misunderstood our place in the **clash of currents**, so they cried that we belong to neither side, and others that we belong exclusively to one side or the other...we are doomed by fate to be the East in the West and the West in the East, to acknowledge only heavenly Jerusalem beyond us, and here on earth–no one.

(Miletić, 1997, p. 208)

"*Zvezdobrojac* is an old Serbian word meaning a talented child looking into the starry sky place from which all brilliant minds of the Serbian science began climbing up the stairs of knowledge...becoming also good persons" (Tašić, 2018, p. 7). Mihailo Pupin, Nikola Tesla and Milutin Milanković are among the group of Serbian zvezdobrojac representatives, who had, in the late 19th century, taken their life-journeys toward America making it possible for their talents to turn into real achievements, becoming significant scientists. Like many before them (scientist Ruđer Bošković in the 18th century, even Saint Sava in the 12th century), so did over the last decades, a large number of talented Serbian youth have to leave, then in the Western countries receive recognition, world medals in mathematics, physics, astronomy and make success in the "real world". At the initiative of the Tesla Science Foundation in Philadelphia, the documentary *Tesla Nation* qualified for an Oscar in 2020. The film depicts 70 famous American Serbs, from the disembarkation of the first Serb on the American soil 200 years ago to the present day, and describes their contribution to the development of humanity embedded in the US history.

For Serbian youngsters, the identification with Tesla (and other zvezdobrojci) is significant. Typically, they leave immediately after graduating from Tesla high-school or from technical colleges (with Tesla statue in front); then fly from the Nikola Tesla Airport, while the atmosphere is saturated with ancestral stories and poetry. Marina Mojović, one of the authors, experienced similar situations when, as a child, she left for New York in a cargo-ship with her parents, both physicians, going to work in the field of science. Characteristically, on the way, poetry and stories were narrated, such as the legend of Tesla's arrival to New York with only four cents, poems of Zmaj and his own poems in his pockets. "What I left was beautiful, artistic and fascinating…; what I encountered was mechanical, rough and unpleasant. Is this America?" (Tesla, [1919]2016).

America actualizing the scientists' dreams

It is a painful path leaving the motherland for the country, of which it is expected to enable dreams come true. It is linked to the belief that America offers possibilities to anyone, wherever born or whatever class, to attain success through skills and hard work, rather than by chance – known as the "American Dream".

The capacity to find the *wings* in order to live far away from one's *roots* and to then cope with traumas of immigration highly depends on the development of communication between the *wings* and the *roots* – and, of course, with the social unconscious. Among the Serbian/American zvezdobrojci, some navigated the social ladder better than the others. Comparisons between Tesla and Pupin, another significant inventor, who immigrated a decade earlier, portray Pupin as more balanced in his social life.

We wish to look into the quality of contact between the two cultures, between the original and the new homeland, which includes the liveliness of the intercourse between the resources from the social unconscious. Pupin was seriously involved in helping his homeland through an engagement in education and finances, but also politically during post-war peace conferences. This engagement seems to be important for a balanced mobility of success, both in work and in life (Pupin, 1923). We will hypothesize that by *flying too high*, and therefore losing the links between *roots and wings*, often also the *wings* may crash.

Heavenly Serbia in the social unconscious of Serbs and Tesla

In biographies, frescoes and poetry, the Serbian kings and rulers were not praised for warfare and conquest, but primarily for their piety, beneficial endowments. A turning point in Serbian history came after the Fall of Tsar Dušan's empire, with the advance of the Ottomans and the Kosovo Battle. Before the Battle, while knowing they faced a much stronger enemy, in the famous address/toast to his knights, Prince Lazar said that it was better to choose "death with honour and sacrifice, than life in shame", and "let us die that we may live forever". Sacrifice for the Christian faith and for Kosovo is experienced as a spiritual victory of choosing *the heavenly kingdom over the earthly*. This has been lyricized in the hymns of victory with joy that God blessed the Serbian people, crowned with a martyr's wreath – signifies the triumph of eternal life over death, justice over injustice, truth over deceit and love over hate and force. This is what made Kosovo remain in the minds of Serbs, as the place where their historic destiny was "determined". Kosovo myth was reignited many times during historical crossroads.

To mention some: during Belgrade protests against the pact with Hitler in 1941, the crowds chanted: "Better grave than slave! Better war than pact". And in Patriarch Gavrilo's words: "The destiny for our nation again questions, to which kingdom we will prefer...if to live, then in sainthood and freedom, to die for it as did many millions of celebrated ancestors of ours". This was followed by the total bombing of Serbia, one of the four in the same century. Elaborations about self-destructiveness, narcissistic and scapegoat traps are, of course, numerous. They often emerge in the Reflective Citizens workshops (Mojović, 2016, 2017, 2019a,b, 2020, 2022).

Returning to Tesla, we ask: how was it possible that, even after having lived as an American citizen for six decades, the forces from the social unconscious had such a strong impact on him? In a vignette from an interview (Tesla, [1899] 1952) we see how Tesla related to Njegoš, the famous Montenegrin ruler, bishop and the greatest nation's poet of the 19th century, when he said: "I hear my Serbs are complaining about something. What do you miss? You have Bishop Njegoš and me, the best, Poetry and Science...Serbs are a mediator-tribe, traders of light energy on Earth. Their stuff doesn't go well lately, and they are worried". Tesla deeply resonated with Njegoš, especially his poem "Microcosm of Light" (which describes the soul as being guided by the *spark of the divine*). However, in the interview, we can also recognize aspects of grandiosity – hubris, with all its challenges. *Flying high*, as either persons or peoples, might bring wide visions, but also downfall. This is, actually, very different from Saint Sava's tradition with humbleness toward fellow people. In the current street protests, Njegoš is again used as a challenge for the social unconscious to disentangle unhelpful from helpful threads, the narcissistic perversions from real humanism. It reminds us of the saying: "Saint Sava saw the human – Tesla stared at the cosmos".

Icarus wings and poetry for coping with the labyrinths of traumas

We will now take a look at *Icarus aspects* in Tesla's stories. They can be found ever since boyhood: once he tried to fly from the roof of the house, fell, and seriously injured himself. Just briefly on the Ancient myth: Icarus, who was trapped in Crete's labyrinth, attempted to escape with wings made from feathers and wax, ignored his father's instructions and warnings of hubris: to fly neither too low nor too high, so that the sea's dampness wouldn't clog his wings nor the sun's heat melt them; he drowned, inspiring the idiom "don't fly too close to the sun". Did Tesla with his *wings* keep an optimal distance between the starry and the earth? His parents did warn him in the good Saint Sava's tradition. Certain detachment from it perhaps came with resistance to go for priesthood. Part of his self might have been split/orphaned from family since birth – "the child of the storm".

Tesla was aware of his excessive tendencies: the story from a winter evening in the mountain, when his boys' gang was letting a snowball dangerously roll, when he remembers a strange *destructive excitement with the forces of nature.* Later, he became involved in gambling, but with great discipline he managed to stop. There were large oscillations throughout his life, but Tesla did strive for harmony. He perceived the universe as having a core from which all strength comes, which is beauty and humility. "When we are able to be in touch with it, we feel strong and our work brings joy, because we are then like one tone in the harmony-of-the-whole" (Tesla, [1899] 1952). It also brought him closer to the mathematician philosopher Pythagoras. There are interesting similarities between these two men – even in their world-views, dietary rules, self-discipline and of course, in their interest in mathematical cosmology, the musical harmony of the universe and the attunement of the human soul to the best vibrations: "The stars in the heavens sing music, if only we had ears to hear" (Pythagoras, 2019). How can we use the sensibility to listen and tune into the wonders of nature, like that the "stone is frozen music" (Pythagoras, 2019), to turn into powers available for human use, waves of stars, electromagnetic or poetic, as were Tesla's devotions?

The region of Serbian Lika was often experienced as a historical labyrinth, thus inspiring strong urges to resolve people's suffering. It is well known that throughout history, the Serbs were, in general, exposed to a lot of social trauma, very much linked to living on the East-West historical-cultural borderland. However, Lika, as part of the Military Frontier/Borderland (Serbs officially settled there in the 15th century to protect Europe from the Turkish invasion, as were Tesla's ancestors), has many additional traumatic layers. The largest atrocities committed against the Serbs happened exactly in this region. That escalated throughout the 20th century, especially horrendously by the Croat Nazi-Ustasha State. Many members of Tesla's family disappeared in Ustasha concentration camps and Tesla himself could have suffered the same fate. Today, Smiljan is no longer populated by people; just gravestones remain beside a statue of Tesla.

The *wings* for science, poetry, spirituality and altruism, which Tesla received from his ancestors, were, perhaps, necessary for him to fly far enough from the labyrinths of the social-political "mud" of the area, and to escape the anticipated horrors to come. In addition to the collective traumas, during his childhood, there were also personal and family traumas. A few times, he almost died. From cholera, he found himself on deathbed, and recovered when his father promised to send him to the best European technical studies instead of the priesthood. Nikola was insecure compared to his older brother Dane, who was considered by everybody to be a real genius. Tragically, Dane was killed in an early accident – a trauma of which the family never fully recovered. Nikola's internal relationship with his dead brother was very complex. Psychoanalysts have written about guilt and other difficult feelings in connection with Tesla's intensive obsessive neurosis, which accompanied him throughout his life (Jerotić, 2002; Nastović, 2010).

Stories about revisiting Lika: when Tesla was lecturing in Paris in 1892, he suddenly got a strong *internal call,* a vision of his mother on a cloud with angelic figures, rushed home and found her on her deathbed. After weeks of solitude recovery in Lika monastery, he visited Belgrade. He was warmly welcomed by the Serbian King Aleksandar Obrenović, officials and writers, and engaged in plans for the electric illumination of the city. As part of the ceremony, Tesla was decorated with Saint Sava's Order, the first he had received for his scientific work. Zmaj, a physician and poet, read his poem, which celebrated Tesla's visit. Deeply touched, Tesla stood up, and kissed the poet's hand, saying: "Gentlemen and brothers! I would not be a Serb and feel Serbian if I failed to think that this night has been one of the happiest and most precious hours of my life!"

Tesla indeed saw poetry as a higher virtue than science and philosophy and felt that it had never abandoned him. Actually, the discovery of AC happened while walking with his friend in Budapest's City Park in 1882 reciting Goethe's *Faust.* The sun was just setting when he uttered the following lines (Tesla, [1919] 2016):

The glow retreats, done is the day of toil, It yonder hastes, new fields of life exploring.

Ah, that no **wing** can lift me from the soil, Upon its track to follow, follow soaring!

While pronouncing these last words, the idea of a rotating magnetic field struck him like lightning. He promptly drew a draft-image in the sand, later presented it in his fundamental patents. Most of his discoveries he made in a similar way, first in a state of reverie, then linking in detail in his mind with knowledge and theory, and then turning into real products. However, the last phase needed a good relation with material reality, including money, which he didn't value enough.

The war of the currents and the clash of cultures "Tesla, You Don't Understand the American Humour"

After studying and working in Graz, and Budapest, Tesla lived in Paris, which he admired for its artistic beauty and he dreamt of bringing more light to the city. He received an invitation to work in Saint Petersburg and almost accepted, but changed his mind after receiving the letter of recommendation for Thomas Edison, the famous American inventor and decided to go to the "land of golden promise". He arrived in New York in 1884. The following day, Tesla already started working for Edison, who praised him for his hard work and excellence in resolving problems, like lightning on steamships and design for direct-current (DC) machines. However, Edison lacked interest in Tesla's own inventions. Differences in their personalities were dramatic. Unlike the highly educated Tesla, Edison was not a man of theory but of practice: he worked over 100 hours a week, and came to all his innovations through trial-and-error. Edison built the first industrial research laboratory ("patent factory") from which he registered over a thousand patents, many made by his employees. With the help of the financier J.P. Morgan, he founded the

Edison Electric Light Company. He knew well how to turn ideas into cold cash and become a multimillionaire.

The clash of personality cultures was obvious. While Tesla was an idealist, not truly enough interested in money, in behavior, he was stylish and sophisticated, highly ethical, Edison was practical, rough and untidy, sometimes manipulative toward his employees, even insulting: he asked Tesla if in his Lika people ate human meat and joked that Smiljan, if existed at all, could not be found on any regular map. This cultural clash impacted many outcomes. Edison tasked Tesla with redesigning DC-generators to be more efficient and threw out the carrot that "there's $50,000 in it for you–if you do it". When Tesla fulfilled the task and asked for the money, Edison said, "Tesla, you don't understand American humor!" Tesla resigned; he ventured out on his own, but continued to hold the legendary Edison in high esteem.

For a while, Tesla was even a ditch-digger. However, businessmen soon sensed the commercial potentials of Tesla's discoveries and financed the birth of the Tesla Electric Company. George Westinghouse was among the first of them. He purchased all of Tesla's patents for a high amount of money, including royalty of $2,5 per horse-power. At this point, Tesla's career was reaching its peak: he registered fundamental patents for poly-phase systems of generating, distribution and exploitation of AC and lectured at the American Institute of Electrical Engineers. At that time, he was described as a handsome man with European manners and education, impeccably dressed, and witty, who kept withdrawing into his spiritual world. He enjoyed a reputation as not only a great inventor but also a philosopher, poet and connoisseur. Mark Twain frequented his laboratory. Serbian King Petar II Karađorđević also visited him.

Tesla often saw himself as a hero from epic poetry or as a knight from Schiller's or Goethe's work. These "hero aspects" or childlike idealism impacted outcomes at some financial crossroads. When Westinghouse was in crises and asking for help, Tesla without hesitation said: "You believed in me when others had no faith", and tore up the contract, sacrificing what today would be at least $250 million. Here, some Serbian features can easily be identified: blind sacrifices for friends and allies, which often hide narcissistic self-destructiveness, with long-lasting consequences, whereby the actual acts are fast forgotten. There exist many sarcastic and bitter jokes about Serbs in these terms, usually ending with "Nobody else is responsible for this, but our own stupidity". Together, Tesla and Westinghouse developed/pushed up AC that proved to be lower in cost for the transmission than Edison's DC. This was dubbed the battle of the currents. However, while AC triumphed as the system of choice, Edison remained rich and famous, while Tesla was forgotten and poor.

Tesla technically supplied the spectacular illumination of the Chicago World Fair exhibition for the 4th centenary of Columbus' discovery. At the fair, Tesla enjoyed playing with the tension between science and magic, to amaze the audience with feats of wonder, such as a wireless electric light and mechanical oscillators, which vibrate thousands of times per second – his high-frequency AC became widely known as "Tesla currents". Another victory in the War of the Currents was the opening of the huge Niagara Falls hydroelectric power-plant, the first large-scale

AC-power plant in the world: of 13 patents, nine belonged to Tesla. His statue is still there to this day. In his experiments at Colorado Springs in 1899, he built the largest oscillating transformer, and discovered the resonant frequency of the Earth's sphere (confirmed to be true in 1960), which became the basis for wireless energy transmission. Tesla envisioned a costless transmission of power from Niagara Falls through the Ionosphere to serve the entire Earth, as well as other forms of wireless communication. He believed that his system could not only distribute electricity around the globe, but also provide worldwide wireless communication. Backed by Morgan, he began building a global communications network with a giant tower on Long Island. Tesla's vision included the exploration of solar and sea energy. He foresaw interplanetary communication and the use of satellites. However, the financial support for his work ceased. The tower was pulled down in 1917 and to this day no scientific reconstruction has been made. Tesla's notes are yet to be deciphered and interpreted.

The Vice President of the Electrical Engineers Institute, Behrend, awarded Tesla (ironically) the Edison medal in 1917, saying:

> Were we to seize and eliminate from our industrial world the results of Mr. Tesla's work, the wheels of industry would cease to turn, our electric cars and trains would stop, our towns would be dark and mills would be idle and dead. His name marks an epoch in the advance of electrical science…God said Let Tesla Be and All was Light!
>
> (Matić, 2015, p. 152)

Tesla materialized a considerable number of his inventions, but many still await future to reveal their full potential. His basic system of radio in 1896 was used by Marconi, who went on to win a Nobel Prize in 1909. Only in 1943 (after Tesla's death) did the US Supreme Court uphold Marconi's patent is invalid, recognizing Tesla's more significant contribution as the inventor of radio; in 1896 Tesla's work on X-rays was published at the same time as Roentgen's, however, it was Roentgen who received all recognition for the invention. In fact, many of his inventions were accredited to others.

Tesla highly appreciated American ideals of freedom, humanity and prosperity. Yet, it remains unclear, if he were aware that eventually his projects for costless energy were not in favor of capitalist growth models and their logic of capital. It is noted that Morgan's decision to drop financing them, was accompanied with his concerns: "What if Tesla is not crazy, but does succeed in making costless energy for all? What will we then sell? Antennas!?"

Tesla in the everyday life of Serbs

Tesla is present all around us. UNESCO declared the year of 2006 as the Year of Tesla (celebrating the 150th anniversary of his birth). Unit of magnetic induction, atom-particle, electric car, hundreds of books and articles, scientific, cultural and spiritual communities bear Tesla's name and he is present in many small talks.

Tesla in a group vignette

A vignette from the author's supervisee from Kosovska Mitrovica, a university town in Kosovo and Metohija: there was an increase in social-political tensions, which, within the group-session itself, brought out strong feelings of helplessness and despair, where many people felt abandoned/forgotten (by the Serbian state, by Europe, the world, students'/citizens' networks, etc.). In addition, there were rumors that university diplomas would be treated as worthless anywhere else. The conductor thought about well-known students' exchange programs in Italy and Spain, where the University was appreciated. He was aware that he was holding different feelings than the others, but decided to stay silent in order for the group to first express their difficulties. However, they stopped relating, began avoiding eye-contact and the silence felt increasingly heavy, almost unbearable. Tesla narrative emerged (there was a student's drawing of Tesla in the room). A: "Tesla was from a village unknown to the world, but he changed the world!" B: "And he had to prove his knowledge in Austria, then in Paris, and America". C: "Don't forget digging trenches". A: "But he didn't lose hope. Many didn't believe him, but some gave him a chance". D: "He cared about money, but only to the extent that it was needed to finance his work. He died poor – he didn't care. And look at us! We are whining because someone should take better care of us!" E:

> We are simply not aware of what we can do. I feel electrified by Tesla's story and it is not a fairytale! He had to fight for what he believed, but he persisted and managed to balance his logical, practical side with the spiritual, without losing human values. What about that documentary we wanted to make? We have all we need, okay, maybe not everything, but at least we have electricity!

Everyone laughed. The group had come back to life.

Some **counter-transference** of the supervisor herself might be worth mentioning: she remembers her anxiety and sadness that the discrimination and denigration of Serbs, with so many losses, especially again there in Kosovo, might activate miserable feelings or manic-narcissistic defenses in this youth group. She felt helplessness and despair, almost unbearable, being transferred onto her during the session. The supervision group was silent for a while, as if there was a need for staying long enough with those feelings. Experience of exclusion of the group-analytic trainees from Kosovo to join the Symposia of the International Group Analytic Society due to inability to get visa for the Western countries, seemed to increase the feelings of helplessness and injustice within the transference/contra-transference processes – as if being left out by the wider professional community as well. For a moment the supervisor even doubted if her work was worth enough for the supervisee, perhaps if not recognized highly enough by some Western "universities". That thought was shared and accepted with interest.

How could the identification with Tesla help?

Although the Western allies from previous wars had in the latest history betrayed Serbs, perhaps in a paradoxical way, hope might especially emerge through the migrant Tesla. Namely, in spite of the denigration/discrimination of Tesla, the fact that he still reached/materialized in America many of his visions might help in transcending the pain of the injustice or of some related scapegoat positions. It brought inspiration and soothing also to the supervisor in her role. Particular memories from international conferences also suddenly became lively and helpful, linked to the exchanges of divergent perspectives touching important meaning, although usually only after a long while. Tesla's energy of persistence, often with spite, holding to the faith, brings alive those layers in the character of Serbs.

Transforming the clashes of cultures into creative encounters

In the social unconscious of Serbs, in line with Tesla, there are various other figures-of-lightening as role-models: from Ancient Svetovid, Saint Vid, Saint Sava, Prince Lazar, etc.

In these terms, the outcomes of our destinies depend much on the good balance between the heavenly and the earthly – certainly for Serbs, but it might have a wider meaning, for all people. For scientific dreams to become true, creative relationships with the faraway cultures/"planets" are usually necessary. The development of ways of communication between cultures is vital, as we have illustrated with the Serbian scientific youth immigrating to America – the *Tesla Nation*. Even if those dreams are well grounded in scientific knowledge and talents, without the practical/financial dimensions, they will remain forgotten and useless. If the connection between *the roots and the wings* is kept alive, the *alternating current* moving between them without obstacles, with a good transmission of contents of meaning, then *clashes of cultures might not lead to crashes* but to creative encounters – commensally containing different worlds. Aspects of the narcissistic over-identification with the starry/heavenly dimension (hubris) might be transformed into humbleness and more easily integrated with the practical.

Emigrants and immigrants experience clashes of cultures on daily bases, challenging us all. In fact, there are many unknown psychosocial areas (of social unconscious) where significant denials, blind spots, etc., can be reached and transformed through inter-cultural mirroring, as it may happen in group-analytic groups, local and international. When zvezdobrojci return to their homeland, enriched with resources from abroad and understanding of U-turns of perspectives, the clashes of course also appear. Integration needs serious work with resistances.

In both our clinical and psychosocial work (in Reflective Citizens Koinonia, local, regional and international) often we encounter Tesla images in the relational matrices. Transference and counter-transference processes related to Tesla need then to be revealed and understood; what is at a particular group moment at the stage. Most often, it is about people's transformative journey from unrecognized miserable positions toward reaching states with altruistic meaning and with faith into humanity – in spite of injustice. Tesla is often linked to the "light" like in the saying: "think only on all the towns in the world that Tesla literally brought lightening into".

Working often together, like when we, the authors, co-conduct our regular large and median groups, we have recognized that two of us often have a valence for different aspects of Tesla in the Serbian character: Marina holding more the *immigrant zvezdobrojac* and Jelica more the *Great Spirit* dimension. In group situations with the 4th ba:I A/M, when in fears of annihilation the oscillations between states of aggregation and massification happen; two of us often get mentioned related to those two major aspects of the *Tesla transference.* Illustration from the recent group situation: A: "All youth are leaving abroad. Soon we'll not have anybody in this country to hold good work!" Heavy silence with fear and paralysis was in the air, then a few stories about illnesses and dying. An older physician:

> Like Tesla unexpectedly found his way through huge troubles so in this corona pandemics, in spite of all, in our Serbian health system, actually, a lot is functioning well. Every day I am working with really fantastic, highly educated and devoted young doctors. They manage unbelievably well in most difficult circumstances!

He keeps on giving examples. G: "Jelica and Marina are also here! Who would expect in these cataclysmic times our group to enlarge with all of you joining from so far away!" B: "Marina used much to travel around, but was always returning and Jelica's wisdom keeps here the vertical contact open". N: "Tesla was able to **see** how all people on Earth are connected in the wide-web and explicitly talked about that!" S:

> The feeling of connectedness, which we get in this group with Jelica and Marina make us feel connected with both the wider external world and among us here. This experience helps us somehow keep managing the difficulties of pandemics with care and persistence, even with so many losses, fears and sadness.

Exiting with zvezdobrojac

Was the *zvezdobrojac-vehicle* a useful lighthouse in the chapter to guide us through the challenges of the theme and to embrace the bigger picture with figure-ground dynamics' occurring on the way? Did it help us to balance: preserve humbleness despite touching on "Great Ideas" – in the endlessness of the unknown, keep us safe-enough from Faustian liquids of our times (Donskis & Bauman, 2016), as well as from "flying too high"? Have we made the chapter a small transitional-home – encouragement to think about and to link social unconscious fields between communities as are the Serbian and the American aspects in Tesla's worlds? We have to leave with many open questions like: Was the monastic aspect of Tesla's life his psychic-retreat for coping with pain of the lonely genius, or with the hidden "child of the storm", eventually orphaned since birth? Perhaps it was indeed the only way to grasp the secrets from the Great Spirit of Invention, as Tesla noted. Is it linked with the "social-psychic-retreats" (Mojović, 2011, 2019a,c) in the socially unconscious character of Serbs in both meanings of circular causality for Tesla-as-a-person and Tesla-as-a-figure in the social matrices? We lend our vehicle here. Anyway, Tesla Zvezdobrojac is there around us.

References

Bendix, R. (1966). A Memoir of My Father. *Canadian Review of Sociology and Anthropology* 2(1): 1–18.

Bion, W. R. (1970). *Attention and Interpretation.* London: Karnac.

Carlson, B. (2013). *Tesla: Inventor of the Electric Age.* Princeton, NJ: Princeton University Press.

Chany, M. (1981). *Man out of Time.* Englewood Cliffs, NJ: Prentice-Hall.

Cvijić, J. (1922 [2011]). *Psihičke osobine Južnih Slovena. Dinarski tip. Lička grupa. Balkansko poluostrvo i Južnoslovenske zemlje.* Beograd: Marso.

Donskis, L. & Bauman, Z. (2016). *Liquid Evil.* Cambridge: Polity Press.

Fenichel, O. (1945). *The Psychoanalytic Theory of Neurosis.* New York: W. W. Norton & Co.

Gerth, H. & Mills, C. W. (1953). *Character and Social Structure: The Psychology of Social Institutions,* pp. xxi, 490. New York: Harcourt, Brace and Company.

Gunderman, R. (2020). *The Man, the Inventor, and the Age of Electricity.* London: Welbeck Publishing Group.

Hopper. E. (2003). *The Social Unconscious.* London & New York: Jessica Kingsley Publisher.

Hopper, E. & Weinberg, H. (eds.) (2011). *The Social Unconscious in Persons, Groups and Societies: Volume I: Mainly Theory.* London: Karnac.

Jerotić, V. (2002). *Darovi naših rođaka 4.* Beograd: Ars libri.

Lomas, R. (1999). *The Man who Invented the Twentieth Century: Nikola Tesla, Forgotten Genius of Electricity.* London: Headline.

Matić, M. (2015). *Tesla.* Novi Sad: Studio Bečkerek.

Miletić, M. (1997). *Brojanice Svetog Save. Povest o ljubavi.* Novi Sad: Beseda.

Mojović, M. (2011). Manifestations of Psychic Retreats in Social Systems. In: Earl Hopper & Haim Weinberg (eds). *Social Unconscious in Persons, Groups and Societies,* pp. 209–234. Karnac: London.

Mojović, M. (2016). Serbian Reflective-Citizens Flourishing in the Leaking Containers. *Group Analysis* 50(5): 370–384.

Mojović, M. (2017). "Untouchable Infant Gangs" in group and social matrices as obstacles to reconciliation. In: G. Ofer (ed.). *A Bridge Over Troubled Water. Conflicts and Reconciliation in Groups and Society,* pp. 119–139. London: Karnac.

Mojović, M. (2019a). Totalitarian and Post-Totalitarian Matrices: Reflective-Citizens Facing Social-Psychic-Retreats. In: Bernd Huppertz (ed.). *Approaches to Psychic Trauma: Theory and Practice,* pp. 159–177. Lanham, MD, Boulder, CO, New York & London: Rowman & Littlefield.

Mojović, M. (2019b). Serbian Reflective-Citizens and the Art of Psycho-Social Listening and Dialogue at the Caesura. *Journal of Psychosocial Studies* 12(1–2) July, 81–95(15).

Mojović, M. (2020). The Balkans on the Reflective-Citizens Couch Unraveling Social-Psychic- Retreats. In: Anna Zajenkowska & Uri Levin (eds.). *The Psychoanalytic and Socio-Cultural Exploration of a Continent: Europe on the Couch,* pp. 175–187. London & New York: Routledge.

Mojović, M. (2022b). Thinking Together in Reflective Citizens. In: Ringer M., Gordon R. and Vandenbussche B. (eds.) *The collective spark: Igniting thinking in groups, teams and the wider world,* pp. 211–224. Gent: Grafische Cel.

Munson, R. (2018). *Tesla: Inventor of the Modern.* New York: W.W. Norton & Co.

Murray, D. (2019). *The Madness of Crowds.* London: Bloomsbury Continuum.

Nastović, I. (2010). *Archetype World of Nikola Tesla.* Novi Sad: Prometej.

Pupin, M. (1923). *From Immigrant to Inventor*. New York & London: Charles Scribner's Sons.

Pythagoras (2019). *The Golden Verses*. Athens: Aiora Press.

Rifkin, J. (2017). *The Third Industrial Revolution*. (Documentary).

Tašić, A. (2018). *Zvezdobrojci: Pupin, Tesla, Milanković*. Beograd: Agape.

Tesla, N. ([1899] 1952). Interview with Nikola Tesla. In: *From Colorado Springs to Long Island: Research Notes, Colorado Springs, 1899–1900, New York, 1900–1901*, p. 244. Belgrade: Nikola Tesla Museum, 2008.

Tesla, N. (1904). Notes on Cabanallas. Patent No.164, 995. In: Jovanović, B. (ed.). *Wireless: The Life, Work and Doctrine of Nikola Tesla* (2016), p. 9. Beograd: Vulkan.

Tesla, N. ([1919] 2016). *My Inventions: The Autobiography*. Novi Sad: Akademska knjiga.

Tesla, N. (1920). Interview. In: Jovanović, B. (ed.). *Wireless: The Life, Work and Doctrine of Nikola Tesla* (2016), p. 324. Beograd: Vulkan.

6 Sex, custom and madness

A case study of the personification of the tripartite matrix of South Africa by a South African psychiatrist

Penelope Busetto

Twenty-one years into the 'new' South Africa, at the 2015 Franschhoek Literary Festival, the 'black' author and panellist Thando Mgqolozana stated, to an audience composed almost entirely of 'white' delegates, that he would no longer take part in literary events in South Africa:

> ... I feel that I'm there to perform for an audience that does not treat me as a literary talent, but as an anthropological subject – as though those people are here to confirm their suspicions that somehow I am inferior to them.
> (Mallinson, 2015)

The audience was dismayed by the suggestion that they might be racists. Most felt shame and embarrassment without quite knowing why.

Mgqolozana was expressing a disquiet and rejecting certain ways of being seen as 'other', as not quite human, that lie malignantly beneath the surface of everyday interactions in South Africa, in spite of far-reaching political changes. This persistent set of beliefs and attitudes has been highlighted across the Western world by the *Black Lives Matter* movement. Insidious racist assumptions continue to haunt contemporary life.

Clearly, there is a pressing need to investigate how racist thought is produced and entangled with non-racist thought. There is, in fact, a need to explore more broadly the shared beliefs that linger across generations, and that are transmitted, unacknowledged and unquestioned.

To this end, I have studied the 1930s archive of Dr BJF Laubscher, a South African psychiatrist and ethnographer who was in charge of the 'Native Wards' at the Komani Mental Hospital in Queenstown in the Eastern Cape between 1934 and 1938, and the author in 1937 of *Sex, Custom and Psychopathology: A Study of South African Pagan Natives*, detailing his ethnographic fieldwork in the Eastern Cape, as well as the psychiatric considerations arising from his work in the hospital. He has often been labelled as a racist.

As a lens through which to understand and unpack his racist legacy, I will make use of the theory of the social unconscious (Hopper, 2003, 2018; Hopper and Weinberg, 2011, 2016, 2017) and the concept of the tripartite matrix (Hopper, 2022) which consists of 'three overlapping and interpenetrating matrices: the foundation matrix

DOI: 10.4324/9781003425915-9

of the wider contextual society, the dynamic matrix of a particular grouping ... and the personal matrices of the members of a particular social entity' (Nitzgen and Hopper, 2017, p. 202). In the case study of Dr BJF Laubscher, the foundation matrix refers to the broader socio-cultural and historical contexts, the dynamic matrix to the discipline of psychiatry and psychoanalysis during the 1930s, and the personal matrix refers to Laubscher's personal and interpersonal world. Of course, these three sub-matrices always interact and intertwine repetitively in terms of what group analysts call a 'dialectical spiral' (Hopper and Weinberg, 2017, Epilogue). What is repressed and made unconscious in one matrix will find expression in another.

Although the three sub-matrices are interwoven, I will attempt to disentangle them by starting with the dynamic matrix: the discipline, psychiatry and how this impacted on Laubscher's thinking through the meanings buried in language that sit at the heart of psychiatry, psychoanalysis and psychology, and his entanglement with Freud and the question of 'the primitive'.

A large amount of research has been done into the history of colonial psychiatry in South Africa (see Swartz, 1996; Parle, 2007; McCulloch, 1995), but little attention has been directed towards the period between the two World Wars, from 1916 to 1938 which is where Laubscher's work is situated. In the first half of the 20th century and up until the 1970s, the number of chronic patients in mental hospitals, not only in South Africa but worldwide, increased exponentially. It was a time of great intensity and fervour as doctors struggled to identify symptoms and syndromes for a developing nosology, to isolate the underlying causes of the newly formulated disorders, to discover treatments and predict outcomes. A new era of medical science was taking shape and psychiatrists, anthropologists, sociologists, philosophers and social scientists grappled not only with practical day-to-day problems of hospitals and patients and their administration, but also with more abstract theoretical questions about the nature of the human subject.

Scientific publications and case records show the psychiatric profession grappling to consolidate its identity as a medical speciality. The scope of psychiatry had broadened and become more scientific since early colonial days. The diagnostic categories such as 'hysteria' and 'melancholia', that had dominated the field until the late 1800s, were being replaced with newer, more scientific, nuanced classifications such as schizophrenia, mood disorders, psychopathy and psychosis, through the pioneering work of Kraepelin (1923), Schneider in 1923 (in Janzarik, 1998) and Bleuler (1911). Karl Jasper's *General Psychopathology,* first published in 1913, advocated a broader understanding of psychopathology that would include phenomenology and existentialism as an essential part of the psychiatric object (Jaspers, 1913). Psychiatry and psychoanalysis were not seen as separate disciplines. Freud was still alive and writing, and his theories of the mind (Freud, 1899, 1901, 1913, 1920) had become part of the psychiatric discourse and armamentarium, driving fierce debate on the question of the origins of mind and mental disorder. Melanie Klein (1932) and Jacques Lacan (1932) were already publishing their first works.

Those working in hospitals around the world outside of Europe and North America were reading about and experimenting with new forms of physical interventions, including the precursors to ECT, but the major breakthroughs in pharmaceutical treatments for mental disorders were still a decade away. The professionalisation of psychiatry and psychology would see its practitioners occupied as advisers in educational policies to the government, in universities and schools, as doctors in the armed forces and as experts in the courts able to judge mental capacity and levels of mental ability.

Increasing numbers of 'culturally other' patients were being admitted to Western-style mental hospitals, and psychiatrists were finding themselves faced with the challenge of helping suffering people without access to their family backgrounds, with no understanding of their social and cultural worlds, or even a shared language in which to talk. Even distinguishing 'normal' behaviour from 'abnormal behaviour', the mentally healthy from the mentally ill, in the absence of any understanding of social norms, was problematic.

Psychiatrists, psychologists and psychoanalysts were increasingly dependent on information gathered by administrators, magistrates, native commissioners, anthropologists and ethnologists working in the field, and attempts were made to connect and share understandings across disciplinary boundaries and cultural differences. As racial tensions grew after the unification of South Africa in 1910 and the Native Land Act of 1913, which severely limited the ownership of land by black persons, there were growing calls for a scientific account of the 'African mind'. In his *Understanding the Native Mind* (1984, p. 26), the historian Saul Dubow writes: "the 'need to understand the native mind' held the undeniable implication that the native mind was somehow of a distinct type. Its recognition as a unique entity therefore entailed the devising of racially-based governmental policies". During the shift in South Africa from 19th-century paternalistic universalism to a policy of growing segregationism, and debates around whether 'the African people should be studied in the context of our common human history or be relegated to a special and inferior category' (Dubow, 1984, p. 14), psychiatry became an increasingly active participant in segregationist discourse.

Saul Dubow states: 'As a broad generalization it would be fair to characterize the general structure of political thought in South Africa as proceeding from within the parameters of nineteenth-century-derived notions of evolutionary progress' (1989). Implicit in this view is an idea of the universality of the 'human race', which was a commonly used synonym for the 'human species'. However, also implicit is the idea that the various 'races' which comprise this human species lie at different stages of development along a continuum between savagery and civilisation.

The concept of the primitive, although older than anthropology, was adopted by it, and the concept became one of the cornerstones of its evolutionary thinking. The term means early, the first, preserving the character of a prior stage in evolutionary or historical development. It is etymologically primary – by definition, it is that which is unanalysable in terms of a specific theory.

Celia Brickman, in her meticulously researched 2018 study, *Race in Psychoanalysis: Aboriginal Populations in the Mind*, traces the genealogy of the term 'primitive' from its earliest use by the European explorers and discoverers across the globe and their observation of human societies very different from their own, through the early colonial period in the Americas and the slave trade where the term began to evoke an idea of inferiority and lack of agency, and became identified with dark skins and immorality. It incorporated many characteristics that the Western world has come to perceive as negative, unwanted and cut off from its own self-consciousness.

Brickman shows how Enlightenment philosophers such as Kant, Rousseau, Hume, Locke and others began to formulate the 'very idea of man' in an attempt to explain both the universality and the difference between themselves and these 'primitives', portraying European 'man' as adult, responsible, rational and scientific. This justified the colonialism and slavery on which the Enlightenment was built.

In the 19th century, the term primitive was adopted by anthropologists and evolutionary theorists when defining the starting point from which, it was increasingly agreed, some peoples, notably white and male, passed in a triumphal march towards civilisation. Contemporary dark-skinned non-European peoples around the world were closely identified with the primitive, those who had been left behind. They were seen as lower on the evolutionary scale and closer to animals, while 'the civilised' were higher, superior, freer from animal instincts, able to live a life of self-control and agency. Women, too, were historically perceived and treated as inferior, the weaker sex, dominated by their animal instincts and unable to live a life of self-control and agency.

Early psychoanalysis both absorbed and contributed to these anthropological ideas, and the concept of the primitive lies at the heart of Freud's foundational thinking about the nature of the human subject. His theory of mind is built on evolutionary principles, according to which certain mental structures and certain ways of thinking, as well as certain cultures, are higher or superior compared to others. In his 1913 book *Totem and Taboo: Some Points of Agreement between the Mental Lives of Savages and Neurotics* (T&T), Freud tries to reach back into the prehistory of humankind, to find the primitive origins of mind, the moment when humankind lifted itself out of a purely animal state governed by instinct, when culture and society began for all humans, no matter how differently their cultures then developed.

According to Freud, the primitive was not only an imaginary, mythological character living in prehistoric times. He writes: 'There are men still living who, as we believe, stand very near to primitive man, far nearer than we do, and whom we therefore regard as his direct heirs and representatives' (Freud, 1913, p. 1). Not only does the term 'primitive' refer to present-day 'natives', the darker-skinned peoples of the world; Freud also posited the idea that primitive thinking is recapitulated in childhood development and in mental disorder. According to this theory, every child repeats all the stages of evolution, both physically and mentally, in order to grow into adulthood. The stages of the child's psycho-sexual and social development are linked to the incest taboo and the Oedipus myth which lie at the heart of psychoanalysis. Freud also believed that an individual's mental growth may become blocked at early developmental stages, perhaps as a consequence of trauma, and may revert to more 'primitive' states in neurosis and psychosis. In this way, he provides an easy slippage between three separate ideas – childhood, mental disorder and savagery – all are described as primitive and by evoking one, all are evoked. In common with several other 19th-century social theorists, Freud extends his evolutionary project to include developmental levels of thinking. He writes:

> The human race, if we are to follow the authorities, have in the course of ages, developed *three (...) systems of thought – three great pictures of the universe*: *animistic (or mythological), religious and scientific.*
>
> (Freud, 1913, p. 77)

These systems of thought do not merely give an explanation of a particular phenomenon, but allow the thinker to grasp the whole universe as a single unity from a single point of view.

According to this theory, 'primitive man' is caught up in animistic thinking, through which he projects his inner world into inanimate objects and events, such as trees or rivers or thunder, and creates a universe peopled by spirits and demons which are seen to be the cause of all natural phenomena and which need to be propitiated via rituals and sacrifices. This animistic system of thinking is followed by a religious phase in which thoughts and feelings are projected into all-powerful parent-like beings which impose laws and judgements and a moral code. This, in turn, is followed by a scientific phase. Freud writes:

> At the animistic stage, men ascribe omnipotence to *themselves*. At the religious stage they transfer it to the gods but do not seriously abandon it themselves, for they reserve the power of influencing the gods in a variety of ways according to their wishes.
>
> (Freud, 1913, p. 88)

Scientific thinking is seen as being at the highest level of development, the end point. Scientific 'man' has:

> reached maturity, has renounced the pleasure principle, adjusted himself to reality and turned to the external world for the object of his desires.
>
> (Freud, 1913)

Because scientific man is in touch with reality, however, he is conscious of his smallness and limitations in the face of the enormity of nature and death, which he accepts. This of course is the 'Western man'.

It is into this intellectual context that Dr BJF Laubscher was thrust after completing his medical and psychiatric studies, and it became entangled with his own personal subjective matrix. Laubscher was born into an Afrikaans-speaking family in 1897 and grew up on a farm north of Cape Town. He studied medicine in Scotland,[1] and specialised in psychiatry. In 1927, Laubscher returned to South Africa and set up a general medical practice. A few years later, he took up a post as a psychiatrist at Valkenberg Mental Hospital, a large state-run psychiatric institution in Cape Town which catered mostly for white and coloured patients.

Hospital records show that he was employed there from 1929 to 1934, working in the acute wards.

The historical folders from Valkenberg from these years portray a curious, ambitious doctor who was publishing papers in scientific and medical journals and trying out all the latest methods of treating his patients. The treatments ranged from metrazol convulsive therapy, to alcohol therapy for catatonia, to psychoanalysis, at a time when there were very few treatment modalities available.

In the hospital case notes written by Laubscher, which sometimes continue for pages, unlike the terse, repetitive, two- or three-line reports by his colleagues, he minutely and imaginatively describes patient presenting symptoms, giving examples of their speech patterns and dreams, outlining their developmental history and attempting to work out a model of the patients' mental functioning based on Freudian meta-concepts such as the unconscious, the ego, the Oedipus complex. He seems to be distinguishing clearly between disorders with a neurological origin, and those with psychogenic, traumatic or developmental aetiology. He also conducts elementary tests to ascertain levels of intelligence and mental development.

In 1933, while at Valkenberg, Laubscher was appointed the Clinical Lecturer in Psychology in the Faculty of Medicine at the University of Cape Town. This was the first time that psychology had been taught at the university. From 1931 onwards, he offered his services as an honorary court psychiatrist to the Juvenile, Criminal and Supreme Courts of Cape Town. In a letter to the Carnegie Trust dated 10th March 1934, he writes:

> Since June 1933 I have personally treated and investigated and recorded over 200 cases of juvenile offenders. One hundred or so were psycho-analysed. The results have been extremely gratifying.

In 1934, he applied to the Carnegie Trust for a travel grant which was awarded on 27th April 1934 and in the same year, Laubscher travelled to America and Europe.

A brief online search shows that the doctors and institutes he visited varied greatly in their approaches to mental disorders, ranging from the psychoanalytic, through the biological and scientific, to the eugenicist. In his book, Laubscher talks about the importance to himself of the experience in Berlin:

> The triad, mental deficiency, epilepsy and schizophrenia, occurring in the inbred pagan families studied, as well as my personal observations of the careful work done at the "Kaiser Wilhelm Institute", Buch, Berlin, have strongly influenced me in seeking the determinants of schizophrenia in the soma.
>
> (Laubscher, 1937, p. 235)

The Kaiser Wilhelm Society was an umbrella organisation consisting of many research units and was implicated in Nazi scientific operations, including the eugenic sterilisation and euthanasia of people identified as 'life unworthy of life', including the criminal, degenerate, dissident, feeble-minded, homosexual, idle, insane and the weak, for elimination from the chain of heredity.

Clearly, something was shifting in the way he was thinking about mental disorder, although he does not seem to be conscious of the implications of the shift. He was no longer conceiving it as emerging from 'childhood years' in terms of developmental and social psychology, which was part of the Freudian project. He now perceived it as located in the organism, a biological thing, which was another part of the Freudian project, an important element of which concerned the genetic origins of unconscious phantasies, which was the basis for assuming the importance of instincts and other innate phenomena. Some of the questions with which Laubscher was preoccupied and with which he later grappled in his book began to be outlined at this point.

In 1935, on his return from his travels, Dr Laubscher accepted a posting as a Senior Psychiatrist, Union Mental Service, at the Komani Mental Hospital in Queenstown in the Eastern Cape, in charge of the native wards. At this point, the entanglement of the third element of the social unconscious, the foundation matrix, or the socio-economic and historical context, will become apparent.

Queenstown lies in an area which is still today known as the Border, which for over a century had been the site of wars and clashes between white settlers and Xhosa tribes which had ended in a disastrous defeat for the amaXhosa. This, compounded by the Land Act of 1913, led to massive poverty, hunger, landlessness and disenfranchisement, as painfully described by Sol Plaatje in his 1916 book *Native Life in South Africa*.

In the rural areas like Queenstown, there was widespread unemployment and hunger. Many young men left for the cities to work on the mines under extraordinarily difficult circumstances, crowded into segregated slums that were simmering with violent crime and labour unrest. Many were unable to cope with the strain caused by urbanisation, separation from their families, tribes and culture, and the extreme poverty and hardship on the mines, and were sent home (Dubow, 1989).

In South Africa, racial segregation was becoming entrenched both in law and in fact through the three Native Bills of 1935[2] which abolished the remaining black franchise in the Cape and confirmed the unequal division of land between blacks and whites. Urban segregation was reinforced by the 1937 Natives Laws Amendment Act which "severely restricted the mobility of the Black population, and also set a limit on 'the size of the African urban population to the bare number needed for 'reasonable labour requirements', allowing the authorities to evict from urban areas Africans who were not engaged in 'ministering to the needs of whites'" (Simons & Simons, 1969, p. 499).

The hospital was opened in 1923 in spacious grounds on the outskirts of Queenstown. It is situated about 30 kilometres from the site of the Bulhoek Massacre which in 1921, two years before the hospital was completed, saw some 200 rural men, women and children protesting over land rights gunned down and killed by police and reservists (Edgar, 2021).

Laubscher took up his post at Komani Mental Hospital in 1935, in charge of the native wards. Not speaking *isiXhosa*, the language of his patients, and unfamiliar with the culture and history of the local people, the *abaThembu*, he had no under-standing of what would be the 'normal', everyday experience and behaviour of a person growing up in this environment, and therefore no sense of what would be deemed to be pathological or abnormal. For three years, while conducting research for his book, Laubscher studied the 'normal' way of life of the *abaThembu* people, their psychopathology and how they conceived of it, personally travelling great distances by car and on foot to gather information from chiefs, healers, magis-trates and native commissioners. He also sent questionnaires to the families of his patients asking for background information.

Sex, Custom and Psychopathology: A Study of South African Pagan Natives was published in 1937. The book was reprinted internationally a further four times over the next 15 years. From *Totem and Taboo*, Laubscher adopts Freud's evolutionary ideas and weaves them into his observations and understandings of the abaThembu patients and their families with a profound racialising effect. The first two-thirds of his book outlines the 'normal' beliefs and development of an individual growing up in this culture. The final one-third of his book deals with his observations on psychopathology, where he differs from Freud.

In the first part of the book, he describes a worldview created socially and cul-turally into which its members are born and in which they live out their lives. He portrays in great detail the *abaTembu* mythological beings and magic, their kin-ship structure, sexual mores and rites of passage, in particular those of puberty (circumcision) which he attempts to relate to the Oedipal complex. He writes:

> The phallic cult which permeates this *culture*, with those *mythological creatures* of evil, is almost an object lesson illustrating Professor Freud's the-ories, and shows that the conceptions of psycho-analysis are not far-fetched when viewed in the light of these mythological beliefs.
>
> (Laubscher, 1937, p. xii)

Laubscher, clearly under the sway of Freud's ideas, introduces the concepts of projection, personification and unconscious forbidden desires, and links them all to infantile thinking:

> The native in his setting reacts to his *unconscious* images and fears as does *the child* to his dreams, and these unconscious impulses, where they fall within the category of forbidden impulses, are transformed into living objects and viewed as mythical beings. Whether he thinks subjectively or objectively, invisible links always bridge his thoughts and experiences, for always ready at hand is his mythical system of beliefs serving as a channel for *projecting his own unconscious forbidden impulses and desires*. The *personification* of these ideas is similar in image and function, because they are conditioned by a *cultural pattern* which accepts them as realities.
>
> (Laubscher, 1937, p. 49)

He proceeds to show how these 'childish' beliefs form the mental world, the mind, of the abaThembu:

> Once these personified images and possibilities of activities have been given a reality value through their acceptance by the social milieu, they are no longer perceived as images of thought but as living objects which, *as the result of the mechanism of projection*, have inherited a world of their own... the native cannot isolate himself from the activities of these creatures, for the world in which these personified symbols live is his mind, and their activities are the activities of his instincts and impulses, which crawl, walk and fly as the *Inyoka, Tikoloshe* and *Impundulu*.
>
> (Laubscher, 1937, p. 49)

This is not physical racism in the usual sense of the concept. Here, he is describing the 'primitive mind' as quite other. He is portraying the symbolic world of the *abaThembu* as a projection, out of touch with reality following Freud's theory of the animistic level of thinking. According to Freud, it is a narcissistic worldview, unconscious of its own projections and closely tied to the basic savage instincts and drives of the Freudian unconscious. Indeed, Laubscher is beginning to imply that the native mind *is* unconscious. The instincts and drives are not repressed but are defended against as if they were real external objects in the world.

By accepting Freud's evolutionary levels of thinking, the way has been opened for Laubscher to express the idea that the abaThembu are pre-rational rather than irrational:

> His reasoning is quite logical once we accept the magical premises; to call his reasoning illogical or prelogical is to confuse logic with truth or reality, for a system of reasoning may be logical but still very far away from the truth; but if logic is meant to imply consistent reasoning from rational premises, then, of course, his reasoning may be described as prelogical.
>
> (Laubscher, 1937, p. 51)

Laubscher describes the difference between his worldview and that of the abaThembu in these terms:

> All this clearly shows how we move in different worlds of thought with the partition of mythology between us. My scientific training and culture has given me one form of reality and his mythology and culture pattern have given him another.
>
> (Laubscher, 1937, p. 221)

He is unable to see, however, that he, like the abaThembu, is completely immersed in his own scientific world which he considers to be superior. According to him, these are separate worlds, and the abaThembu world is greatly inferior.

By focusing on the prehistory of the abaThembu, Laubscher is able to completely ignore, virtually to deny and to disavow, the recent violent history of colonisation, exploitation and disenfranchisement. He describes the abaThembu as living out of time, constantly repeating the original unchanging patterns of social behaviour. Laubscher again invokes evolutionary theory to explain that 'the native' must evolve towards the higher level of civilisation exemplified by the whites.

> It is understood that the native will have to shed his customs in the course of his social evolution, but this should rather be a process of growing out of them by gradually changing them to suit the new conditions of his new social orders, than removing or prohibiting them by just but perhaps not wise legal action.
>
> (Laubscher, 1937, p. 88)

In terms of mental disorder and illness, he agrees with much of Freud's thinking. The normal 'native mind' is closer to the 'primitive' stirrings which psychoanalysis recognises as the unconscious of the civilised mind. But because the 'native' is primitive, 'he' is closer to the unrepressed instincts and drives. In *Totem and Taboo*, Freud likens the savage mind to that of a civilised person suffering from Obsessive Compulsive Disorder, OCD. Laubscher picks up and repeats this thread in the following passage:

> The native's attitude and reactions towards witchcraft have some analogy to the thinking and acting of the compulsive neurotic patient. Both are struggling against the dynamic expressions of forbidden impulses. The obsessional neurotic is defending himself against the impulses from his own mind, while the native is defending himself against impulses from the world of mythical beings. We know that the obsessional neurotic is continually making compromises with his unconscious desires, as well as sacrifices and ceremonials. A study of the various pagan customs and sacrifices shows this same factor of atonement towards the *Izinyanya* (ancestors, my translation), which together with the mores of this culture, correspond to the superego or moral conscience of the obsessional neurotic patient. This similarity is further observed in the magical power that words have for the obsessional neurotic. In this respect do the phobias and obsessions in European patients serve as clinical illustrations of the native's defence reactions against witchcraft.
>
> (Laubscher, 1937, p. 51)

In fact he believes that repression is not really a part of 'native' mental activity at all since there is no separate unconscious:

> In the type of psychoneurotic under discussion, it is an individual matter peculiar to the experiences of the person and is portrayed in symptoms as a conflict between the instinctive infantile urges and the later acquired moral components of the mind, whereas in the pagan native it is the instinctive

infantile needs in conflict with the dictates of patriarchal law and tribal moral customs. But the guilt feelings underlying both forms of reaction remain the same and, in the native culture, it is the problem of a people wherein all share.

(Laubscher, 1937, p. 52)

Thus, the 'native' is seen as not having subjective moral feelings, which are typical of the Western mind, but only moral obligations imposed by tribal culture. For Laubscher, the 'native' has no real agency or individuality and is immature:

This belief forms the basis of his immature differentiation between subject and object relationships. In fact, it is the emotional and dynamic value of his beliefs that leads to this defective appreciation of subject and object relationships. If such a description is permissible, this condition appears to me, to consist in his defective discrimination being due to a fusion of his ego with objective reality. The comprehension of rational relationships as known to us has but a faint glimmer in his psychology.

(Laubscher, 1937, p. 56)

Laubscher has thus provided a 'scientific' explanation, haunted by Freudian meta-concepts, to justify a description of 'the native' as trapped in a world of his own making, filled with monstrous creatures of evil which he must placate. He portrays this person as immature, unconscious, without any subjective moral compass, behaving like a person suffering from OCD for whom reason is simply 'a faint glimmer'. He compares this to 'the civilised man' who is able to distinguish between subjective and objective relationships through reason, and is able to control his impulses and have agency in the world.

Laubscher's work, based on the 'socio-biology' of Freud, Darwin, Fraser, Jung and others, was, in Hopper's terms, 'a matter of his unconscious personification of the saturation of the dynamic matrix of the profession of psychiatry and its institutions by the foundation matrix of the contextual society'. However, his work was used to justify political and economic racism in the build-up to apartheid. Laubscher's ideas sounded so reasonable and so scientific. Unfortunately, these ideas had significant influence on the thinking of judges, educators and administrators in their work. It should be acknowledged that the racism of apartheid in South Africa was an extreme version of political processes and racist ideologies which were common throughout the world. Professions and the practitioners of them are hardly insulated from the unconscious constraints and restraints of the foundation matrix of the contextual society.

Note

1 It seems probable that he studied towards a Triple Qualification, which was a licence to practice medicine granted jointly by the Royal College of Physicians of Edinburgh, the Royal College of Surgeons of Edinburgh and the Faculty of Physicians and Surgeons of Glasgow. (Correspondence with Alistair Tough, University of Glasgow Archive Services 2013)

2 https://www.SAHistory.org.za/archive/Chap-3/ "In 1935 the Union Government confronted the country with what were called the Three 'Native Bills', or, as we knew them, the notorious Hertzog Bills, which were to 'settle the Native Question once and for all'- according to the rulers' way of thinking. The need for this drive to 'settle the Native Question' did not spring out of the fertile brain of some politician. It had its roots in the economic and political conditions of the country".

References

Bleuler, E (1911) *Dementia Praecox oder Gruppe der Schizophrenien.* Leipzig: Deiticke, translated by J Zinkin *as Dementia Praecox: Or, the Group of Schizophrenias*, published by International University Press, New York (1952).

Brickman, C (2018) *Race in Psychoanalysis: Aboriginal Populations in the Mind.* London and New York: Routledge.

Dubow, S (1984) *Understanding the Native Mind: Anthropology, Cultural Adaptation, Elaboration of a Segregationist Discourse in South Africa, c. 1920–1936*, Seminar Paper, University of Cape Town.

Dubow, S (1989) *Racial Segregation and the Origins of Apartheid in South Africa 1919–1936.* Palgrave Macmillan, London.

Edgar, RR (2021) *The Finger of God: Enoch Mgijima, the Israelites, and the Bulhoek Massacre in South Africa.* Charlottesville, VA: University of Virginia Press.

Freud, S (1899) *The Interpretation of Dreams*, translated by James Strachey (1981). The Standard Edition of the Complete Psychological Works of Sigmund Freud, Volume IV. London: Hogarth Press.

Freud, S (1901) *The Psychopathology of Everyday Life*, translated by James Strachey (1981). The Standard Edition of the Complete Psychological Works of Sigmund Freud, Volume VI. London: Hogarth Press.

Freud, S (1913) *Totem and Taboo: Some Points of Agreement between the Mental Lives of Savages and Neurotics*, translated by James Strachey (1953). London: Routledge & Kegan Paul Ltd.

Freud, S (1920) *Beyond the Pleasure Principle*, translated by James Strachey (1981). The Standard Edition of the Complete Psychological Works of Sigmund Freud, Volume XVIII. London: Hogarth Press.

Hopper, E (2003) *The Social Unconscious: Selected Papers.* London: Jessica Kingsley.

Hopper, E (2018) Notes on the Concept of the Social Unconscious in Group Analysis. *Group*, 42, 2, 99–118.

Hopper, E (2022) "Notes" on the theory and concept of the fourth basic assumption in the unconscious life of groups and group-like social systems: Incohesion: Aggregation/ Massification or (ba) I:A/M. In C. Penna (In Press) *From Crowd Psychology to Large Groups: Investigations on the Social Unconscious* (pp. 176–208). London: Routledge.

Hopper, E & Weinberg, H (eds.) (2011) *The Social Unconscious in Persons, Groups and Societies: Volume 1: Mainly Theory.* London: Karnac.

Hopper, E & Weinberg, H (eds.) (2016) *The Social Unconscious in Persons, Groups and Societies: Volume 2: Mainly Foundation Matrices.* London: Karnac.

Hopper, E & Weinberg, H (eds.) (2017) *The Social Unconscious in Persons, Groups and Societies: Volume 3: The Foundation Matrix Extended and Reconfigured.* London: Karnac.

Janzarik, W (1998) Jaspers, Kurt Schneider and the Heidelberg School of Psychiatry. *History of Psychiatry* Jun, 9(34 Pt 2), 241–252.

Jaspers, K (1913) *Allgemeine Psychopathologie translated as General Psychopathology by* Hoenig, J. and Hamilton, M.W., Manchester: University Press (1963). Pages 1–5, 138–140, 556–562.

Klein, M (1932) *The Psycho-Analysis of Children.* Penguin Vintage Classics (1997).

Kraepelin, E (1923) *Clinical Psychiatry: A Textbook for Students and Physicians.* Abstracted from the 7th German edition of *Lehrbuch der Psychiatrie,* by A. Ross Diefendorf, Macmillan, London, New York, digitized by University of Wisconsin. https://babel.hathitrust. org/cgi/pt?id=wu.89097730584&view=1up&seq=9

Lacan, J (1932) *De la psychose paranoïaque dans ses rapports avec la personnalité, suivi de Premiers écrits sur la paranoïa.* Paris: Éditions du Seuil, (1975).

Laubscher, BJF (1937) *Sex, Custom and Psychopathology: A Study of South African Pagan Natives.* London: Routledge & Sons.

Mallinson, T (2015) "Thando Mgqolozana: The Audience Does Not Treat Me as a Literary Talent, but as an Anthropological Subject." *The Daily Vox,* 13 May 2015. https://www. thedailyvox.co.za/thando-mgqolozana-the-audience-does-not-treat-me-as-a-literary-talent-but-as-an-anthropological-subject/

McCulloch, J (1995) Colonial Psychiatry and "The African Mind". Cambridge University Press, Cambridge, England.

Nitzgen, D, & Hopper, E (2017) The Concepts of the Social Unconscious and of the Matrix in the Work of S. H. Foulkes. In E. Hopper & H. Weinberg (Eds.) *The Social Unconscious in Persons, Groups, and Societies: Volume 3: The Foundation Matrix Extended and Re-Configured.* London: Karnac.

Parle, J (2007) *States of Mind: Searching for Mental Health in Natal and Zululand, 1868–1918.* Scottsville: University of KwaZulu-Natal Press.

Plaatje, Sol.T. (2016) *Native Life in South Africa,* P.S. King & Son Ltd, London, this edition with Foreword by Kader Asmal by Picador Africa, Northlands South Africa (2007).

Simons, HJ, & Simons, RE (1969) *Class and Colour in South Africa, 1850–1950.* England: Penguin Books Ltd.

Swartz, S. (1996). Colonialism and the production of psychiatric knowledge in the Cape, 1891–1920. PhD Thesis, University of Cape Town.

Part III

Personifications and clinical work

7 Transference, countertransference, and the social unconscious

The bastion in clinical figurations in tripartite matrices

Carla Penna

Introduction

Psychoanalytic and group-analytic theory and technique are shaped by clinical observations, which offer insights into the development of intrapsychic, intersubjective, and trans-subjective processes of persons and persons in interaction. However, in their daily practice, clinicians do not always take into account the way the societal context, especially under traumatic situations, influences, shapes, and reshapes theory and technique (Hopper, 2003a, p. 103). In this sense, discussions on the social unconscious in clinical work meets what Foulkes (1948) announced when he affirmed that "the old juxtaposition of an inside and outside world, constitution and environment, individual and society, phantasy and reality, body and mind and so on, are untenable" (p. 10). It means that individual persons cannot be separated from their contexts: "We cannot isolate biological, social, cultural and economic factors" (Foulkes, 1975, p. 37). The new perspective proposed by Foulkes highlights the importance, almost as an urgency, of taking seriously "total situations" (Foulkes, 1948) in clinical work, allowing the exploration of socially unconscious dimensions of human interactions. The idea of the social unconscious refers to:

> the social, cultural, and communicational constraints and restraints of which people are to varying degrees unconscious. The social unconscious emphasizes the shared anxieties, fantasies, defences, myths, and memories of the members of a social system... The field theory of the social unconscious includes its sociality, relationality, transpersonality, transgenerationality, and collectivity.
>
> (Hopper & Weinberg, 2017, p. xxii)

One of the main difficulties of the social unconscious project is to present and discuss clinical evidence of the restraints and constraints of social unconscious processes. It is still a challenge for group analysts to present clinical illustrations that consider the connection established between "psychic facts and the

DOI: 10.4324/9781003425915-11

social-historical facts" (Hopper, 2003a) in a way personal unconscious feelings, fantasies, and defences can through processes of equivalence (Hopper, 2003a, p. 100) find their corollaries in the psychodynamics of the family, groups, and society.

In this chapter, we examine socially unconscious clinical perspectives from Latin American conceptualizations of the psychoanalytical field theory (Baranger & Baranger, 2008, 2009; Tubert-Oklander, 2007, 2011, 2017). They present especial affinities with group-analytic thinking, bringing concepts that contribute to the exploration of clinical aspects of the social unconscious. The most recent development on the social unconscious theory extended and reconfigured the concept of matrix in terms of tripartite matrices (Hopper & Weinberg, 2017). The new proposed model for the concept of matrix allows the exploration of specific figurations (Elias, 1984) co-created by personal, dynamic, and foundation matrices. These developments reshaped the concept of matrix, now "firmly *rooted* or *grounded* in both historical time and space, and in *interpersonal* and *transpersonal* space" (Nitzgen & Hopper, 2017, p. 11). They introduced to group-analytic theory, especially to clinical work, a four-dimensional time/space outlook to explore the social unconscious in the realms of tripartite matrices through systems theory and/or field theory (Hopper & Weinberg, 2017).

Latin American field theory

Gestalt theory and Kurt Lewin's (1947) social field theory lie in the roots of the main analytic group approaches; however, the way these postulations influenced the theories developed by Bion, Foulkes, Pichon-Rivière, and Kaës differs. The idea of social field also played an important role in psychoanalytic theory and practice, not only in the study of the transference-countertransference relationship, but also in the development, under John Rickman's influence, of new ideas on countertransference (Heimann, 1950; Money-Kyrle, 1956) and on Bion's later work (Hinshelwood, 2018). In Latin America, the Gestalt theory, Lewin's social field theory (1947), and Maurice Merleau-Ponty's (1945) phenomenology also influenced the psychoanalytic and analytic group theories formulated by Pichon-Rivière, José Bleger, Henrick Racker, Madeleine and Willy Baranger and Jorge Mario Mom in the 1950s and 1960s. The idea of an "analytic situation as a dynamic field", as configured in 1961–1962 by the Barangers (2008), explores the unconscious dynamic of the psychoanalytic field. Their work extended the analyst's observations regarding the intersubjectivity co-created by the analyst-patient and their transference-countertransference relationships at the analytic room. Through the characterization of the analytic situation as a dynamic bi-personal field, we can observe the interplay of processes of projective and introjective identifications and counteridentifications. We can also see the emergence of a new gestalt built through mutual identifications and shared unconscious phantasies co-created by the analytic pair (Baranger & Baranger, 2008, p. 809).

The analytic situation comprises, among several properties (Baranger & Baranger, 2009, p. 2): (a) conscious and unconscious, verbal and non-verbal communications in a bi-personal field; (b) the totality of phenomena involved in the analytic situation in terms of process and non-process as described by Bleger (1967, 2013); (c) the use of the transference-countertransference relationships, as well as the resistance-counteresistance interplay as a technical tool (Penna, 2008; Racker, 1960). Although connected to Kleinian theory, the field theory allows for exploring the unconscious dimensions created in the analytic field, revealing a spatial, temporal, and asymmetric functional structure comprised by the analyst-patient relationship. The analytic situation involves two persons, but it is only bi-personal at the level of ordinary perception, when it acquires a triangular character underlined by "a third, absent-present part, that represents the oedipal triangle" (Baranger & Baranger, 2008, p. 795). Thus, "the analytic couple is a trio, one of whose members is physically absent and experientially present" (p. 798). In this sense, "the bipersonal situation is also a multipersonal relationship" (Baranger & Baranger, 2009, p. 2).

However, the Barangers did not extend their conceptualizations beyond the limits of the analytic office nor included on their views the socio, cultural, political, geographical, ecological, dimensions (Tubert-Oklander, 2017, p. 195). This task had been undertaken by Foulkes (1948) and group-analytic authors who drew attention to the importance of "total situations„ and by Pichon-Rivière and his co-workers, such as José Bleger, David Liberman, and Edgardo Rolla, who in the 1950s and 1960s discussed a more holistic process theory of the analytic treatment centred on Pichon-Rivière's concept of spiral process[1] (Baranger, 1979, p. 45; Losso, de Setton & Scharff, 2017; Pichon-Rivière, 1958).

Clinical figurations

The group-analytic international community makes possible to get in contact with the clinical practice of several countries where sociocultural differences concerning the group-analytic situation – such as communication, interaction, group-specific factors, dynamic administration, setting and group composition – are apparent. Sometimes, these differences are noticed only by comparison. However, the way each group matrix experiences the particularities of the *habitus*[2] (Elias, 1939) of their own foundation matrix (Hopper & Weinberg, 2017) is unconscious in various degrees, just as the interplay between the tripartite matrices on their daily work. These differences refer us to the realm of the social unconscious in clinical practice. Thus, in the group-analytic group, features of the foundation matrices, like race, gender, social class, socioeconomic structure, power relations, language, and transgenerationality, social unconsciously influence the dynamic matrix relationships and the personal matrices of group participants, including the convener (Hopper & Weinberg, 2011, 2016, 2017). That is, embedded in the soil of particular foundation matrices, denial, disavowals, fantasies, myths, styles of thinking and communication (Hopper, 2003b), as well as different forms of experiencing personal and social suffering revolve and evolve in group matrices.

In clinical practice, social unconscious contents remain most of the time out of the conscious, not only denied, repressed, or disavowed, but also sometimes as if they were almost encapsulated (Hopper, 2003a), "in retreat" (Steiner, 1993) in the analytic field. The unawareness of the socially unconscious co-constructions immobilizes, blinds, and even splits the contents out of the individual session and out of the psychodynamic of the group matrix. Nevertheless, these contents remain inside the analytic field, waiting for the "point of urgency"[3] (Baranger, 1993; Pichon-Rivière, 1971) where the unconscious contents are ready to emerge in the session, as an insight to be interpreted (Churcher, 2008, p. 791), reconfiguring the field and twisting the rotation of the dialectic spiral of the session. The point of urgency reveals an unconscious fantasy[4] co-created by the "communication from unconscious to unconscious" (Baranger & Baranger, 2008, p. 805) between the analytic pair. In this sense, the Barangers (2008, p. 806) states:

> With these restrictions in mind, we can only conceive of the basic phantasy of the session – the point of urgency – as a phantasy in a couple (in analytic group psychotherapy, the appropriate expression is "group phantasy"). The basic phantasy of the session is not the mere understanding of the patient's phantasy by the analyst, but something that is constructed in a couple relationship.

However, these contents can remain immobilized and split, but still present in the field. It means that, in the bi-personal situation, this impairment can hinder the treatment, crystallizing the spiral process of the dynamic field mainly when "the patient's attempted splitting meets the analyst's unconscious complicity or a blind spot" (Baranger & Baranger, 2009, p. 8). In this direction, the Barangers (2008) introduced the concept of *baluarte*/bastion to discuss "the unconscious refuge of powerful phantasies of omnipotence" (p. 814) that the patient makes use of in analysis to resist and avoid confrontation with "states of extreme helplessness, vulnerability and despair" (p. 814).

The bastion is also connected to patients who do not want to put at risk the gratification obtained through pathological activities. In other patients, it relates to the maintenance of a sense of intellectual or moral superiority, richness, social class, and even to a specific ideology (p. 814). Others need to keep untouched their relationship with an idealized object of love, their love for an Oedipal rival, or even an ambivalent love towards the rival.

The concept was initially related to intersubjective resistances/counter-resistance collusions in the analytic pair interplay (Racker, 1960) and was explored by Bleger (1967) in his work on the psychoanalytic frame. The idea of bastion can be understood "as a retreat where omnipotent unconscious phantasies remain protected in a bulwark" (Churcher, 2008, p. 791). However, in connection to the bi-personal unconscious fantasies co-created by analyst and patient, the bastion can be defined as a gestalt, as a product of the field, a "dyadic fantasy" (Tubert-Oklander, 2007, p. 123) co-created by the analytic pair (Cassorla, 2018).

Therefore, we suggest that the kernel of social unconscious restraints and constraints in clinical work lies in the blind spots engendered by the unconscious fantasies created between the analyst and the patient in the field. In a group-analytic group, these blind spots can be translated as the presence of unconscious collusions co-created by the members of the group that remain split, denied, and untouched. Such considerations allow us to understand the "bastion" from a transpersonal perspective as a "socially unconscious group collusion" that rests silenced, disavowed, and encapsulated, as a "static foreign object" (Baranger, Baranger & Mom 2009, p. 66) in the group matrix (Hopper & Weinberg, 2017). Bastions can certainly be associated with group-analytic explorations as black holes (Doron, 2017) in clinical work and with the creation of social psychic retreats (Mojovic, 2011) in groups and society.

Although split and preserved against intrusion and experiences of pain, as in a "fortress", a bastion is never absent in the field, and "varies enormously from one person to another" (Baranger & Baranger, 2008, p. 814), and certainly from one group matrix to the other. Moreover, we believe that the bastion is not only connected to unconscious fantasies, or even to "a group phantasy" (p. 806). It is also connected to Hopper's (1991) work on encapsulations and his subsequent conceptualization of a fourth basic assumption theory – Incohesion: Aggregation/ Massification – in the traumatic experiences in the unconscious life of groups and group-like social systems (Hopper, 2003b). In this regard, a bastion seems to protect against experiences of failed dependency, the defences associated with them, and the acknowledgement of massification as a defence against aggregation, which is itself a development of social psychic retreats.

Consequently, we can suggest that a "group bastion" is like a socially unconscious area associated with the group's tripartite matrix, in which fantasies, defences, disavowals, myths, and collective or transgenerational memories probably connected to historical, structural trauma or chosen traumas or glories (Volkan, 2004) lie unconsciously in the foundation matrix in particular. It means that social unconscious contents rest as unconscious collusions in blind spots/areas, which, as bastions, remain untouched, out of sight, and out of the transference-countertransference relationships in the group matrix and in the overlapping worlds of analyst and patient or of group analyst and group (Puget, & Wender,1982). The bastion remains as "an immobilized structure that is slowing down or paralysing the process" (Baranger, Baranger & Mom, 2009, p. 65).

However, the absent presence of these repressed or disavowed contents waits for the point of urgency to emerge – sometimes through an enactment – in the multipersonal group field. The "fall of the bastion" might be at first experienced as catastrophic, but through interpretation and intensive analytic work it may eventually lead to a positive enrichment, bringing insight and integration to the field (Baranger & Baranger, 2008, p. 816). Therefore, group interactions are retaken and the formerly paralysed nucleus in the "group bastion" is reintegrated. This change within the field allows for recovering and reappropriating the meaning of the socially unconscious contents that had been alienated, denied, and disavowed in the group matrix. In this sense, the insight restores the group-analytic field, overcoming split areas, bringing awareness of socially unconscious processes, new meanings, and movement to the group matrix. The convener's ability to be attuned to their countertransference/counter-resistance, developing an attitude of listening, of suspended attention, of second look (Baranger, Baranger & Mom, 2009, p. 65) to communications within the field is fundamental. This attitude brings insight and change to a previously impaired communication, expanding exchange to different levels of communication in the group's tripartite matrices. In the next section, we explore and illustrate the social unconscious vicissitudes through a clinical vignette.

Clinical illustration

Below follows a brief illustration from a Brazilian out-patient group-analytic group held at the psychiatric ward of a university hospital in Rio de Janeiro. It was a small group composed of disadvantaged female patients, highly traumatized by different dimensions of failed dependency and real threats of annihilation, with life stories marked by poverty, abandonment, adoption, abuse, and violence.

Ana: "You know, doctor, I suffered a lot. I lost hope and I am depressed. I don't know what to do with my daughter. She often disappears for two or three days and, when she comes back, she behaves as if nothing had happened…"

Rosa: "I wish I had three daughters like yours! I have no one. I was happy until I was fifteen, living with a family I thought was mine. Then, during a party, my mother got drunk and told me I was adopted. I got crazy! I ran away and got ran over. I tried to kill myself, but I ended up hospitalized for one year. When I left the hospital, I didn't want to see my family. I came to Rio de Janeiro to live on my own, but I wanted to build a family. Four months ago, I lost my new-born daughter and my womb. And now…" (She cries.)

Ana: "I am adopted too, and I have been mistreated. I was poor. I didn't have any shoes. They used to beat me so hard that I fainted often. I never knew why I was being beaten up. I have already been through tough times in life, but I don't accept being mistreated by my own daughter. I do everything for her…"

Norma: "I don't know… I was not in the mood to speak, but after hearing what was said here, I begin to feel hope. I think something good can come out of this group. We have to believe, to value ourselves. I have hope…"

Discussion

This group has met for four years, once a week, until its termination. The group sessions were permeated by psychic suffering, experiences of helplessness, pathological and regressive states. Throughout our intensive work, the group matrix began to experience more lively interactions and a sense of deep cohesion, fostered by communication and a mutual support has been built. This more positive dynamic, which lasted until the end of the process, was triggered by an episode that reconfigured the tripartite matrices interplay in the group field.

On one occasion, I was stuck in a staff meeting and arrived late for a session. Coincidentally, the room where the group usually met was taken by another therapist and her client. My group managed to kick them out, starting a near riot in ward lobby, so that they could re-occupy "their" territory/group room. When I arrived, my patients were already working on their own.

At first glance, this episode can be seen as a typical organizational problem in an out-patient psychiatric ward that interfered in the group setting. At that time, I understood it as a sign that the group as a whole was more mature and able to fight for their "rights", instead of reexperiencing and re-enacting abusive situations.

My experience with groups of disadvantaged patients in Brazil had previously shown me that group analysis is a fundamental tool to treat this population (Penna, 2012). These patients are, in general, surrounded by precariousness. They live invisible and voiceless lives in the margins of society. In this sense, group analysis is an ally in their "struggles for recognition" (Honneth, 1996), both in the personal and public spheres. The group matrix has provided the group with a safe space for communication, resonance, mirroring, exchange, and support (Foulkes, 1948). Moreover, it fostered a sense of community, of citizenship – *Koinonia* (de Maré, Piper & Thompson, 1991).

The "group riot" at the ward lobby unveiled uncontained anxieties connected to the patients' helplessness as regards experiences of failed dependency in a situation in which my absence and the rupture in the setting, at least in their fantasy, meant a real threat of annihilation to the group or its continuation at the out-patient psychiatric ward. This episode revealed the psychodynamics between the personal matrices and the group's dynamic matrix.

Taking into account the social unconscious of Brazilians and the features of its foundation matrix (Hopper & Weinberg, 2017; Penna, 2016), other dimensions of that group's "riot" can be analysed.

As opposed to my patients, I come from an advantaged background, and during my role as the convener in the group, their traumatic experiences and psychosocial hardships had a deep impact on my countertransference. In groups, the transference-countertransference relationship is always intense and influences the group field in different dimensions. By that time, I considered my countertransference as "normal", as a result of the "appropriate oscillation in the analyst between projective and introjective identification" (*apud* Cassorla, 2018, p. 64; Bion, 1962; Money-Kyrle, 1956). However, my countertransference was marked by a sense of compassion regarding the patients' difficult lives and by my uneasiness, derived from my perception that the Brazilian government does not address social inequalities. In this respect, the creation of sort of "phantastic collusion" – the interplay of projections between caregivers and patients, in which only the roles of health and illness, helpful and helpless are on offer (Main, 1975, p. 61) – was a hidden presence/content in the group matrix interactions.

A "group bastion", a "socially unconscious group collusion", has been created between the patients and I. Although split, it was clearly grounded on the Brazilian sociocultural context. That is, the features of the Brazilian foundation matrix – patriarchal relationships, power relations, class struggles, social guilt, structural racism, and the discourses about these relations, typical of the former colonies (Penna, 2016; Souza, 2018) – remained socially unconscious, fomenting the creation of a "group bastion". An unconscious "phantastic collusion", rooted in the Brazilian socio-structural inequalities, was being enacted in the group field. The bastion hosted an "involuntary and unconscious complicity" (Baranger, Baranger, & Mom, 2009, p. 65) between the convener and group members that silently interfered and impaired progress. Convener and patients in their transference-countertransference, in their resistance and counter-resistance relationship (Hopper, 2007a,b; Penna, 2008; Racker, 1960), were socially unconsciously enacting in the group matrix field, as in a nutshell, the structural traumatic experiences of the unconscious life of Brazilian foundation matrix. They were personifying fixed roles, the ideal types available and ever-present in the socioeconomic structures of the Brazilian foundation matrix (Penna, 2016). In this sense, the bastion had led to a crystallization of the field, giving space to a "shared fantasy assembly" among its members when it attributed "a stereotyped imaginary role to each" (Baranger, Baranger, & Mom, 2009, p. 66).

The "group riot" functioned as a "point of urgency" for important transformations in the field. It allowed the revelation of "the group bastion", of the "group unconscious collusion" that had role-sucked the convener and the patients for stereotyped roles in the transference-counter transference interplay. Polarized personifications (Hopper, 2003b) between caregiver/patient, health/illness, potency/impotency, richness/deprivation, as well as "fantasies of illness and fantasies of cure" (Pichon-Rivière, 1971), were impairing the group process. Until that moment, the group matrix, including the convener, was trapped in a socially unconscious discursive formation forged by centuries of patriarchalism in terms of interclass relationships. The group matrix was captured by apparatuses of power (Penna, 2016) that engender the discourses that usually divide social classes in Brazil (Souza, 2018), attributing social categorizations and states of mind to both. In other words, through an interplay of projective and introjective identifications, the group matrix enacted those psychosocial struggles. My social guilt was being translated and acted out in the group matrix through excessive concern regarding "the fragility and helplessness" of my patients. However, "the group's riot" dismantled the phantastic collusion, surprising both the group members and I. The strength of Eros and the bonding the treatment created transformed the process. Despite their personal difficulties, the patients were able to fight for the "group space" in the ward. In doing so, they revealed the "group bastion", allowing a new figuration for the tripartite matrices of/in the group field.

After the incident, our interactions improved, giving room for more communication and less polarized relationships. We could discuss how the episode transformed their perceptions about themselves inside and outside the matrix. Some were pleased to observe their pro-activity and "power". After that, they slowly move from victimhood and impotence to a more positive attitude towards life. In psychoanalytic terms, we can state that the quality of group interactions gradually shifted from a paranoid-schizoid to a depressive position, from monologue to dialogue. After my "absence" in the session, the group started to de-idealize me and empathically recognize me as a person with failures and difficulties. Yet, my privileged social status has never been mentioned or considered as a topic for discussion in the group. The "fall of the bastion" made possible to reveal an important feature of Brazilian social unconscious – co-created in our *habitus*, and unconsciously present in the realms of the Brazilian tripartite matrices – enabling the group to develop more horizontal and mature interactions. In this regard, the group's spiral process was recovered and the realms of the tripartite matrix found renewed figurations and new spiral turns. Cohesion was enhanced and a mutual recognition of their sufferings, as well as of their capacities, allowed for identifying and creating what Mendes Leal named as a new "internal relational matrix" (Neto & França, 2021). However, we wonder if the group has not developed a sort of "healing" group illusion (Anzieu, 1984).

Traumatic experiences in this group were extreme. Most of the time, a tendency to massification fulfilled the field, relegating to the background a deeper investigation of the total situation, especially the impact of socio-historical context, racial and social class issues. In this respect, "the fantasy of cure as the unconscious goal of the analytic process" (Pichon-Rivière, 1971) seems to have dominated the interactions, despite the awareness of the inevitability of the interdependencies between persons, groups, and the society in the location of psychic disturbances (Foulkes, 1948). In retrospect, taking into account afterwardsness/ *Nachträglichkeit* processes (Faimberg, 2005), the analysis of the clinical vignette is a construction/reconstruction of a core moment in a small group work. However, this manoeuvre revealed the very nature of investigations on social unconscious processes. It meant that to grasp social unconscious processes in clinical work, we need to transcend schemes of reference and thinking, distance ourselves from taken-for-granted views, even ideologies, and discourses on behalf of deeper analytic sensibilities and skills – such as binocular vision, reverie, and negative capability (Bion, 1962). Therefore, it is necessary to clear the listening, "listening to listening" (Faimberg, 2005), learning to listen with "the fourth ear" (Horwitz, 2014) to capture the capillary forms in which social unconscious processes emerge in the analytic field.

It means that the analyst/group analyst must listen to the unconscious (Baranger, 1993). However, as Eizirik (2009, p. xiv) noticed:

> What does the analyst listen to? The analyst listens to something other than what he is being told. But to imagine that he seeks a latent content that exists behind the manifest content would be to reify something dynamic. The unconscious is not *behind*: it is elsewhere.

This statement, from the psychoanalytic framework, is consistent with the group-analytic observation that the social unconscious is "not *located* in any *one* part of the group matrix. Instead, it has to be *located* in all of them" (Nitzgen and Hopper, 2017, p. 16; italics in original). Therefore, explorations on the theory and practice of the social unconscious focus on the different tones, undertones, and silences present in the personal and transpersonal interactions of the group field.

Notes

1 The intuition of the "spiral process" was sketched in Freud's letters to Fliess (May 1897 in Freud, 1892–1899, p. 251), but the idea was expanded by Pichon-Rivière (Baranger & Baranger, 2008, p. 820). Pichon-Rivière's (1958) conception of the analytic process as a "spiral process" dates back to 1954–1958 and understands the analytic situation as a unity, as a whole. The theory of the "spiral process" is based on Kleinian concepts; however, it brings an innovative perspective by designating a dialectic view of the analytic treatment connected to temporality. Thus, the analytic session comprises all temporal dimensions, both the past, which is repeated in the present analytic situation, and the future, which opens prospectively. "*Hic et Nunc et Mecum*", Pichon-Rivière says – here, now with me – but he adds, "as far away and long ago" and also "as in the future and somewhere else" (Pichon-Rivière, *apud* Baranger, 1979, p. 49). The progressions and regressions in the analytic session, the return to the past and go forward to the future without a beginning or a predetermined end, reveal the presence of a superposition of curves in the spiral. The spiral process has its roots in archaic configurations predating the differentiation for the subject of his existence in mind, body, and world, his interrelated and constitutive areas (Losso, de Setton & Scharf, 2017). It shows Socratic (non-Hegelian) dialectics between repetition and non-repetition of events in the patient's life in the session (Baranger, 1979, p. 49). The "spiral process" defines the analytic process, observing the individual session or the group-analytic session from a three-dimensional perspective, and addresses the temporal development of the analytic process, "the dialectic of history and temporality" (p. 52).
2 The concept of *habitus* (Elias, 1939) designates the way in which unconscious ingrained habits and dispositions shape how individuals internalize, perceive, think, and react to/ in the social world. These taken-for-granted aspects are shared by people from the same group/background – social class, religion, nationality, ethnicity, education, language – in a particular society/foundation matrix.
3 Pichon-Rivière defines the point of urgency as the moment in the session when something is about to emerge from the analysand's unconscious. Madeleine Baranger considers the point of urgency to be a moment in the functioning of the field "when the structure of the dialogue and the underlying structure (the basic unconscious fantasy of the field) can come together and give rise to insight and interpretation" (Baranger, 1993, p. 95). The analyst's work consists of selecting the interpretation point of urgency in the material, whether this is provided by the patient through verbal and non-verbal forms of communication. The comprehension of the analytic session as spiral dialectic processes grasps the point of urgency of the session, and through its interpretation produces a new structure with a new point of urgency, that is, in turn, interpretable, guaranteeing insight and growth (Baranger, 1993, p. 95).
4 The use of the psychoanalytic terms "unconscious phantasy" and "unconscious fantasy" varies according to the different versions and translations the Baranger's works into English. We use these terms as cited by the authors consulted for this chapter. In the English version of the "Analytic situation as a dynamic field", published in the *International Journal of Psycho-analysis*, the term unconscious phantasy was used; however, in further publications and versions, the term of choice was unconscious fantasy. The journal's policy is to use "phantasy" when referring to an unconscious representation of an instinctual impulse, and "fantasy" when referring to an imaginative construction. This distinction is usually misunderstood and some psychoanalysts quite mistakenly have begun to assume that "phantasy" is used in psychoanalysis, whereas "fantasy" is used in general.

References

Anzieu, D. (1984). *The Group and the Unconscious*. London: Routledge & Kegan Paul.
Baranger, M. (1993). The mind of the analyst: From listening to interpretation. In: M. Baranger & W. Baranger (Eds.) (2009). *The Work of Confluence. Listening and Interpreting in the Psychoanalytic Field* (pp. 89–106). London: Karnac.

Baranger, M. & Baranger W. (2009). *The Work of Confluence. Listening and Interpreting in the Psychoanalytic Field*. London: Karnac.

Baranger, W. (1979). Spiral process and the dynamic field. In: M. Baranger & W. Baranger (Eds.) (2009). *The Work of Confluence. Listening and Interpreting in the Psychoanalytic Field* (pp. 45–62). London: Karnac.

Baranger, W. & Baranger, M. (2008). The analytic situation as a dynamic field. *International Journal of Psycho-Analysis*, 89: 795–836 (originally published in Spanish in 1961–1962).

Baranger, W., Baranger, M. & Mom, J. (2009). Process and non-process in analytic work. In: M. Baranger & W. Baranger (Eds.) *The Work of Confluence. Listening and Interpreting in the Psychoanalytic Field* (pp. 63–88). London: Karnac.

Bion, W. (1962). *Learning from Experience*. London: Karnac.

Bleger, J. (1967). Psycho-analysis of the psycho-analytic frame. *International Journal of Psycho-Analysis*, 48: 511–519.

Bleger, J. (2013). *Symbiosis and Ambiguity. A Psychoanalytic Study.* London: Karnac (originally published in 1967).

Cassorla, R. (2018). *The Psychoanalyst, the Theatre of Dreams and the Clinic of Enactment* (pp. 63–74). London: Routledge.

Churcher, J. (2008). Introductory notes for the English translation of 'The Analytic Situation as a Dynamic Field' from Willy Baranger & Madeleine Baranger. *International Journal of Psychoanalysis*, 89: 795–836.

de Maré, P., Piper, R. & Thompson, S. (1991). *Koinonia: From Hate Through Dialogue to Culture in the Large Group*. London: Karnac.

Doron, Y. (2017). "Black holes" as a collective defence against shared fears of annihilation in a small therapy group and in its contextual society. In: E. Hopper & H. Weinberg (Eds.). *The Social Unconscious in Persons, Groups, and Societies. Vol. 3. The Foundation Matrix Extended and Re-configured* (pp. 151–162). London: Karnac.

Eizirik, C. (2009). Foreword. In: M. Baranger & W. Baranger (Eds.) (2009). *The Work of Confluence. Listening and Interpreting in the Psychoanalytic Field* (pp. xi–xv). London: Karnac.

Elias, N. (1939). *The Civilizing Process.* Oxford: Blackwell, 2000.

Elias, N. (1984). *What Is Sociology?* New York: Columbia University Press.

Faimberg, H. (2005). *The Telescoping of Generations. Listening to Narcissistic Links between Generations.* London: Routledge.

Foulkes, S. H. (1948). *Introduction to Group-Analytic Psychotherapy*. London: Karnac, 1983.

Foulkes, S. H. (1975). *Group Analytic Psychotherapy: Methods and Principles*. London: Karnac.

Heimann, P. (1950). On countertransference. *International Journal of Psycho-Analysis*, 31: 81–84.

Hinshelwood, R. (2018). John Rickman behind the scenes: The influence of Lewin's field theory on practice, countertransference, and W.R. Bion. *International Journal of Psycho-Analysis*, 99 (6): 1409–1423.

Honneth, A. (1996). *Struggle for Recognition: The Moral Grammar of Social Conflicts*. Cambridge: Polity.

Hopper, E. (1991). Encapsulation as a defence against the fear of annihilation. *International Journal of Psychoanalysis*, 72 (4): 607–624.

Hopper, E. (2003a). *Social Unconscious: Selected Papers*. London: Jessica Kingsley.

Hopper, E. (2003b). *Traumatic Experiences in the Unconscious Life of Groups: The Fourth Basic Assumption: Incohesion: Aggregation/Massification*. London: Jessica Kingsley.

Hopper, E. (2007a) Theoretical and conceptual notes concerning transference and counter-transference processes in groups and by groups, and the social unconscious: Part I. *Group Analysis*, 40 (1): 29–42.

Hopper, E. (2007b) Theoretical and conceptual notes concerning transference and countertransference processes in groups and by groups, and the social unconscious: Part I. *Group Analysis,* 40 (2): 285–300.

Hopper, E. & Weinberg, H. (2011). *The Social Unconscious in Persons, Groups and Societies. Vol. 1. Mainly Theory.* London: Karnac.

Hopper, E. & Weinberg, H. (2016). *The Social Unconscious in Persons, Groups and Societies. Vol. 2. Foundation Matrices.* London: Karnac.

Hopper, E. & Weinberg, H. (2017). *The Social Unconscious in Persons, Groups and Societies. Vol. 3. The Foundation Matrices Extended and Reconfigured.* London: Karnac.

Horwitz, L. (2014). *Listening with the Fourth Ear. Unconscious Dynamics in Analytic Group Psychotherapy.* London: Karnac.

Lewin, K. (1947). *Field Theory in Social Sciences.* New York: Harper & Brothers.

Losso, R., de Setton, L & Scharff, D. (2017) *The Linked Self in Psychoanalysis. The Pionnering Work of Enrique Pichon Rivière.* London: Karnac.

Main, T. (1975). Some psychodynamics of large groups. In: L. Kreeger (Ed.) *The Large Group.* (pp.57–86). London: Karnac.

Merleau-Ponty, M. (1945). *Phenomenology of Perception.* New York: Routledge, 2002.

Mojovic, M. (2011). Manifestations of psychic retreats in social systems. In: E. Hopper & H. Weinberg (Eds.) *The Social Unconscious in Persons, Groups and Societies. Vol. 1. Mainly Theory* (pp. 209–232). London: Karnac.

Money-Kyrle, R. (1956). Normal Counter-Transference and Some of Its Deviations. *International Journal of Psycho-Analysis,* 37: 360–366.

Neto, I. M. & França, M. (2021). *The Portuguese School of Group Analysis: Towards a Unified and Integrated Approach to Theory research and Clinical Work.* London: Routledge.

Nitzgen, D. & Hopper, E. (2017). The concepts on the social unconscious and of the matrix in the work of Foulkes. In: Hopper, E. & Weinberg, H. (Eds.) *The Social Unconscious in Persons, Groups and Societies. Vol. 3. The Foundation Matrices Extended and Reconfigured* (pp. 3–26). London: Karnac.

Penna, C. (2008). Counterresistance: Its manifestations and impact on group intervention and management. Chapter 21. In: S. Fehr (Ed.) *101 Interventions in Group Therapy* (pp. 111–115). New York: Taylor & Francis.

Penna, C. (2012). Group analytic psychotherapy with low-income patients in Brazil. *Clinical and Social Work Journal,* 40: 412–420.

Penna, C. (2016). Reflections upon Brazilian social unconscious. In: E. Hopper & H. Weinberg (Eds.). *The Social Unconscious in Persons, Groups, and Societies, Vol. 2. Mainly Foundation Matrices* (pp. 139–158). London: Karnac.

Pichon-Rivière, E. (1958). Referential schema and dialectical spiral process as a basis to a problem of the past. *International Journal of Psycho-Analysis,* 39: 294 [abstract].

Pichon-Rivière, E. (1971). *El proceso grupal. Del psicoanálisis a la psicologíasocial (1)* [*The Group Process: From Psychoanalysis to Social Psychology (1)*]. Buenos Aires: Nueva Visión.

Puget, J. & Wender, L. (1982). Analista y paciente en mundos superpuestos. *Psicoanálisis* 3 (1): 503–521.

Racker, H. (1960). *Transference and Counter-Transference.* London: Karnac, 1982.

Souza, J. (2018). *A Classe Média no Espelho.* [*The Middle-Class in the Mirror*]. Rio de Janeiro: Estação Brasil.

Steiner, J. (1993). *Psychic Retreats: Pathological organizations in Psychotic, Neurotic and Borderline Patients.* London: Routledge.

Tubert-Oklander, J. (2007). The whole and the parts: Working in the analytic field. *Psychoanalytic Dialogues,* 17 (1): 115–132.

Tubert-Oklander, J. (2011). Enrique Pichon-Rivière: The social unconscious in the Latin American tradition in group analysis. In: E. Hopper & H. Weinberg (Eds.) *The Social Unconscious in Persons, Groups and Societies. Vol. 1. Mainly Theory* (pp. 45–70). London: Karnac.

Tubert Oklander, J. (2017). Field theories and process theories. In: K. Montana, R. Cassorla and G. Civitarese (Eds.) *Advances in Contemporary Psychoanalytic Field Theory. Concept and Future Development* (pp. 191–200). London: Routledge.

Volkan, V. (2004). *Blind Trust: Large Groups and Their Leaders in Times of Crisis and Terror.* Charlottesville, VA: Pitchstone.

8 Recognizing codes of superiority in clinical work

Social unconscious, racism, sexism, and other elements of intersectionality

Kavita Avula

As an Indian-American female psychologist, my intersecting identities have impacted the way in which I have experienced the field of group psychotherapy in the United States. Location of the self and the naming of salient identities can be meaningful in the clinical encounter (Watts-Jones, 2010). When I walk into a process group as a Brown woman, I know that people are making assumptions about me based on their perception of me – my skin color, hair color, facial features, and other visible aspects of my identity. This is true for any group member, but for Black, Brown, Indigenous, and other People of Color (BBIPOC), chances are people will assess us in a biased or limiting way due to race-based stereotyping (Crenshaw, 1989; Gump, 2010).

Social systems of oppression are woven into the fabric of society in ways that often go unnoticed, making us habitually unaware. Bias, whether conscious or unconscious, exists in each of us, even the most open-minded and socially aware. Unconscious bias refers to the attitudes or stereotypes that affect our understanding, actions, and decisions without our conscious awareness. These biases include both favorable and unfavorable assessments that are activated involuntarily and unconsciously. As a result, members of historically marginalized groups who seek mental health care may be relegated to generalized categories around race, gender, and other markers of identities, instead of being seen as persons located in complex systems with even more complex histories.

Developed in a social context of racism and misogyny, the fields of group analysis and group psychology have been dominated by White and male clinicians with notable exceptions such as Agazarian, Glatzer, Durkin, Alonso, Kauff, Azima, and Sharpe as well as others in the United States and Europe. Haen and Thomas (2018) state that "the historical record of people of color has largely been omitted from the cultural history by which Americans are educated." This absence contributes to the transmission of racism across generations, for members of all races. Specifically, this absence is reflected in clinical training programs and the attendant racial aggressions and enactments that inevitably arise within them. Even the discussion of race is often referred to along a Black/White binary, and there are far fewer mentions in the literature to bi- or multi-racial practitioners or clients (Mendez, 2015).

DOI: 10.4324/9781003425915-12

Research has documented that racism, discrimination, and other forms of mistreatment can result in chronic stress and other trauma responses leading to mental and physical health problems, lowering productivity, and negatively affecting problem-solving abilities (Hart, 2019; Sue et al., 2009). Hart (2019) aptly alerts us:

> seemingly minor instances of bias or discrimination can lead to posttraumatic reactions…a "minor," interpersonal incident can seem slight, yet the emotional toll may be great.
>
> (p. 2)

This chapter will examine unconscious bias, how it manifests, and its impact on members of target or marginalized populations. Left unacknowledged, racism and sexism are perpetuated group after group, ironically bringing about the very opposite of the healing we profess to deliver for our clients.

Sue et al. (2019) underscore the importance of beginning the process of "disrupting, dismantling, and disarming the constant onslaught of micro- and macroaggressions," and our challenge is how to do that while also retaining integrity to our theoretical orientations (p. 128). Social scientists have proposed that inaction occurs due to a myriad of factors, including the invisible nature of bias, the perception of an incident as innocuous, diffusion of responsibility, fear of repercussions, and the paralysis that results from not knowing what to do (Sue et al., 2019). As group leaders, we do our best to help our clients and develop our clinical acumen through auxiliary training and education. The idea that we may unintentionally harm our clients, or colleagues, can feel extremely difficult to reconcile with our desire to do good. For this reason, it is important to acknowledge not only the bias embedded in our foundational and dynamic matrices, but also the unconscious bias within ourselves. It penetrates all realms and dimensions of the tripartite matrix. Each of us has intersectional identities, including age, ability, race, ethnicity, citizenship, nationality, sexual orientation, social class, gender, and many more areas (Crenshaw, 1989). We are advantaged in some social memberships, and we are disadvantaged in others. It is reductionist to categorize people as either biased or not biased. While we may be most acutely aware of the biases that affect us and those we love, understanding the intersectionality of our identities may foster a sense of togetherness over an us-versus-them divide.

Our societies are structured to benefit specific groups, whether directly through legislation or indirectly, and implicitly, through cultural messaging. Bias, microaggressions, and other oppressive forces originate in these systems of superiority (Sue et al., 2009). White supremacy is a system of superiority that privileges White communities' needs over the needs of BBIPOC communities. Patriarchy is a system of superiority that advantages men over women, genderqueer, transgender, gender-non-conforming, and non-binary individuals. By taking action to address these codes of unconscious superiority, we can cultivate a humane, socially just mentality as we deliver excellent clinical care. Making a lifelong commitment to learning and growing is far more useful than believing that cultural competence, as it is often referred to, is even attainable, although this process might evoke resistance in those that benefit from their privileged social statuses. We can improve individual and group-therapeutic experiences for BBIPOC members by intentionally trying to understand and relax our defenses against bias, recognizing bias by paying attention to subtleties, acting in alignment with this recognition, and learning to embody real allyship.

Taking steps to recognize unconscious bias

Fors (2018) states that "the list of religions, myths, fairy tales, and monarchies in which power and privilege are seen as directly sent from a god or as a reward for good behavior is long"(p. 14). The message from these cultural sources is that superiority and, consequently, inferiority are deserved states. Whether it is the Black child who is sent to detention regularly; or the group therapist who centers White voices sending implicit messages about who is superior and who is inferior; instances occur all the time in our families, schools, jobs, the media, legal and penal systems, and psychotherapy groups that implicitly and explicitly communicate superiority. Unexamined biases can lead to enactments recreating the problematic scenes that we as healers strive to address. Experiences that subject group members to the same unconscious dynamic time and time again require members to relive what is familiar, and often harmful. By amplifying awareness, we can make unconscious representations of oppression more identifiable with the goal of equipping individual and group psychotherapists with the ability to recognize, with intention to act, what is oppressive. Without this deliberate effort, racial, heteronormative, and gendered re-enactments will continue to occur in therapy groups and professional organizations.

Within organizations, this oppressive dynamic can occur among colleagues. When I was in graduate school, I attended my first A.K. Rice conference. I was one of six women in a small group. At one point, a cisgender man in the group counted the women in the group, pointing at each woman. When he got to me, he skipped me entirely. When he stated the number of women in the room, it was one less than the total number of women. He had not counted me, insinuating that I do not count. As a graduate student, I could not find my voice – I was frozen. The other women looked at each other, puzzled, until one challenged him by stating the actual number of women in the group. He responded in a matter-of-fact tone, *"Oh, I tend to sexualize younger women, so I don't count her."* The women either raised their eyebrows or rolled their eyes and did not say more about it. The silence of the women, most of whom were older than myself, was confusing to say the least. I felt discounted, minimized, and undermined by the women in their silence, and this was perhaps more harmful to me than the dismissiveness of the male member. Moreover, the group facilitator did not intervene. The leader's inaction had a diminishing effect on me, and their silence created *unsafety*. Left on my own by the facilitator and my group members, I confronted the aggressor during a break to let him know that he could not discount me. The one-on-one interaction was important to me. I feared that if I addressed the male more directly in the group, I risked a gendered enactment (i.e., further sexism) where my personhood and my voice would again be made invisible. I knew I was on safer ground one-on-one than in an apolitical group space that was created without consideration for how to protect members with marginalized identities from further oppression, including woman-on-woman misogyny.

In my first years of practice, I experienced another example of supremacy at work, this time, originating in my client. I was taken aback when one of my male clients left me a voice message requesting that I wear the same outfit the following week to our session. In the message, the client commented on how he appreciated my figure-hugging skirt and boots. Twenty years later, I still remember the plaid, below-the-knee, fuchsia wool skirt and the black turtleneck paired with the black boots that I was wearing at that session. I remember how I questioned if I should ever wear them again. Raised in an Indian family, I was taught to be self-conscious about my body and for many years wore loose clothing. I wanted to ignore the heart of the issue by concealing my body under loose-fitting outfits, but I knew I had to do the more difficult work of directly addressing the client's inappropriate and offensive comment.

As a contemporary psychodynamic relational psychologist, I take a more active stance with my clients than a very traditional analyst would do. I consulted with a senior psychologist and together we saw this as a boundary violation that warranted being addressed prior to the next session. As the target of this violating request, I felt safer making an inter-session contact. If the client felt that his comment was appropriate, who knows what he would do next, given that he was twice my size and we were alone in a closed room together. After consultation, I called him and told him that his request was inappropriate, that we would discuss this in his next session, and that, in order to continue our work, he would need to do the work to understand why his comments were inappropriate and refrain from making similar comments again. He agreed. I made the choice to go against the grain of psychodynamic theory because it felt essential to hold my ground and speak what needed to be spoken, while also guaranteeing my safety. I continued to work with this client on his sex addiction and strained marriage without further incident. However, this interaction contributed to my second-guessing my clothing choices for some years to come.

Recognizing how unconscious bias manifests and how it may be interrupted

Racism and sexism are intimidating concepts. The language we use to dialogue on these topics is essential. Language can shape the way in which a topic is understood, defended against, or embraced. Unconscious codes of superiority uphold racist and misogynistic dynamics while undermining, invisibilizing, diminishing, and killing off members of marginalized groups. The term *targets of oppression* will be used to emphasize what is done to members of marginalized groups. The word *minority* can be imprecise, though many marginalized group members have claimed and prefer this term. Although the number of people of color is expected to surpass the number of white-bodied individuals in the near future, even as a "minority," members of White society will likely still hold structural power and continue to enjoy unearned privileges.

Similarly, the term *agents of oppression* will be used to denote members of privileged groups who can act out of bias. This term places an emphasis on agency and action rather than pathologizing the person committing these acts as the oppressor.

Microaggressions are everyday slights, indignities, putdowns, and offensive behaviors that members of marginalized or target groups endure (Sue et al., 2019). They can be conscious or unconscious, which means that some people are aware of their bias, while others are not. The *micro* in microaggressions is misleading. Coined by Pierce in the 1970s and expanded on by Sue and Sue in the 1990s, the term was meant to refer to the multiple daily occurrences of these slights, not to their insignificance. To the contrary, the slights of microaggressions are recognized to be quite harmful and can have significant health impacts, as discussed above.

As members of a helping profession, therapists often become defensive when a microaggression is brought to our attention. Given our role, we might feel insulted, as if we were being personally accused of deliberate, intentional discrimination, rather than speaking or acting from an unconscious shared dynamic embedded in our societies. As therapists intent on dedicating our lives to healing, it runs counter to our experience of ourselves and our positive self-image. In addition, we might conflate taking responsibility with feeling guilt about our unconscious bias. The manner in which some agents try to draw our attention to our unconscious racism can evoke more rage and the hidden guilt behind it because the delivery comes across with tones of superiority. Instead of assuming responsibility and taking action, we therapists unwittingly perpetuate more harm.

White supremacy can be misunderstood as a conscious, deliberate discrimination against target groups by extreme racists. Instead, as a metaphor, it is often referred to as the water we are all swimming in, not the few sharks in the water. We are unconsciously socialized to see members of certain social groups as inferior. The important concepts of internalized racism and internalized misogyny are relevant. Even the members of target groups are unconsciously socialized into seeing their own group as inferior. This explains why people of color and women can defend and even perpetuate racism and misogyny.

The national, and later global, chorus calling for an end to racism is both remarkable and depressing. Racism is a prejudice against someone based on race that is reinforced by systems of power (Uluo, 2018). Although an important aspect of the social unconscious, racism has not been sufficiently discussed in psychoanalytic or psychological theories. Lee (2005), an Asian clinician, describes how the indoctrination of therapists allows them to bypass issues of oppression and race in the clinical encounter. He maintains that the focus in many training programs has been on the presenting problem rather than on the oppression clients face and on the social context of this oppression.

In the field of psychology, there has been an evolving understanding of how to deal with difference, including ethnic background. Much of this literature has shared generalized information about cultural groups, with the unintended impact of fostering stereotypes instead of understanding within-group differences. Our clients who are members of marginalized groups want and need to be known as individual persons. They want to be seen for who they are, not categorized into sweeping generalizations or stereotypes. It is important to ask open-ended questions and to contain our biases, giving us a chance to think about them more deeply.

Starting with the moment we greet our clients and the subtle or overt ways we respond to information they provide, we are showing our biases. I recall my eyes lighting up when a client referenced their Palestinian heritage only to find that the client knew little about the situation in Palestine and identified more as an American. Similarly, when a former Israeli special police force member walked into my office, I had to work to contain my biases and in particular my non-verbal body language as a person who was interrogated by Israeli soldiers in Palestine and detained by soldiers at the Tel Aviv airport. I had to work to be open to hearing and believing his experience while addressing my own biases through self-work and learning/unlearning.

I did some of this work at group conferences where I shared my limited experience with Israelis in my small groups that often had Jewish members. It has only been through connecting more directly with Israelis and having vulnerable conversations that I have grown and amplified my experiences, undoing the fear that I had learned at the checkpoints in Palestine. In a recent implicit bias training group that I co-lead, I was deeply moved to hear an Israeli member share how meaningful and grounding her time in the army was. She opened up about the impact of the Holocaust on her father, and how both had gone to visit the Christian woman who hid him and cared for him as a baby for three years during the war. That our stories could co-exist in the same group, each story honored as valid, was healing for everyone in the group. My choice to use self-disclosure as one of the leaders of the group was necessary. Omniscience is not possible, and no one is exempt from enacting bias; self-disclosure was a way for me to model this.

The therapeutic value of *cultural humility* similarly embraces the therapeutic alliance as primary and is grounded in a commitment to being open, self-aware, and letting go of the need to be correct or all-knowing. Cultural humility does not suggest an absence of microaggressions or cultural errors. Rather, it centers the more helpful frame that the therapist may more readily recover in the face of these inevitable slights (Moster, Hook, Captari, Davis and DeBlaere, 2017). This capacity enhances the lifelong motivation to learn and critically examine our own cultural awareness and ability to cultivate interpersonal respect, as well as develop mutual collaborations that address power imbalances, and an inclusive-oriented stance that welcomes new information.

As a presenter on this topic for 20 years, I make mistakes frequently. Contrary to what some therapists may think, the goal is not to avoid mistakes or microaggressions altogether. Instead, we can accept that we will constantly make microaggressions, offending our clients and colleagues; if we know mistakes are a given, then we will be all the more ready to focus on repair. There is no way to avoid oppression. The forces are already within us, operating unconsciously. If we can embrace that this process is occurring within us already, we can be vigilant and not only invite, but also be gracious in the face of feedback. We can be ready to work on examining our impact instead of explaining away our intent. To show up, to listen, to keep showing up to work toward repair as agents of oppression is useful.

However, it is also important to understand and respect that the target of oppression may walk away and leave the group that does not serve them. What is a healthy, skillful choice for the target can often be misinterpreted and pathologized, as once *drapetomania* referred to the so-called "disorder" causing slaves to run away from their masters. Though group therapists often ask members to return to group to work through conflict, it may help to think about the wider structural systems of oppression that inform this way of thinking. Often, we inadvertently reinforce biases and cause harm to the target group member, while focusing on the needs of the rest of the group, and even the leader, by endorsing this form of process. In actuality, it may be more powerful, and corrective, to support the target member in their courage to leave.

Organizational example: interrupting racial re-enactments

Ijeoma Uluo (2018) states that racial oppression is harder to see than the abuse of a loved one because the abuser is not limited to one person and encompasses the surrounding world.

> Being a person of color in a white-dominated society is like being in an abusive relationship with the world. Every day is a new little hurt, a new little dehumanization. We walk around flinching, still in pain from the last hurt and dreading the next. But when we say "this is hurting us," a spotlight is shown on the freshest hurt, the bruise just forming: "Look at how small it is, and I'm sure there is a good reason for it. Why are you making such a big deal about it?"
>
> (p. 19)

As the authority figure, the group leader disseminates unspoken rules for what is acceptable and what is not. If, however, unconscious racism and sexism permeate all levels of the tripartite matrix, affecting both the oppressed and the oppressive, we will find them in our social systems, our therapy groups, and ourselves. When the matrix is racist, misogynistic, and biased, the group will re-enact the same oppressions that characterize the contextual society.

Agent skills

The framework that I often use to understand oppressive enactments was developed by Dr. Leticia Nieto et al. (2010) who describes skill sets, one for targets of oppression and one for agents. Nieto delineates skill sets that are *holarchical*, meaning that in order to have access to the next skill, the first skill must be mastered. For agents, the skills include indifference, distancing, inclusion, awareness, and allyship.

The Agent Skills Model

As Agents develop anti-oppressive consciousness, they build better skills for understanding and responding to oppression. This development is a holarchical sequence of skills sets, as shown below. Each of these skill sets represents some tools for dealing with oppression. As we move toward Allyship, we have more and better tools to work with

Experience of Allyship Awareness

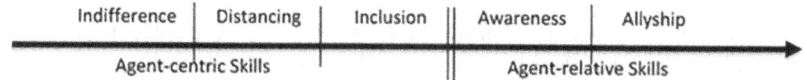

Figure 8.1 The Agent Skills Model from Beyond Inclusion, Beyond Empowerment (Nieto et al., 2010).

The initial agent skill of *indifference* refers to the times when members of the dominant or privileged group do not have significant contact with members of the marginalized group, so they are often indifferent about that group. The *distancing* skill may occur when there is increased contact with members of the target group; it can include distancing up, out, or down. *Distancing up* refers to glorifying or exoticizing groups (e.g. "Asian women are exotic."); *distancing out* is holding the group at arm's distance (e.g. "I have nothing against the gay community as long as they don't come into our neighborhood."); and *distancing down* includes overt racism or using racial epithets.

The *inclusion* skill means simply involving more members of the marginalized group without making any actual change. For example, many organizations hire more people of color under the guise of inclusivity without doing anything to shift the structural racism that exists. In Figure 8.1, a double line is seen after inclusion, indicating that the skills prior to that line are agent-centered, while the skills after the line are agent-relative. The first skill to the right of the double line is *awareness*. Nieto et al. (2010) states that it can be experienced as disorienting or disturbing when the vastness and the pervasiveness of oppression, and privilege, begin to come into focus. This often occurs when we have a loved one who is a member of the target group and something occurs that shocks us, propelling us into awareness on a different level. Sometimes being in a different context can bring codes of superiority into focus.

The skill of *allyship* involves agents of oppression using their influence to talk to other agents of oppression to become liberated. We can use agent skills to interrupt oppression, to shift the racist and misogynistic matrix to one that is more diverse, just, and inclusive. Agents can learn to step back, listening to and believing targets about their experience. Agents should do their own work instead of further burdening targets of oppression.

Case example

I was recently invited to do a diversity, equity, and inclusion facilitation for an organization. The facilitation team consisted of a Black facilitator, a White facilitator, and myself, a Brown facilitator. We offered three two and a half hour long facilitations. Each session began with a brief plenary didactice, then shifted to small groups lead by each of us, and culminated in a large group. Unsurprisingly, the large group is where the most hostility emerged. The following interaction occurred in the second of the three large groups.

A member of the large group objected to the term *White supremacy*, asking to call it by another, less intense name. This is a common request for groups who are newer to discuss concepts of power and privilege. She proceeded to make her case that she is not a White supremacist by using the conditional language of "if I were to call the Black facilitator a..."; however, instead of using a general term to describe this, she actually used the racial slur. In her attempt to deny White supremacy, she performed it without being aware of it. By so doing, she directly insulted my colleague bringing into focus whose needs and well-being are prioritized.

When these types of encounters occur, pitting one group leader or member's emotional well-being against another's, the group leader has to make a choice. Because racial re-enactments can reinforce codes of superiority, I made the decision to step out of the conventional frame and chose to be more authentic, using self-disclosure as a tool for "calling in" (Tran, 2013). Given that this was a training on oppression awareness, it made sense to me to model how to prioritize the target group leader's well-being over the White group participants' needs. As I saw it, we were there to not just talk about how to interrupt oppression but demonstrate how to do it, even if it was done clumsily.

In an effort to express coalition, in which members of target groups stand in solidarity against an anti-Black statement, I decided to make an intervention that jolted the group into accessing the next agent skill set, one that is often deeply unsettling, of awareness. I let the group know that this language was not acceptable, conditional or not. Letting go of my need to be the good leader that is admired by the group, I shared what I felt in a transparent and candid manner, uncharacteristic of most traditional psychodynamic therapists. It was not merely an emotional "acting-in." I opted to allow my anger to be seen by the group rather than be complicit with supremacy. Lorde (1981) aptly states:

> My response to racism is anger. I have lived with that anger, on that anger, beneath that anger, on top of that anger, ignoring that anger, feeding up on that anger, learning to use that anger before it laid my visions to waste, for most of my life. Once I did it in silence afraid of the weight of that anger. My fear of that anger taught me nothing. Your fear of that anger will teach you nothing [...].

> (p. 278)

Inaction can mean colluding with the privileged group's codes of superiority, in this case, White supremacy. I knew the mostly White group would see my coalition as "acting out," which meant that they might engage in derailing and more readily dismiss me as inexperienced, dysregulated, or as breaking the frame. I imagine that there might have been some "tone police" among the White attendees who did not appreciate the tone of my intervention. While my anger was justified, when White fragility is present, it can feel like the target has to make a choice between showing warranted anger and holding onto credibility with the group.

If I were to do this facilitation again, I would place the onus of the work on the group rather than rushing them to a realization stemming from my anger and impatience. For example, I could say,

> Let's slow down, something really significant is happening here, something potentially dehumanizing, that I know this group probably does not consciously intend. Can we do the hard work as a group to unpack this while also working together to embrace humility?

This may have guided the group more skillfully while also serving as a reminder to myself and my team. However, when a racial slur is used live in a diversity, equity, and inclusion training – and in this group, there were several such slurs – it seems that would be the place, if any, to be able to model contextually appropriate and rational anger. In the end, while some of the group may have written me off as an unskilled facilitator, there were many in the group who grew as a result of the overall facilitation, and I felt stronger in my dignity and integrity knowing that I did not stand by in the face of racial injustice. The lack of awareness in those who hold key unexamined agent identities should not be mistaken for a problem located in the targets of oppression.

Target skills

Target skills are a set of skills for targets of oppression to use. To the left of the double line, the skills of survival and confusion are agent-centric and the skills to the right are agent-relative (see Figure 8.2). The *survival* skill allows targets to stay alive by conforming to agent expectations either by moving, thinking, and talking like an agent or by unconsciously attempting to make agents more comfortable. These skills are operational, and when they are working well enough, they bring the experience of danger down. The shift into using the *confusion* skills arises when survival skills become very reliable. Confusion may involve presenting oneself in the way that agents expect at times and at other times not. The confusion emerges when there is a sense that something is not right.

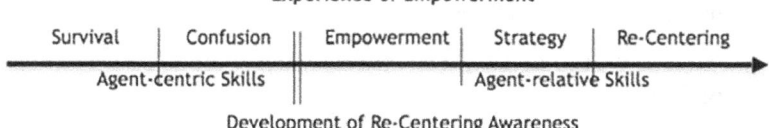

Figure 8.2 Target Skills Set from Beyond Inclusion, Beyond Empowerment (Nieto et al., 2010).

Empowerment takes a great deal of energy and can feel like responding to a life-threatening situation. Acquiring this skill often requires access to empowered target-only spaces. When using empowerment skills, targets seek to talk about the experience of oppression in many different situations. This skill helps to mobilize groups to resist oppression though often not without an enormous emotional toll. Though it feels liberating to speak out, it can also be exhausting, excessively taxing, and ultimately depleting. We only have so much to give to all that life demands of us. Since this toll is not sustainable, the next skill, *strategy*, shifts the target into evaluating how to conserve energy by evaluating first what works. In strategy, the target chooses when to take action, protecting and conserving energy for ourselves and our families, and choosing to act when it really matters. Finally, targets can use the *re-centering* skill which becomes accessible when targets are able to access true inner power, collaborating with other targets and ally agents, and working to change systems of oppression in skillful, humanizing ways.

Training group example: expanding the boundaries of psychoanalysis

Many group therapists join training groups that meet intensively several times a year. I am one of two BBIPOC members in a group of 15. Like many group leaders since George Floyd's murder, the leader of my group – a White woman – is making an effort to talk more about race. She shares articles on race and centers the topic. She works to draw in more people of color using Nieto's inclusion skill (2010). Striving for a social justice framework, she has expanded on her modern analytic framework to ask the group how she is doing in this effort. I was able to share my lack of faith in her, knowing that she serves on a faculty that, with a single exception, is all White. By asking the question, she makes it possible for me to answer it in the group and not seek contact outside. Her painful awareness shifted her into skills that centered my needs as a target of oppression. Atypically for a traditional analyst, she asked what she could do. I told her she needed to figure it out, that it was not my work to do, that I did not want to pay money to attend a group where I also have to educate the members and the leader. To my surprise, she registered for one of my time-limited implicit bias groups. Though it is unusual for a leader to join one of their group member's groups, this turn-taking felt exactly right. She knew I had an expertise that she does not have, and I believe my case made sense to her. I felt so touched and respected that she was willing to expand the traditional boundaries to make way for my leadership. Her humility, combined with action, is emblematic of how we can make progress in the realm of healing racialized trauma. We disclosed our relationship at some point in the course of both groups at junctures that felt right to both of us.

Concluding thoughts

In order to challenge dominant therapeutic paradigms and advocate for real structural change, mental health clinicians must shift how we think about the clinical encounter by incorporating a social justice framework that goes beyond raising awareness and actively engages issues of power relations, equity, and institutional oppression. The psychodynamic tenet that therapy sessions are an apolitical space is counter to creating an alliance that places a high value on social justice (Hopper, 2003). Clients do not come to therapy on equal footing. Equity means that we adjust how we respond to our clients and one another by taking into account barriers experienced by persons from marginalized groups. Instead of exploring oppression *only* as subjective –which risks dehumanizing therapists, clients, and colleagues – there may be a place to step in more actively, directly doing our part as a profession committed to healing, exerting our power to raise awareness and recognizing what is both subjective *and* systemic.

Recognizing racism and sexism as codes of superiority in our social systems will help us adapt our current group theories and models of group leadership. Traditional psychotherapeutic models are based on the needs of the White community. Contemporary psychodynamic mental health professionals who embrace social justice embrace a more active stance in addition to the interpretative one characteristic of traditional psychodynamic work. Unrecognized structural oppression harms our group members and colleagues instead of healing them. If we are willing to be wrong, to feel shame and guilt, and to do something about the conditions that caused them, including respecting the healthy departure of target group members from groups that do not serve them, we can work to counter the unwritten codes of superiority that underlie our individual and group interactions. When codes of superiority are actively internally and externally confronted, and clinicians respond to microaggressions or other harms with curiosity, acceptance, thoughtfulness, interior excavation, and warmth, the possibilities for healing become amplified.

References

Crenshaw, K. (1989). Demarginalizing the intersection of race and sex: A Black feminist critique of antidiscrimination doctrine, feminist theory and antiracist politics. *The University of Chicago Legal Forum*, 1989(1), 139–167.

Fors, M. (2018). *A grammar of power in psychotherapy: Exploring the dynamics of privilege*. Self-published by American Psychological Association in Washington, D.C.

AU: Please provide the publisher location for Reference "Fors (2018)."

Gump, J. P. (2010). Reality matters: The shadow of trauma on African American subjectivity. *Psychoanalytic Psychology, 27*(1), 42–54.

Haen, C. and Thomas, N. (2018). Holding history: Undoing racial unconsciousness in groups. *International Journal of Group Psychotherapy, 68*(4), 498–520.

Hart, A. (2019). The discriminatory gesture: A psychoanalytic consideration of posttraumatic reactions to incidents of racial discrimination. *Social Work*, 1–19. *Psychoanalytic Social Work*, 26 (1) 5–24. Published by the American Psychological Association in Washington, D.C.

Hopper, E. (2003). *The social unconscious: Selected papers*. Jessica Kingsley Publishers. London.

Lee, L. J. (2005). *Taking of the mask: Breaking the silence – the art of naming racism in the therapy room*. In M. Rastogi & E. Wieling (Eds) *Voices of Color: First-person Accounts of Ethnic Minority Therapists*, 91–115. London: Sage Publications.

Lorde, A. (1981). The uses of anger. *Women's Studies Quarterly, 25*(1), 278–285.

Mendez, T. (2015). 'My sister tried to kill me': Enactment and foreclosure in a mixed-race dyad. *Psychodynamic Psychiatry, 43*(2), 229–241.

Mosher, D. K., Hook, J. N., Captari, L. E., Davis, D. E., DeBlaere, C. (2017). Cultural humility: A therapeutic framework for engaging diverse clients. *Practice Innovations, 2*(4), 221–233.

Nieto, L., Boyer, M., Goodwin, L., Johnson, G. R. & Smith, L. C. (2010). *Beyond inclusion, beyond empowerment: A developmental strategy to liberate everyone.* Cuetzpalin. Olympia, WA.

Sue, D. W., Alsaidi, S., Awad, M. N., Glaeser, E., Calle, C. Z. & Mendez, N. (2019). Disarming racial microaggressions: Microintervention strategies for targets, white allies, and bystanders. *American Psychologist, 76*(1), 128–142.

Sue, D. W., Lin, A. I., Torino, G. C., Capodilupo, C. M., Rivera, D. P. (2009). Racial microaggressions and difficult dialogues on race in the classroom. *Cultural, Diversity, and Ethnic Minority Psychology, 15*(2), 183–190.

Tran, N. L. (2013). Calling in: A less disposable way of holding each other accountable. BGDblog.org

Uluo, Ijeoma. (2018). *So you want to talk about race.* Seal Press. New York.

Watts-Jones. (2010). Location of self: Opening the door to dialogue on intersectionality in the therapy process. *Family Process, 49*(3), 405–420.

9 The white mirror

Face to face with racism in group analysis

Anne Aiyegbusi

Introduction

This chapter describes a form of racialized group mirroring I've called the white mirror. I understand the white mirror to be a defensive structure, primarily functioning to prevent white group members, including the conductor(s) from coming face to face with the reality of racism and the enduring racial trauma experienced by Black communities. While functioning as a form of dissociation preventing any contact with pain associated with racial trauma, it simultaneously mirrors racist stereotypes for Black group members to internalize in their position as the location of disturbance. As a Black group analyst, I have experienced and observed this process in numerous group settings, frequently from the receiving end.

I suggest that the white mirror may be understood as a vestigial trauma response with roots as far back as the invention of 'race'. It has been generationally transmitted into the present day through racialized sedimentation in the social unconscious. The white mirror emerges in an exacerbated way within the amplified space of analytic groups when there is ethnically diverse membership. I believe it is inevitable and even essential that racism emerges in groups as a manifestation of the combined social unconscious of members, including the conductor(s). This potentially offers opportunities for reparation and healing. However, when narratives of racism are instead pushed to one side, regarded as a peripheral issue of concern only to minority Black or other members of colour, it is reasonable to suggest that systems of denial and disavowal involving segregation, ghettoization and/or colonization are being replicated within groups. These negative social psychic retreats reflect the unconscious restraints and constraints of the foundation matrix of the contextual society within the dynamic matrices of the groups within them (Hopper, this volume; Mojovic, 2011).

The trauma of racism

It is impossible to disentangle trauma from racism. The former can be considered implicit in the latter. Indeed, racism carries with it the weight of multiple forms of bodily, social, psychological, intergenerational and attachment trauma (Carter and Pieterse, 2020; De Gruy, Menakem, 2017; Stoute, 2021; Volkan, 2020).

DOI: 10.4324/9781003425915-13

Herman (1992) emphasizes the need for clear theoretical frameworks when working therapeutically with trauma, especially phenomenologically complex forms. Effective theoretical frameworks are required to contain a central dynamic implicit to trauma which is the ubiquitous tension between truth telling and denial (Herman, 1992). This tension is a battlefield upon which the centuries-long story of racial trauma has been enacted and re-enacted. In this context, such a battlefield can be understood in terms of transgenerational traumatogenic processes that will unconsciously affect the descendants of both the victims and the perpetrators of racial atrocity (Menakem, 2017). So, facing the truth of racism including its traumatic sequelae has too often remained in socio-political, psychological and bodily battle with the need to seize comfort by denying its history, presence and impacts.

Where there is ethnically diverse membership, the truth/denial dynamic appears like a raw nerve in the amplified environment of a group-analytic matrix. It is typically struck by details of racism being verbalized and brought into open field by a minority Black group member. An excruciating affect is predicted and swiftly defended against by mobilization of the white mirror. DiAngelo's (2011) concept of white fragility may be helpful in understanding the defensive function of the white mirror. DiAngelo suggests that people racialized as white lack stamina to reflect on their whiteness because they have never had to. Therefore, when white racism is described, the white mirror manoeuvre is activated as a protective mechanism. This has the effect of intensifying racialized hurt felt by the Black victim who may also be left to bear what others, including the conductor(s), cannot.

It feels safe to say that Black group members will have at the very least experienced cumulative racial trauma by repeated othering, micro aggressions, casual abuses and identification with the historic and real-time assaults and murders of Black people shown on repeated loops of celluloid footage. Most likely though, severe incidents of racial trauma will have been personally experienced and/or generationally transmitted. Feelings associated with those experiences will inevitably be stirred up by membership of an analytic group encultured as white. However, words spoken about them will be rendered void by mobilization of the white mirror, reflecting back to the Black person a viscerally punishing, disorienting experience of isolation and error to be internalized. It leaves the minority Black group member reeling with no anchor, no touchstone or point of reference available with which to re-stabilize. Relationally, the experience concurs with Garland's (1998) description of how traumatic events disrupt a person's sense of object constancy, continuity, predictability and safety in the world.

The white mirror

Mirroring

Mirroring has been described by a number of analytic writers. As Zinkin (1982) states, these writers can be broadly divided into two camps. In the first camp are those who emphasize the positive, beneficial elements of mirroring while in the second camp are those who call attention to negative, damaging aspects. Winnicott

(1971) described mirroring in healthy child development whereby the infant first experiences themselves through the empathic mirror of their mother's face. In an extension of this positive position, Foulkes (1984) described mirror reaction as one of the original group-specific factors, explaining how it is fundamental to self-development whereby group members experience themselves through the way they are seen by and the impact they have on other members. Schlapobersky (2016) describes mirroring as a process whereby previously inaccessible parts of the self are revealed through what is reflected back by others. Group members are able to see themselves as they are seen which from a therapeutic perspective offers the possibility of improved self-awareness and growth (Garland, 1980; Pines, 1982). Also, through mirroring, group members can learn from other members about how to address aspects of life they find difficult. In an elaboration of mirroring within the group-analytic context, Foulkes and Anthony (1965) describe how different group members provide unique mirror images. This effectively provides the individual with 'a hall of mirrors' (P150) experience consisting of multiple examples of previously hidden parts of the self, requiring exploration and navigation. The role of the conductor includes functioning as a mirror for individual group members and the group as a whole, shedding light on aspects of people or group events in the service of therapeutic progress (Pines, 1982).

Those who write about the negative or destructive potential of mirroring explain how it can go very wrong and serve anti-therapeutic purposes. Garland (1983: 128) states that when what is 'recognized' in the mirror is actually false, it can be damaging. This is in keeping with the concept of the false self which Winnicott (1960) has described as a disturbing aspect of early mirroring. Due to failed attunement, a child dissociates from their real self, unconsciously masquerading in the persona their mother or wider social setting requires of them. Lacan's (1977) mirror stage describes a period between 6 and 18 months when a child recognizes themselves in the mirror as an object to be observed with necessary alienation before they are able to reconcile with their subjectivity. Malignant mirroring, meanwhile, involves unconsciously identifying unrecognized and disavowed parts of the self in another and then attacking them (Zinkin, 1983). This often manifests in malignantly mirrored pairs becoming locked in preoccupied but nonreflective conflict within a group with each functioning as a distorting mirror to the other (Zinkin, 1992). Zinkin (1983, 1992) describes this situation as one of the few times the conductor needs to intervene in a determined manner, removing the malignancy. Importantly, Zinkin (1992) emphasizes the containing task of the group as being to integrate within it the constellation of opposite qualities that have become lodged between the malignantly mirrored pair. Weinberg and Toder (2004) described the different types of malignant mirroring and summarized that Foulkes did not take into consideration the ability of the specific patient to tolerate mirroring. One of the types of malignant mirroring Weinberg and Toder (2004) describe is 'the all-knowing mirror' (P501) whereby the group unconsciously provides an undifferentiated, distorting mirror, usually falsely presented as a truth. The group does this because of a need to scapegoat and project aggression onto a single group member whose reaction, according to Weinberg and Toder (2004: 501), will be '*defensive or fragmented or she/he withdraws from the group'*. Dalal (2002) reflects on the essential developmental phase of seeing the self through the eyes of another. This process becomes damaging when a Black person experiences themselves through the racist gaze in which case *'he is torn asunder and becomes an object to himself'* (Dalal, 2002: 97).

The white mirror is mobilized in groups to prevent Black members from reflecting details of white racism into the group. In a secondary manoeuvre, it forcefully mirrors into minority Black minds, disavowed projections that are shaped and saturated with racist content. Projections are primarily experienced in the form of stereotypes, usually permutations of criminalization, sexualization and/or demotion as Wekker (2016) has identified. In their inevitable role as the location of disturbance, the Black person will be pressured into internalizing this mirrored racist imagery.

Racist history and aetiology of the white mirror

Our shared social unconscious is key to contextualizing how the white mirror manifests in present-day analytic groups. It is a medium for trauma including that which is generationally transmitted and explains the ways in which racial trauma emerges in group settings (Hopper 2003). It is necessary to face up to the history of racism and race in order to recognize how historical traumatic experience is reproduced in groups. It is also necessary to recognize the entrenched, stubborn and highly tenacious nature of racism, including its capability to adapt to changing circumstances and locations. As such, mirroring manoeuvres feature prominently within all strategies operating to oppress and dominate. The following section aims to clarify the origins and persistence of anti-Black racism:

Slavery and American racism

In considering what of the past is with us today that needs to be unconsciously dissociated and turned away from, denied, silenced, segregated and/or converted, the author Ta-Nehisi Coates (2015) is explicit about the history of white dehumanization and criminal dominion over the Black body and how it was gained by:

> …the flaying of backs, the chaining of limbs; the strangling of dissidents, the destruction of families; the rape of mothers, the sale of children!
>
> (P8)

Inculcated within white supremacist mentality were psychic strategies to manage the trauma of perpetrating violent atrocity, so involvement in such barbarity was denied, with savagery attributed to the victim. Yancy (2017) captures the essence of racialized gaslighting and the mind control therein whereby the perpetrator's disavowed characteristics were converted and perceived as embodied by the victim:

> …whites accused slaves of being what the 'masters' really were; hateful, brutal and godless …
>
> (P156)

W.E.B. Du Bois (1903/1994) conceptualized double consciousness as a racialized form of dissonance. He described how Black people were required to manage their own self-consciousness as well as the degraded, inferior and guilty version of themselves that was constantly and forcefully mirrored into their minds by the more powerful whites. Under the threat of annihilatory violence, the position could not be challenged.

The mirror metaphor has been much used in discussions around the dynamics of racism. Baldwin (1985: 410) referred to the colour of his skin as '*a most disagreeable mirror*', forever reminding white Americans of atrocities committed to secure their privilege. As Hopper (2023) has noted, he also described how the '*Negro problem*' was a function of white Americans going to great lengths not to be seen as they were while at the same time being desperate to be seen as they were and freed from the 'tyranny' of the white mirror (Baldwin 1963: 81).

Colonization

The carving up and colonization of Africa by Europeans for material gain by stripping the continent of its rich natural resources, while denigrating and dehumanizing its citizens was another racist atrocity. Azu-Okeke (2003) describes the wholesale trashing and subordinating of all aspects of his indigenous Nigerian culture in favour of that of British colonizers'. Colonized victims internalized the colonizers' perspective of their relationship which in a persisting internalized way came to form a model for the relationship between Black and white people with Black inferior and denigrated, while white was superior and in power (Azu-Okeke, 2003; Blackwell, 2003; Dalal, 2002). Importantly, the colonized Black person emerged from this relation with a divided self (Blackwell, 2003). That is, a white self which attempted to reflect a persona that was acceptable to the colonizer by representing their culture positively in every possible way. The white self was separated off from a Black self, the latter being devalued, debased and regarded as inferior.

Fanon (1952) was explicit in articulating the psychological phenomenology of racist mirroring. Fuelled by their phantasies and projections during interpersonal interactions, the colonizer mentally converted the colonized into something dehumanized, guilty and inferior. This distortion was then felt to be forcefully mirrored back into the mind of the Black person for self-redefinition. Fanon (1952: 10) called this '*a zone of nonbeing*' and described how, through interpersonal contact with white people, he was constantly being returned (or mirrored) back to himself in a different form:

> My body was given back to me sprawled out, distorted, recoloured, clad in mourning in that white winter day. The Negro is an animal, the Negro is bad, the Negro is mean, the Negro is ugly;...

> (P113)

Fanon (1952) explained that only when in the company of other Black people did he not have to experience himself in this mirrored back way.

Post-colonial context

Frosh (2013) in writing about the post-colonial context describes the predatory nature of an interpersonal process culminating in racialized mirroring through:

> … a search for a mirror that will reflect **difference**. The white subject needs the Black to define itself; and it desires the Black as the repository of those necessary things – above all sexuality – which it has repudiated out of anxiety and self- loathing.
>
> (P148)

Hook (2012) explains how if Black people respond authentically to their reflection in the white mirror by challenging it, a sense of personal integrity may be retained but as a result they will be treated as a bad person, objectified and ultimately silenced. Alternatively, they may behave falsely to appease white people and so be treated as a good person with subjectivity and able to speak but only in the 'master's voice'. There may be some variations to post-colonial societal configurations. For example, Penna (2016), in reflecting on the Brazilian social unconscious, describes a more co-created community.

Post-war immigration

In the 1940s, the British government called on people from the colonies for help to re-build the post-war state. As a result, Black people arrived on British soil believing that they would be welcomed by the 'mother country', given all they had contributed. Instead, they were met with the colour bar, hostility, abuse and in a clear message that they were not felt to belong here, repeatedly told to 'go back home!'

No Blacks, no dogs, no Irish!

The now infamous signs on rooms and properties to let in the post-war era stating 'no Blacks, no dogs, no Irish' communicated clearly the exclusion and vilification of Black bodies and that absolutely no gratitude was felt. It is worth noting that until large numbers of actual Black people arrived in the country, Catholic Irish people had occupied a colonized and denigrated ethnic position with echoes of Black equivalency. Open racism was expressed by some British politicians with the exemplar being Enoch Powell's 1968 'Rivers of Blood' speech delivered to a conservative party meeting in Birmingham. He called for repatriation of Black immigrants following his white constituents' repeated expressions of complaint and fear about becoming overtaken by 'coloured people' after the colour bar was lifted. These projective fears were most evident in one prediction that, '*in 15 or 20 years the Black man will have the whip hand over the white man*'. Although roundly applauded within his constituency for speaking out, Powell was ejected from his front bench seat in parliament for this. However, racism towards Black and Brown people has continued in Britain, the bulk of it covert, structural and continuing to be vehemently denied even as it is perpetrated.

Criminalization

The excessive criminalization of Black people is another consequence of unconscious historical sedimentation from a time when white people required a defence against recognizing the many forms of criminality involved in their plunder of Black bodies (Sartwell, 1998; Watson, 2013; Yancy, 2017). Distorting the Black reflection towards guilt serves the unconscious purpose of maintaining white innocence. This concurs with Butler's (1993) thesis about how four police officers who were clearly seen on film surrounding and clubbing a prostrate and defenceless Rodney King in the streets of Los Angeles were freed by a mainly white jury who, despite viewing the footage, upheld the police officers' defence of fearing for their lives. This is the white mirror at work. As a result, the Black victim was seen as the perpetrator and the white perpetrators were seen as victims. Black skin is experienced synonymously with guilt leading to areas where Black people live being overpoliced and constantly targeted (Andrews, 2018). Intermittently, when police brutality overwhelms a community, uprisings occur. In which case, as Anderson (2016) states, the public focus is on Black rage, while the underlying white rage embedded in structures upholding systemic racism remains invisible.

The criminalization of Black people, including automatic assumptions of guilt is deeply embedded in the racialized social unconscious of Western cultures. In Britain, it can be seen in the disproportionate stopping and searching of Black people and in widely unequal rates of incarceration (Lammy, 2017). It was clearly described in the circumstances of Stephen Lawrence, a Black British teenager who was stabbed to death by a gang of white racists in London in 1992. What is unusual about Stephen's death is that it was later subject to a public inquiry. The inquiry found that institutionalized racism in London's Metropolitan Police Service underlay a catalogue of errors which ultimately led to Stephen's killers remaining free. Even as Stephen lay dead on a pavement, police officers were unable to perceive him as a victim. His traumatized friend who had outrun the murderous mob and witnessed Stephen being killed by them was afforded no care. He was interrogated as though both he and Stephen were criminals and somehow implicated in the crime (Macpherson report, 1999). Again, through epidermalization, on sight of Black skin (Fanon, 1952), police officers were unable to conceptualize victims, only perpetrators.

Windrush scandal

Some 70 years after HMT Empire Windrush arrived at Tilbury Dock carrying the first wave of Caribbean people, the British government introduced their policy of creating a 'hostile environment' for people supposedly living here illegally. Children of the 'Windrush generation' who had come to Britain with their parents became embroiled as this policy was implemented. Wrongly denied their rights to live in Britain, many lost everything, were held in immigration detention centres and deported 'back' to countries they had no knowledge of. This generation included older adults who even when severely ill were refused access to the very

National Health Service their parents had helped build. The social repetition of racial trauma is evident in creating a hostile environment, of harmful accusations of wrongdoing, of vilification on the grounds of skin colour and determination to segregate and exclude. A repetition of the confiscation and disposal of Black bodies by imperial whiteness which featured in earlier racist atrocity is also seen. These are examples of the re-enactments of racial trauma fuelling a constant battle which also manifests in analytic groups which can be understood in terms of the tripartite matrix (Hopper, this volume; Nitzgen & Hopper 2017).

Emergence of the white mirror in an analytic group – case example

'Sticks and stones might break bones but the "n word" really hurts'

In an analytic group, one member, Christian, is a forensic psychologist. He is 35, British-born of Caribbean heritage. He is the only Black group member. Addressing the group, Christian says that he feels he needs to talk about his experiences at work. He says that he is repeatedly racially abused by white patients. He doesn't feel his managers take it seriously enough as they say the patients are mentally ill so there isn't really anything to be done. He has reported some incidents to the police. On these occasions, patients have chanted at him for prolonged periods, called him 'fucking monkey' or used the 'n word'. The police have acknowledged that this language and the hostility with which it was directed at Christian are unlawful in the UK, fulfilling criteria for hate crimes. However, on each occasion, it was deemed not to be in the public interest to charge the patients as they were already legally detained in a secure facility. A fellow group member, Kinga, immediately asks Christian what 'the n word' stands for. Kinga says she is not from the UK and claims not to be familiar with the term. Christian explained that the word is so abusive and traumatizing to him that he doesn't want to say it in full and nor does he want to hear it in full within the group but suffice to say that it is an abhorrent racial slur as well as a taboo word and that if Kinga still wishes to know what 'n word' stands for, it can easily be googled. Some other group members take issue with this, as does the conductor. They ask how they are supposed to talk about racism when they are not even allowed to hear about or say particular words. Two group members have a conversation between themselves about how they cannot imagine any slur making them actually feel *'traumatized'*. While the group expresses feelings about Christian's 'embargo' on full use of a racial slur which he has explained feeling traumatized by and which no other member of the group is subjected to, he is reeling with significant emotional pain and deep physical discomfort. His anxiety has escalated during the conversation and he feels on the verge of a panic attack. He feels claustrophobic and his heart is pounding so hard that he can literally feel each beat of it in his ears. Christian struggles to tell the group that he now feels the same as he does on his ward, surrounded by white people who expect him to tolerate no end of abuse. It seems to him that they do not feel his humanity to be equal to theirs and that they don't feel any need to consider his feelings while he is expected to accommodate to theirs no matter how much it might hurt or harm him.

Once Christian spoke about his experience of racism and objected to full articulation of 'n word' within the group, the scenario was repeated in subsequent sessions. Christian never felt that he was able to convey the enormity of his racial trauma to the group. He felt that he was being worn down and that declining to degrade himself by submitting to use a dehumanizing term of abuse within the intimate space of an analytic group had placed him in a catch 22. If he agrees to the 'n word' being used in full, he will be party to his own debasement and re-trauma. If he doesn't, he remains alienated from other group members under an unbearably intense yet erasing scrutiny. Further, Christian feels instinctively that the group is unconsciously trying to pressurize him to anger or even violence. When he voices this, he is accused of projecting his rage onto them. Concluding that the group was actually damaging to him, Christian left prematurely and sought out a Black therapist.

Discussion of case example

In attempting to use his therapy group to explore and process his racial trauma, Christian found himself caught up in a trap brought about by white mirror mobilization. Rather than receiving support in the form of empathy or compassion from the group, his distress was escalated as white group members dissociated from it, leaving his emotional wounds open while focusing on a very tool used to inflict them on this occasion. A tool used to inflict Christian's wounds was described by him as 'n word' which, in keeping with the unparalleled traumatic history the deliberately dehumanizing construct emerged from, is rarely spoken in full nowadays, unless with intent to abuse. The exception being when Black people have tried to soften its impact by reclaiming the term. However, just as racism cannot be disentangled from trauma, 'n word' cannot be disentangled from either, including when internalized.

A number of Black scholars have written about the 'n word'. In fact, Baldwin (1963/2017) spoke to the degradation integral to the 'n word' construct when he impelled white Americans to search inside themselves for an answer as to why they invented it, suggesting that the future of the country depended on it. Akala (2018: 255) also referred to 'n word' as '*a fictional subhuman creation of the white racist imagination*' that was used to justify the worst and most enduring, terrorizing atrocity in human history. Anderson (2011) speaks to the 'n word' moment as a terror Black people live with, ever aware that a profoundly stripping and degrading othering experience can be brought about at any time, without warning, usually while in spaces identified (until the 'n word' moment) as safe enough. An example would be an analytic group whereby sufficient depth of intimacy and emotional security is required for psychosocial reparations. Oluo (2018) speaks to the desire of some white people to say 'n word' in its explicit form despite being informed just how unbearable a Black person would find that. Oluo (2018) suggests that the correct action would be to try to understand what lies behind the desire to use a word synonymous with annihilation and deep debasement.

In the clinical example provided, the time and energy devoted by the group to their desire for Christian to either say the 'n word' in its entirety himself rather than the more acceptable abbreviation, or to submit to the white group members saying it was a function of the white mirror. While dissociated from the trauma of his racial victimization, they worked together, in a malignantly, 'all knowing' (Weinberg and Toder 2004) manner to overpower him, effectively fetishizing the tool of his torment in the process. By the unconscious activation of a vestigial trauma response designed to maintain complete emotional distance from the horror of racial trauma, the group projected its full, shared and generational impact into Christian, including and especially bodily sequelae. As such, the specular consequence was of Christian experiencing himself as endangered and dehumanized within the group, much as he did on the end of racial abuse by psychotic forensic patients within his workplace and much as generations of Black people have felt while subjugated to white supremacist regimes throughout history. With no hope of change in sight, he had little option but to leave the group.

Reflection on the role of the conductor

While the struggle to work effectively with racism within analytic groups has its roots in systemic factors, including the training of group analysts, it is important to consider the positionality of the conductor in this clinical example. A number of authors have described the inevitability of racial trauma being reproduced in analytic groups (Aiyegbusi, 2021a; Kent, 2021; Kinouani, 2020b; Stevenson, 2020), observing that the role of the conductor is to actively intervene (Aiyegbusi, 2021b; Kent, 2021; Stevenson, 2020). In this case example, the point at which the conductor could have most effectively intervened was at the point of white mirror mobilization. That is, instead of actively joining in with this manoeuvre and escalating Christian's distress, the conductor's role was to offer containment by functioning as a mirror for the whole group. The ideal point of intervention by the conductor would have been when Christian was allocated the role of perpetrator of racism rather than someone who was distressed as a result of being victimized by it. In keeping with Zinkin's (1992) thesis, the task was for the group to integrate the shared nature of racialized trauma. The conductor could have begun this process by questioning why this group seemed unable to empathize with Christian's distress and in fact appeared determined to add to it by further traumatizing him.

Conclusion

A potentially destructive form of mirroring, the white mirror is in keeping with numerous forms of mirror phenomena that analytic authors have described. It can be understood as an archaic trauma response of denial and disavowal which is mobilized as the group social unconscious reacts to the threat of the reality of white racism being revealed within the group matrix typically by a minority Black group member describing their racial trauma. It serves to maintain a way of remaining removed from the pain of racial trauma. Furthermore, the white mirror re-traumatizes Black group members by overpowering them, erasing their attempts to talk about their experiences while simultaneously projecting racist stereotypes into them to internalize as the location of disturbance. A representative case example has been employed to demonstrate how this happens, causing such distress in the Black group member that their only option is to leave the group. I would suggest that this is a common occurrence and as such it behooves group analysts to recognize how it manifests in groups, while they also work towards establishing clinical practices to work effectively with it. Guidance may be found in Zinkin's (1992) observation about the distortion integral to malignant mirroring whereby he describes the task of the group as being to integrate into it the polarized positions held by the mirroring pair, in order to achieve a higher level of group development. Achieving this, when the white mirror is mobilized, would require the group to integrate the shared nature of racialized trauma, including sequelae of their generational histories as victim, perpetrator or beneficiary.

References

Aiyegbusi, A. (2021a) The White Mirror: Face to Face with Racism in Group Analysis. Part 1 – Mainly Theory. *Group Analysis*. 54 (3) PP402–420.

Aiyegbusi, A. (2021b) The White Mirror: Face to Face with Racism in Group Analysis. Part 2 – Mainly Practice. *Group Analysis*. 54 (3) PP421–436.

Akala (2018) *Natives : Race and Class in the Ruins of Empire*. London. Two Roads.

Anderson, C. (2016) *White Rage: The Unspoken Truth of Our Racial Divide*. London. Bloomsbury.

Anderson, E. (2011) *The Cosmopolitan Canopy: Race and Civility in Everyday Life*. New York. Norton.

Andrews, K. (2018) *Back to Black: Retelling Black Radicalism for the 21st Century*. London. Zed Books.

Azu-Okeke, O. (2003) Response to Lecture by Dick Blackwell. *Group Analysis*. 36 (4) PP465–476.

Baldwin, J. (1963) *The Fire Next Time*. London. Penguin Books.

Baldwin, J. (1963/2017) *I Am Not Your Negro*. London. Penguin Modern Classics.

Baldwin, J. (1985) White Man's Guilt. In: The Price of the Ticket. Collected Non Fiction 1948–1985. New York. St Martin's Marek. PP409–414.

Blackwell, D. (2003) Colonialism and Globalization: A Group-Analytic Perspective. 27th Foulkes Annual Lecture. *Group Analysis*. 36 (4) PP445–463.

Butler, J. (1993) Endangered/Endangering: Schematic Racism and White Paranoia. In: *Reading Rodney King: Reading Urban Uprising*. Cooding-Williams, R. (ed). New York. Routledge. PP15–22.

Carter, R, T. & Pieterse, A, L. (2020) *Measuring the Effects of Racism. Guidelines for the Assessment and Treatment of Race-Based Traumatic Stress Injury*. New York. Columbia.

Coates, T. (2015) *Between the World and Me*. Melbourne. Text Publishing.

Dalal, F. (2002) Race, Colour and the Process of Racialization. New Perspectives from Group Analysis, Psychoanalysis and Sociology. Hove. Brunner-Routledge.

De Gruy, J. (2017) *Post Traumatic Slave Syndrome*. USA. JDGP.

DiAngelo, R. (2011) White Fragility. *International Journal of Critical Pedagogy*. 3 (3) PP54–70.

Du Bois, W. E. B. (1903/1994) *The Souls of Black Folk.* New York. Dover.

Fanon, F. (1952) *Black Skin: White Masks.* London. Pluto.

Foulkes, S. H. (1984) *Therapeutic Group Analysis.* London. Karnac.

Foulkes, S. H. & Anthony, J. (1965) *Group Psychotherapy: The Psychoanalytic Approach.* London. Karnac.

Frosh, S. (2013) Psychoanalysis, Colonialism, Racism. *Journal of Theoretical and Philosophical Psychology.* 33 (3) PP141–154.

Garland, C. (1980) Face to Face. *Group Analysis.* 13 (1) PP42–43.

Garland, C. (1983) Discussion of Paper by Louis Zinkin. *Group Analysis.* 16 (2) PP126–129.

Garland, C. (1998) *Understanding Trauma: A Psychoanalytical Approach.* London. Duckworth.

Herman, J, L. (1992) *Trauma and Recovery. From Domestic Abuse to Political Terror.* New York. Basis Books.

Hook, D. (2012) *A Critical Psychology of the Postcolonial: The Mind of Apartheid.* London. Routledge.

Hopper, E. (2003) *The Social Unconscious: Selected Papers.* London. JKP.

Hopper, E. (2023) A Hopeful Memoir of the 'Baldwin/Buckley debate' in 1965, in Cambridge, England. IAGP The Forum, Volume 11, September.

Kent, J. (2021) Scapegoating and the 'Angry Black Woman'. *Group Analysis.* 54 (3) PP354–371.

Kinouani, G. (2020b) Silencing, Power and Racial Trauma in Groups. *Group Analysis.* 53 (2) PP145–161.

Lacan, J. (1977) The Mirror Stage as Formative of the Functioning of the I. In: *Ecrits: A Selection* (P1–8). London. Tavistock/Routledge.

Lammy, D. (2017) *The Lammy Review: An Independent Review into the Treatment of, and Outcomes for, Black, Asian and Minority Ethnic Individuals in the Criminal Justice System.* London. Her Majesty's Government.

Macpherson, W. (1999) *Independent Report of the Stephen Lawrence Inquiry.* London. Home Office.

Manakem, R. (2017) *My Grandmother's Hands: Racialized Trauma and the Pathway to Mending Our Hearts and Bodies.* Las Vegas. Central Recovery Press.

Mojovic, M. (2011) Manifestations of Psychic Retreats in Social Systems. In: *The Social Unconscious in Persons, Groups and Societies: Vol 1. Mainly Theory* (PP209–234). Hopper, E. & Weinberg, H. (eds). London. Karnac.

Nitzgen, D. & Hopper, E. (2017) The Concepts of the Social Unconscious and of the Matrix in the Work of S.H. Foulkes. In: *The Social Unconscious in Persons, Groups and Societies: Vol 3. The Foundation Matrix Extended and Re-Configured* (PP3–26). Hopper, E. & Weinberg, H. (eds). London. Karnac.

Oluo, I. (2018) *So You Want to Talk about Race?* New York. Seal Press.

Penna, C. (2016) Reflections Upon Brazilian Social Unconscious. In *The Social Unconscious in Persons, Groups and Societies: Vol 2. Mainly Foundation Matrices* (PP139–158). Hopper, E. & Weinberg, H. (eds). London. Karnac.

Pines, M. (1982) 6th Annual Foulkes Lecture. Reflections on Mirroring. *Group Analysis.* 15 (2) PPS1–S26.

Sartwell, C. (1998) *Act Like you Know: African – American Autobiography and White Identity.* Chicago, IL. University of Chicago Press.

Schlapobersky, J, R. (2016) *From the Couch to the Circle. Group-Analytic Psychotherapy in Practice.* London. Routledge.

Stevenson, S. (2020) Psychodynamic Intersectionality and the Positionality of the Group Analyst : The Tension Between Analytic Neutrality and Inter-Subjectivity. *Group Analysis.* 53 (4) PP498–514.

Stoute, B. J. (2021) Black Rage: The Psychic Adaptation to the Trauma of Oppression. *Journal of the American Psychoanalytic Association.* 69 (5) DOI 10.1177/00030651211055762

Volkan, V, D. (2020) *Large-Group Psychology. Racism, Societal Divisions, Narcissistic Leaders and Who We Are Now.* Oxford. Phoenix.

Watson, V, T. (2013) *The Souls of White Folk : African-American Writers Theorize Whiteness.* Jackson, MS. University of Mississippi Press.

Weinberg, H. & Toder, M. (2004) The Hall of Mirrors in Small, Large and Virtual Groups. *Group Analysis.* 37 (4) PP492–507.

Wekker, G. (2016) *White Innocence : Paradoxes of Colonialism and Race.* Durham, NC. Duke University Press.

Winnicott, D, W. (1960/1984) Ego Distortion in Terms of True and False Self. In: *The Maturational Process and The Facilitating Environment.* London. Karnac. PP140–152.

Winnicott, D, W. (1971) Chapter 9: Mirror-Role of Mother and Family in Child Development. In: *Playing & Reality* (PP149–159). Winnicott, D. W. (ed). London. Tavistock.

Yancy, G. (2017) *Black Bodies, White Gazes. The Continuing Significance of Race in America.* Second Edition. London. Rowman and Littlefield.

Zinkin, L. (1982) Invited Discussion on Malcolm Pines' Lecture: M. Rita, M. Leal & Louis Zinkin. *Group Analysis*. 15 (2), PPS29–32.

Zinkin, L. (1983) Malignant Mirroring. *Group Analysis.* 16 (2) PP113–126.

Zinkin, L. (1992) Borderline Distortions of Mirroring in the Group. *Group Analysis.* 25, PP27–31.

Part IV

Topics

Section A
Envy & Gender

10 "They envy us" – privilege and power relations in the social unconscious

Avi Berman

In this chapter, I intend to deal with envy as an aspect of social unconscious (Hopper & Weinberg, 2011). I suggest that the feeling of envy can arise in one person, in a group of people or even in an entire society or nation. At the same time, envy, because of its painful quality and its bad reputation, may be disowned and repressed out of people's consciousness. Unconscious envy still affects attitudes and behavior within a society and between societies. I offer an analysis of these options.

The discourse about the social unconscious' aspect of Envy argues both explicitly and implicitly that some verbal contents, motives, emotions and wishes of people who belong to a certain society are denied or concealed and absent from explicit discourse. However, when these materials are openly addressed, they may evoke a sense of surprise, which may be hopefully followed by recognition. The emotion of envy in people's inner world is liable to be repressed to the (personal and social) unconscious. The psychoanalytic dominant attitude about envy draws mainly on Klein (1957), who views envy as an elementary and unavoidable emotion in the context of the child's relation to its mother. According to Klein's terminology, Envy is a destructive emotion. "Envy is the angry feeling that another person possesses and enjoys something desirable – the envious impulse being to take it away or spoil it" (1957, p. 181). Envy is almost always regarded as a reprehensible emotion and is thus rejected and disowned by most people and, as we shall soon see, by entire societies. (Envy, according to the Kleinian terminology, deals with the romantic triangle and based on the fear of losing what one already has. Envy is regarded as immature but passionate emotion, while envy is considered to be evil).

Envy is an "abject emotion" which cannot be attributed to either me or you. Thus, those who envy are always "they" and never "us." Those "unenvious" people see themselves as morally superior in a way, among other things, because they feel themselves to be "untainted" by this grave emotion. The envious others are considered immoral and ill-intentioned. As such, it is instantly grounded in the division into us and them (Berman et al., 2000). "We are the objects of other people's envy and its potential victims."

Observations of children and babies (for example, Frankel & Sherik, 1977) suggest that envy is in everyone and remains with us (with certain changes) throughout our lives.

DOI: 10.4324/9781003425915-16

I choose to begin with the central tenets of the age-old cultural tradition regarding envy. In order to understand the social *unconscious* about envy, we ought first to familiarize ourselves with the social *conscious* about it – and with those views which are explicit and known. The assertion that envy is destructive was accepted in Christian culture (especially European) as an axiom that does not require additional thought. This axiom states that envy in another person is destructive, and only destructive. One should consider this radical statement, since its significance is that if the emotion is not destructive, then it is not envy, but something else. In this sense, the Kleinian claim that envy is designed to harm, rob or destroy the good object (Klein, 1957) was conceived by means of a cultural context that is over a millennium old. Let us first examine the concept of the seven deadly sins and the notion of casting an evil eye.

The word "envy" originates in the Latin *Invidia*, which means looking at another person with the evil eye (Raufman & Weinberg, 2017). The eye is the fundamental organ of envy. The eye sees differences; it sees the gap between what you have and what I do not. The evil eye seeks out these differences and thus resents the other's possessions (their property, status, qualities and relationships) and happiness. Casting an evil eye entails the wish to rob and destroy and therefore amounts to a curse. This is soon joined by an ethical and moral reaction, seeing as the evil eye wishes to harm the other, whose crime was nothing more than exercising their right to enjoy the fruits of their labor and what they were able to achieve and establish through great efforts. Is this not sinful?

Eventually, the condemnation of envy crystallized in its definition as a sin in catholic Christianity (Bloomfield, 1952). The roots of the definition of envy as a sin in Christianity are attributed to St. Augustine's *Confessions*.[1] In his confessions, Augustine attested that, throughout his youth, he had been a mindless and careless "playboy." At a certain moment, he was fortunate to have a religious experience in which he encountered the grace of god, which had utterly transformed his understanding of his place in the world. "The grace of god" had made all the difference. Augustin's message runs as follows:

> god gives you everything – life, love and the ability to subsist and to thrive. And you, the one who envies, turn your back on these wonderful gifts and, instead of acknowledging god's generosity and being grateful, you turn your back on God and contrive to take the possessions of your fellow man. That is sinful and therefore envy is a sin.

Between the 3rd and 6th centuries, various lists were compiled naming cardinal sins that were known as "deadly sins." The notion of a "deadly sin" did not necessarily refer to sins punished by execution (though in many cases this had been the sinner's fate). Committing a deadly sin meant that the sinner was sent to hell. The number seven gained a certain degree of sanctity. In all the lists enumerating the seven deadly sins, envy was given a place of honor. The list that is widely accepted today is the one made by St. Gregorius (Gregory) who lived in the 6th century, trumping all other competing lists in the context of a political struggle within the ranks of the church. In the 13th century, the list was reformulated by Thomas Aquinas (Bloomfield, 1952).

Here then is the triumphant list of seven deadly sins according to Gregorius' doctrine: Gluttony (Latin – Gula), Greed (Latin – Avaritia), Envy (Latin – Invidia), Lust (Latin – Luxuria), Pride (Latin – Superbia), Sloth (Lain – Acedia), Wrath (Latin – Ira).

In a way, the 6th century had been a century of catastrophes. A series of volcanic eruptions around 540 AD caused a rise in mortality rates in Europe and Constantinople. This was also related to an outbreak of the plague in Constantinople and the Byzantine Empire. These events led to the economic decline of the Byzantine Empire which, due to its influential position as a significant buying force in the Middle East, caused other regions to decline and gradually led to the dwindling of local cultures within the empire and beyond it. A great number of people, many of them sick and poor, immigrated to wealthier cities in hopes of a better life. These catastrophes and the plight of these masses led to an encounter between social classes which had thus far remained more segregated.

I propose exploring the possible connection between this inter-class encounter and the consolidation of the list of seven deadly sins. I suggest that the definition of these sins was influenced and inspired by the members of the privileged class when confronted by those of the lower classes. In my view, the definition of these sins was meant to discipline the lower classes and restrain their wishes for comparing their lot with that of other classes. From now on, they are not allowed to covet, to desire or to feel angry. They must work (as laborers) in the mansions of the upper classes and their laziness will henceforth be considered a sin. They must be humble and unassuming, because pride, too, is now a sin. And envy? Envying the lot of the upper classes, an emotion which may incite them to "rob and destroy" – that is one of the gravest sins of all, "the envious impulse being to take it away or spoil it," as Klein put it (1957, p. 181) – may express the dread of the privileged classes of the distressed and angry under-privileged people who became oppressed by them. I suggest that the fear of the envious may culminate to the point of social class' annihilation anxiety.

In other words, I would argue that the definition of envy as a sin is not only a theological statement nor even a mere warning about interpersonal relationships. It is a statement made, in the context of a class-based society, by the members of the privileged class as a manifestation of social power relations and designed to preserve the rights and supremacy of this class. This position has been disguised as a religious position. Its disguise has been so successful that it has become, in my view, one of the most important contents of the social unconscious regarding envy. It is a content that is denied by everyone. As envy has become so condemned and disowned, the members of the privileged class attribute it to those others who seek to deprive them of their lawful rights. Under the discipline imposed by the seven deadly sins, they may present themselves as god-fearing and contented. Meanwhile, the members of the lower class may prefer their meager existence to being accused of harboring envy. The combination of these two positions sustains a state in which envy is rejected by either side, constantly attributed to someone else and becomes a persecutory possibility. Social power relations unconsciously utilize envy and its definition as a sin in order to preserve the privileges of the stronger class.

One of the key aspects of the social unconscious of envy involves the denial of the domineering behavior of the members of the privileged class, project their envy onto "Them," manifest in accusing members of other classes of envying them. This domineering position may cause members of other classes to assume an apologetic and self-humbling stance in response to such accusations. The tendency to try and prove that they are not envious may lead them to identify with this projection. This complementary aspect is also part of the social unconscious involving envy. In terms of Foucault about Power/Knowledge, the Seven Sins thesis is presented as a form of theological truth. This presentation preserves the power relations between the privileged and the under-privileged in favor of the stronger (Foucault, 1980).

The division (split) into "Us" and "Them," as it may be expressed in a split into classes, may be regarded as the unconscious result of the underlying Aggregation/Massification basic assumption (Hopper, 2003). This split may be formed as an unconscious reaction to anxiety in situations of envy within a society. The helplessness of the lower class (and in some cases – of both classes) can provoke and heighten anxiety. Envy, besides being a response to the assets of the upper class, can "make sense" for anxieties and feelings of helplessness, and serve as a defense mechanism against them. Helplessness, envy and division into groups can promote rebellious reactions. Within this world of tensions, the concept of the Seven Sins may constitute a cultural theological umbrella under which they all seem to agree on condemning envy and maintaining social stability. Hence, the social dimension of the concept of the Seven Sins may serve as a form of Massification defense mechanism.

Entitlement

Frankel and Sherik's (1977) observations indicate that outbursts of envy stem from an innate desire. Before children appear to envy someone, they seem to want something very much, to treat it as if it is their own and as if they are perfectly entitled to it, merely because they have chosen it. When another child wants to take this chosen object away from them, they react with rage and belligerence. Naturally, this "intruder" child may feel, in the exact same way, that this object was chosen by her (him) and that they are thus (also) unquestionably entitled to possess it. Children first present with envy when adults dictate the laws of possession: "Danny is going to keep this nice red truck. It's his truck. Very soon we will be saying bye-bye to Danny and his truck and go home. Back home you have your own toys." This is what mother and father say and, from this moment on, the child can no longer simply take what they want. There are rules and there is ownership; the laws of possession create frustration and envy.

If we are able to eschew for a moment the bleak Kleinian argument that envy is derived from the death drive, we may find a great deal of vitality in the child's experience of intensely wanting to choose and have what they like and of feeling perfectly entitled to do so. From this perspective, envy and vitality may be transformed eventually into more constructive behaviors than "rob and destroy" motivations.

Entitlement is the professional term for such experiences of "deserving something." The term was proposed by White (1963) and can be viewed as an innate experience. When a new-born baby cries, this can be seen as a kind of complaint – designed to be heard by its mother (parents) – demanding to receive (what it feels to be) proper care. Its complaint contains expectations of entitlement. If this experience is not impaired in the context of their primary relationships, the baby grows up feeling that he has certain unquestionable rights. This feeling will make it easier for children to feel equal to their peers and exercise their rights in accordance to their society's norms. However, if their experience of entitlement becomes impaired at some point in their life, they will no longer feel "deserving" and may suppress their desires and react to conflicts of interests with submission and resignation.

In my view, envy is grounded in desire and desire is grounded in a primary and un-impinged experience of entitlement. This is where these themes converge into the main idea of this chapter. The envy grounded in the experience of entitlement may jeopardize society's power balance. It may cause people to feel that they deserve more, leading them to threaten other groups. One of the most effective defenses against this danger is actively impairing this fundamental experience. People who do not feel that they deserve more will not act in order to obtain more. Moreover, when the impairment of this experience is sufficiently severe – the person will not feel envy altogether; they will accept their lack of entitlement and abandon their plight. Internal social struggles may often entail the kind of domineering oppression manifest in physical injury, incarceration and the creation of poverty and starvation (as when slavery was rampant in the United States). However, there are subtler ways of denying people's sense of entitlement and rights: the portrayal of envy as a sin and of those who envy as sinners may end up diminishing the ambition of those who might be accused of being envious. Such people may embrace this social-religious message and turn their frugality into an ideal and an achievement. The privileged members of society are safer the more they deny the experience of entitlement of those around them.

The group dimension of Envy

Even though the emotion of envy is denied and attributed to the other, envy between groups may behave differently than that between individuals. I would like to refer, first of all, to envy between individuals and its possible elaboration.

As an individual, I can confess my own envy: right now, I envy those who are not obliged to write this chapter at this time of night. They must be enjoying their vacation. They must have plenty of time and money. While in a bad mood, I envy people who are a generation younger than me. I envy the opportunities afforded by their young age. I envy people who live in more peaceful countries than the one I live in.

In the past, I had no idea that I was envious. Where I might have felt envy, I felt injustice and anger instead. The objects of my envy seemed to me to be stained in some way or another: either they had gained what is theirs through dishonest means or mad ambition or they appeared arrogant and condescending.

There came a moment when I realized that I am, indeed, envious and that my raging internal criticism of those who have achieved more than I have was designed to hide this emotion, which I had experienced as hostile and shameful, from myself. In fact, only when I entered group therapy was I able to make peace with envy. I attribute this change mostly to the group's conductor, who apparently was not deterred by envy and had no need to deny it.

At some point, one of the members, Debbie, criticized another member, Dina. Debbie had reservation about Dina's choice of clothes as well as her way of talking: "your clothes are extravagant and your voice is too feminine, too high. And you speak too freely in this group, too." Dina, the "extravagant member" fell completely silent and became withdrawn. The tension in the room was rising and the entire group felt that Dina's withdrawal was expressing a pain that could not yet be verbalized. During this moment, it seemed that Debbie was surprisingly taking Dina's place: she became more active and spoke freely, addressing some of the uncomfortable members and engaging them in conversation. This is when the conductor intervened:

> I think, Debbie, that you are envious of Dina. You're pretending to pass a moral judgement of Dina's extroverted behavior, seemingly accusing her of actually flirting with men in the group. But deep down, maybe you want to be just like her but are too afraid.

This is when Dina came back to life:

> what I find most suspicious is that you mentioned my voice. I didn't choose my voice and if it's too high, there's nothing I can do about it. And I speak freely because that what I came here for. I want to be who I am and, if that comes with a price, well, I'm willing to pay it.

Dina broke into tears. Apparently, she was not that prepared to be hurt in the group. Nevertheless, her words left quite an impression on me. I found the conductor's interpretation accurate and to the point: the envy hitherto disguised as righteousness was clearly visible. To my surprise, I felt relived as well as curious. This is when the conductor added: "Debbie's envy is the group voice for the envy that is hiding in the room – that probably belongs to everyone."

When that particular emotion came up in the group, I became one envier among many. It is the emotional resonance which became possible in that group that allowed most of us to engage in a confessional discourse. One member told another that she envied her because of how attractive she looked and of her ability to bravely and directly approach whoever she wished. Someone told the conductor that he envied her ability to stand her ground, even as one against many, and to express herself in a free and straightforward manner. When it was my turn, I addressed two of the male members in the room and spoke of envying what I perceived as their "unapologetic masculinity." One of them immediately replied, saying that my hesitant and seemingly shy conduct is more effective in gaining women's favors than most of his own attempts. Another member told me that he envied me for being taller than him. Throughout his entire life, he has been suffering from feelings of inferiority because he was short. We discovered that each of us envied someone and something and, at the same time, was the object of someone else's envy. The gradually accumulating sensation was that this boat of envy, which we were all in, is no more threatening than any other emotion. Envy became humanized.

(I am a firm believer in group therapy as the most fruitful process for working through envy, due to the mutuality and the exchange made possible in group-analytic psychotherapy.)

Let us consider the personal working through taken by several members of the group I attended. First, the admission of envy resonated and created a mutuality that was expressed in more and more confessions. For this reason, envy did not give rise to shame. Rather, it urged us to share and take part, while feeling relieved that we are free of the unwavering condemnation envy normally evokes. I believe that the crucial factor in this process of working through in the group was that, through the support of the conductor and the other members, the working through of envy was directed to an internal locus of control for each of the members. What became most important for the members was neither resignation nor the motivation to sabotage the other's achievements but rather the wish to measure up, by self-fulfilling one's abilities inspired by one's chosen envied other. Throughout the months following this exceptional and moving session, it was evident that most of the enviers have taken some steps toward realizing their personal goals. The experience of envy, accompanied by an ongoing interpersonal relationship with the object of envy, turned into inspiration for self-actualization. One member's envy of another's attractiveness had encouraged her to lose weight (quite painstakingly: she started running every evening and worked her way up to running five kilometers each day). Someone who envied the conductor adopted a more direct and bold facilitation style. Personally, I was unhappy with my "hesitant and ostensibly shy conduct" in my relations with women. Following the response of the object of my own envy, I found that this current pattern had seductive and feminine undertones and I abandoned it in favor of a more direct approach. The member who envied me for being tall went on to share with the group the feelings of inferiority that he experienced after the session. He transformed his inferiority into professional achievements. He also shared that his level of shame has decreased; that he had dared to approach a woman that he liked and the two started a relationship.

My personal perspective, which I have just shared, converges into one main general insight: most people (probably everyone) feel envy at some point or another, without acknowledging it, admitting it or attributing it to themselves. They know that other people envy and they despise, fear and oppose whoever they see as envious, while they feel themselves to be free of envy. However, when envy is openly and mutually shared, it helps the envious to leave their shame behind and to reexamine their desires and the ways they measure up (or not) to others. Eventually they turn back to themselves, focusing inwardly. I have noticed that on such occasions, the wish for self-actualization grows stronger and overtakes wishes (and fantasies) about hurting or robbing the other. In many cases, these circumstances transform envy into inspiration for personal development.

It seems to me that envy between groups (like social classes, nations and religions) creates different processes. In general, I wish to argue that envy between groups "chooses" the aggregation pole in the Aggregation-Massification basic assumption (Hopper, 2003). Moreover, while the working through of envy (if it ever occurs) on the individual level contains the potential for growth through envy, inter-group envy might easily become projective and antagonistic and end up in inter-groups conflicts.

I type the words "they envy us" into a search engine. In response, I immediately receive dozens of quotes from various sources, in which these words serve to highlight a central message of "us and them." Following are several incidental examples:

> "The NASA terrorists are super-jelly of us". "This Mussolini, of whom everyone envies us…". "They hate each other and they're miserable and they're jealous of us and they want us to hate each other too". "The oboes are isolated, envied… and disliked" "People envy us, they call us 'The Dream Team.'" "Maybe people just regard things as criminal, because they envy their success?" "They envy the young, and they want to avoid them or denigrate them whenever possible." "The secular do not hate us. They envy us." "They envy us because we're mortal." "Everything that was argued against us is a lie. There are people who has their interests. They are envious of our way of our community and they try to offend us".

All these examples present a clear division into "us and them," in which envy is attributed to "them" and formulated as an accusation and a crime committed against the "us" group. In accordance with the notions presented in this chapter, I would like to argue that any stable group affiliation reinforces the experience of entitlement for its members. The group processes of resonance, mirroring and exchange relations make group members feel that they are worth more and that they deserve more. In every area of life, any member perceived as valuable becomes pertinent to the reflection of others in their image. In self-psychology terms (Kohut, 1971), any valued quality in one of the members (masculine or feminine attractiveness, boldness, generosity, intelligence) and any achievement in the group or in external reality are idealized by others. Klein considers "idealization" as reaction-formation in front of painful envious feelings. Hence idealization serves as a mechanism of defense against such a pain. Mutual idealization within the "Us" group utilizes this defense mechanism on a large scale. Alongside this, the experience of belonging and the creation of "us" as an idealized aspect may be internalized by others. Qualities and achievements become the shared property of all other members. As a result, as mentioned above, stable group affiliation magnifies its members' experience of entitlement.

Nevertheless, there is a difference between interpersonal and inter-group behaviors. In my view, the individual experience of entitlement is potentially transformed into personal development and the wish to measure up. The group experience of entitlement may lead group members (especially when under the effects of aggre-gation-massification processes) to behave in ways that are condescending and aggressive toward groups perceived as inferior.

At the same time, I believe an unconscious social struggle is being waged in the minds of people of both classes. The privileged class strives to diminish the lower class' sense of entitlement; while the latter seeks to preserve it. In some situations, the lower class indeed submits (at least temporarily) to the mind-shaping dictates of the upper class. Let us consider racism for a moment: a Dutch priest gives a ser-mon to his congregation in South Africa. "It is God," so he says, "who decreed that whites are superior to blacks. We will not disobey him." For a time, black people might have embraced these faiths of white people.

Who are these foreigners who want to immigrate to our country? They are poor and hungry people from Eastern Europe – those who have been oppressed under the communist regime and "don't fit" in terms of education and freedom of thought. Everything they know about us has been stirring up their envy and their aspirations. They come to take; to settle down on the vein of life we have spent decades culti-vating and, no less – to obfuscate that which makes us unique.

I suggest that the split into "Us" and "Them" includes here a sense of defining "Us" as opposed to "Non-Us" (parallel to "Me" as opposed to "Not-me"), rejecting by that the others' ("Theirs") sense of entitlement. It seems that "Status Rigidity" (Weber, 2015) may become more strict and oppressive under the "Us" conviction of entitlement that stems from envy of the defenses against it.

As a matter of fact, developed countries which accept immigrants are more pros-perous because most immigrants are highly motivated to work for relatively low wages in order to make a living. However, when we look at xenophobia through the perspective of projected envy and the fear of the envious other, its irrational nature begins to make sense.

The members of the upper class seek to preserve and increase their sense of entitlement. The construction of any group's unique identity requires the develop-ment of myth and ideology.

I would like to mention the notion of penis envy, as it was conceptualized by Freud back in the day. The basic idea is that men have a penis while women lack it. He has it and she does not. For this reason – and this is the heart of the matter – she is destined to envy him. This envy may lead her normally to bear children as a replacement for the absent penis, or become vengeful, as an abnormal solution (Freud, 1925). Oftentimes, the little girl finds her place through submission and resignation and embraces passivity as part of her identity.

Horney was the first to attribute this psychoanalytic thesis with motives related to male dominance (1926). She quotes Simmel who views the relations between men and women throughout history as master-slave relations. Simmel notes that it is the master's privilege not to be constantly preoccupied with being the master, while the position of the slave never lets them forget their status (Quinn, 1987). The feminist movement in psychoanalysis has been able to uncover the notion of penis envy as a manifestation of patriarchal supremacy (Mitchell, 1974), utterly undermining its validity and importance. It seems that in other social fields, the social unconscious concerned with preserving the power of the privileged class by attributing envy to others is still in effect.

I would argue that accusing the "them" group of feeling envy and proclaiming that one's group has been wronged may sometime become part of a victimhood ideology at the group or national level. In another paper (Berman, 2010), I propose that such victimhood may help establish various kinds of group ideology (including nationalism and class warfare).

I view victimhood as a component of both personal and group identities. It may originally be a reaction to some trauma in the group or individual's historical past. Victimhood may also form as a group and even national position. In such circumstances, the victimized national position relies on ideology and myth. Four components are in play in both individual and national victimhood: (1) The demand that the wrongs committed against us and our "victim status" are acknowledged. (2) The displacement of anger from a past enemy to some present group. (3) The translation of suffering into a domineering attitude and a demand for compensation. (4) An exemption from concern. In my view, an accusation along the lines of "they envy us" may become part of a victimhood ideology and link itself to myths as part of the national history. Victimhood-based national positions that are reinforced by envy may, in my opinion, create a group-national experience of entitlement that entails the wish for compensation and the exemption from concern toward members of the other group. This may lead to the emergence of social-national views that justify exclusion, discrimination and disenfranchisement. As an example, consider the following biblical story, which features an accusation of envy and a budding victimhood-based ideology.

Then Isaac sowed in that land, and reaped in the same year a hundredfold; and the Lord blessed him. The man began to prosper, and continued prospering until he became very prosperous; for he had possessions of flocks and possessions of herds and a great number of servants. So the Philistines envied him. Now the Philistines had stopped up all the wells which his father's servants had dug in the days of Abraham his father, and they had filled them with earth. And Abimelech said to Isaac, "Go away from us, for you are much mightier than we." And Isaac departed thence, and pitched his tent in the valley of Gerar, and dwelt there. And Isaac dug again the wells of water which they had dug in the days of Abraham his father, for the Philistines had stopped them up after the death of Abraham. He called them by the names which his father had called them. Also Isaac's servants dug in the valley, and found a well of running water there. But the herdsmen of Gerar quarreled with Isaac's herdsmen, saying, "The water is ours." So he called the name of the well Esek [meaning 'argument'], because they quarreled with him. Then they dug another well, and they quarreled over that one also. So he called its name Sitnah [meaning 'hostility']. And he moved from there and dug another well, and they did not quarrel over it. So he called its name Rehoboth [meaning 'wide open space'], because he said, "For now the Lord has made room for us, and we shall be fruitful in the land."

(Genesis, 26, 12–23; New King James Version)

Isaac is presented as a peace-loving victim of the Philistines' envy. He himself does not envy. He is the victim of the Philistines, whose envy drives him away from his territory. Avoiding confrontation, he eventually finds another plot of land that is far from their reach. Later on, however, his very peace-loving conduct is presented as a manifestation of the wrong he suffered: Isaac is portrayed as the victim, the Philistines as invaders and their envy as a destructive force. Conquering the land and fighting the Philistines are thereby justified. The experience of entitlement of the ancient Hebrews is formulated and reinforced through the biblical narrative.

Conclusion

Envy also has a group-social-national aspect that is manifest in inter-group relations. This group affiliation reinforces the members' experience of entitlement. The conjunction of this experience with envy may lead to envy-driven development. Indeed, it is demonstrable that individuals are capable of transforming envy into inspiration for personal development, self-actualization and measuring up. In contrast, when the group experience of entitlement coincides with envy, this may bring about a hostile and belligerent attitude toward other groups.

My central argument is that the domineering behavior that stems from envy remains unconscious. Envy is always attributed to others: "they envy us." The responses to the danger posed by such envious others are both conscious and ideologically justified. However, I find that the wish to preserve the privilege of the upper class by accusing others of being envious is a key component of the social unconscious involving envy. While most of us social scientists are far from naïve, there may be room for hope (like in the early days of psychoanalysis) that the uncovering of the unconscious will replace conflict with negotiation between people and sub-groups.

Note

1 The text of ST. Augustine's confessions is available on the internet: www.concordane. com/augustine.htm

References

Berman, A. (2010). "Post-Traumatic Victimhood. Victimhood." In: *Vengefulness and the Culture of Forgiveness* (pp. 3–62). I. Ulric, A. Berman and M. Berger (eds). New York, Nova Science Publishers Inc.

Berman, A., M. Berger, and D. Gutmann (2000). "The Division into Us and Them as a Universal Social Structure." *Mind and Human Interaction* 11: 53–72.

Bloomfield, M. W. (1952). *The Seven Deadly Sins.* Michigan, Michigan State University Press.

Foucault, M. (1980). "Truth and Power." In: *Power/Knowlege*. C. Gordon (ed.). Breighton, Harvester: 107–133.

Frankel, S. and I. Sherik (1977). "Observation on the Development of Normal Envy." *Psychoanalytic Study of the Child* 32: 257–281.

Freud, S. (1925). "Some Physical Consequences of the Anatomical Distinction Between the Sexes." *Standard Edition* 19: 241–258. London, Hogarth.

Hopper, E. (2003). *Traumatic Experience in the Unconscious Life of Groups. The Fourth Basic Assumption: Incohision: Aggregation/Massification or (ba) I:A/M*. London, Jessica Kingsley.

Hopper, E. and H. Weinberg, Eds. (2011). *The Social Unconscious in Persons, Groups and Societies*. London, Karnc Books.

Klein, M. (1957 (1997)). *Envy and Gratitude*. London, Vintage.

Kohut, H. (1971). *The Analysis of the Self: A Systematic Approach to the Psychoanalytic Treatment of Narcissistic Personality Disorders*. Madison, CT, Int. Universities Press.

Mitchell, J. (1974). *Psychoanalysis and Feminism*. New York, Pantheon.

Quinn, S. A. (1987). *A mind of her Own: The life of Karen Horney*. New York, Summit Books.

Raufman, R. and H. Weinberg (2017). *Fairy Tales and the Social Unconscious: The Hidden Language*. London, Karnac.

Weber, M. (2015). "The Types of Legitimate Domination." In: *Sociological Theory in the Classical Era: Text and Readings*. L. Desfor-Edles and S. Appelrouth (eds). Sage: 217–223. Los Angeles: London.

White, R. (1963). *Ego and Reality in Psychoanalytic Theory*. New York, International University Press.

11 Bigenderality,[1] bisexuality, foundation matrix and the social unconscious

Gila Ofer

In this chapter, I propose an approach of looking at both gender and sex as parts of our foundation matrix that are usually socially unconscious. Furthermore, I regard them as an aspect of experience that moves between fluidity and fixity, between being both genders and both sexes at one time, and differentiating them at other times. The title of the chapter denotes bigenderality (endnote 1) and bisexuality to indicate that the two are part of this complex experience.

In this chapter, I use bigenderality (or bigender) and bisexuality (or bisexual) since I refer to both of them as they appear in our social unconscious. The concept of bisexuality relates to male and female (biological) denotations, whereas masculine and feminine are socially constructed gender denotations. "Psychic bigenderality" is distinguished from "psychic bisexuality," just as sexual identities differ from gender identities. (I do not refer in the chapter to "object choice," which is a term that usually refers to the sex of the object to whom one is attracted and "chooses.") In a simple way, my approach can be presented in the following two-dimensional matrix (Figure 11.1):

	Femininity	masculinity
Male\	M+f+m	M+m
Female	F+f	F+f+m

Figure 11.1 Two-Dimensional Matrix of Psychic Bigenderality and Bisexuality.

I refer to the term "foundation matrix" as part of the tripartite matrix: the foundation matrix, the dynamic matrix and the personal matrix. The tripartite matrix includes individual persons and groups as one single, inseparable process in which biological, social, cultural and economic factors meet and merge. It exists on a few levels of space and time; and it includes all dimensions of communication – the verbal and nonverbal. Part of this matrix can be more static and parts of it can be more flexible and fluid (Scholtz, 2011). Quite often in the literature, the "social unconscious" is used in order to refer to the social, cultural and communicational constraints and restraints of which people are to varying degrees unconscious (Hopper, 2003; Hopper and Weinberg, 2011). However, we

DOI: 10.4324/9781003425915-17

should keep in mind that "the unconscious mind of a person is always a socially unconscious mind, in the same way that it is always a neuro-physiologically unconscious mind" (Hopper, 2018). While the foundation matrix is shared by all members of the society, the personal internalizations of certain social patterns and processes during a particular period of time bring about some changes which are unique to that person. But also the foundation matrix of the contextual society is enacted in the dynamic matrix of the group via the personal matrices of the participants.

The culturally biased stereotypes of men and women – since the days of hunters and gatherers, free seed sowers and raising children – these are the stereotypes that are planted in our social unconscious, stemming from the foundation matrix. We continue to relate to them and grow in their light. These stereotypical male and female figures that have existed in our culture from time immemorial have a major impact on the creation of our gendered sense of self (Seaglow and Hopper, 1973). Among the many other factors affecting our gendered self are language and technology (Rose, 2002). The interrelationship of linguistic usage, technologies and gender are formed and reformed in our social unconscious with regard to desire and passion.

However, side by side with distinct male and female stereotypes in our foundation matrix, we can also point at the existence of bisexuality and the wish for potentiating this bisexuality. Evolutional sources of bisexuality exist in nature in the world of animals and plants. Some organisms are hermaphrodites who own both female and male organs. In varying degrees, people are biologically androgens or hermaphrodites (this is one reason why we are psychically bisexual but more precisely "bigender"). This is true on chemical, hormonal, embryological and developmental levels. Biological bisexuality contributes to the existence of bisexual fantasies and wishes in our unconscious mind(s).

The study of the unconscious is a complex task that can be performed both directly and indirectly. The direct aspect is performed through clinical work with individuals and in small and large groups. The indirect aspect – by analyzing various elements such as mythology, history, cultural customs and institutions, literature, art and movies, which indirectly reflect, structure, express and resonate the various dimensions of the unconscious.

Let us start by referring to the indirect aspect: if we look at Greek mythology, we already have a few references to bisexuality. **Tiresias**, in Greek mythology, a blind Theban seer, the son of one of Athena's favorites, the nymph Chariclo, is a participant in several well-known legends. Tiresias played an active part in the tragic events involving Laius, the king of Thebes, and his son Oedipus. He is also known for having been in Hades, and for having lived for seven or nine generations. Besides longevity, another of Tiresias's features involves his having lived as a man, then as a woman, and then as a man again. Reportedly, he had been turned into a woman as the result of having struck and wounded mating snakes. When Tiresias returned to the site of the transformation seven years later to see if the "spell" could be reversed, Tiresias did indeed see the same snakes coupling and was changed back into a man.

Another famous reference to bisexuality in the Greek mythology is Aristophanes' speech in Plato's Symposium (360 BC). **Aristophanes'** speech comes in the form of a myth. He explains that long ago there were three types of human beings: male, female and androgynous, a form made up of male and female elements. They were all round shaped, with four hands and four legs each, two faces, and two sets of sexual organs, much like two human beings stuck together. Having so many limbs, they were very fast and strong. The male kind came from the sun, the female was an offspring of the earth, and the androgynous of the moon. Being so strong they tried to ascend to heaven to attack the gods. Zeus and the other gods decided against wiping them out, as that would rid them of receiving worship and sacrifices. Zeus proposed cutting them in half, reducing their strength and increasing their number, resulting in more worship and sacrifice, all of which benefitted the gods. He did so and Apollo turned each person's head toward the wound as a reminder of the cut, which was healed by drawing skin at what is now called the stomach, fastened at the navel. Now each half longed for its other half, and they would hug, wanting to grow together. This caused some to die from hunger and idleness as they would do nothing else. As they were dying out, Zeus took pity and moved their genitals to the front. Before, these were outside, casting seeds in the ground, rather than in each other, to make children. Now, reproduction would occur inside the woman, "by the man in the woman." Previously, when the androgynous hugged, they would have children and when male embraced male, they would enjoy intercourse.

The paradox of bisexuality vis-á-vis binary sexes is also illustrated in the Bible, which more or less starts out with two versions of the creation of man and woman. The first one is one image to both:

1:26 Then God said, "Let us make mankind in our image, after our likeness, so they may rule over the fish of the sea and the birds of the air, over the cattle, and over all the earth, and over all the creatures that move on the earth."

1:27 God created mankind in his own image, in the image of God he created them, male and female he created them.

The second version is two distinct man and woman:

2:7 The Lord God formed the man from the soil of the ground and breathed into his nostrils the breath of life, and the man became a living being.

2:18 The Lord God said, "It is not good for the man to be alone.... So the Lord God caused the man to fall into a deep sleep; and while he was asleep, he took part of the man's side and closed up the place with flesh".

2:22 Then the Lord God made a woman from the part he had taken out of the man, and he brought her to the man.

2:23 Then the man said, "This one at last is bone of my bones and flesh of my flesh; this one will be called 'woman,' for she was taken out of man."

The wish for sameness and the wish for difference, the wish for bisexuality and the wish for different sexes are both manifested here. The first version of creation in the Bible envisions man and woman as equal and the same. In the second version, the woman is created in order to be man's helpmeet – here she is second to him, not like him, and since this difference is inscribed in a patriarchal context, she is, hence, inferior to him. The fact that the woman is the person who gives birth to children is occluded. Here is further evidence for the fight against impotence and the defensive wish for omnipotence: the first pregnancy in the world is a man's pregnancy and the woman is a bone of his bones and flesh of his flesh: man is superior to woman. The fight against impotence is a major issue at hand. The role of this rendition of human creation is, it would appear, to deny the phallic mother. At the same time, though, it is also a denial of the primal scene and the oedipal constellation, that is to say: it denies the fact that a couple is needed for conceiving a child, thus making it seem as if a man by himself suffices (Britton, 1989).

The binary division into men versus women began with the most prominent difference between the two sub-groups of humanity. Myths and legends everywhere resonate this difference, whether in the story of the creation of Adam and Eve in the Bible or in Hindu mythology (in the Matsuya Purana, the most popular and complete of all the puranas), which tells that lord Brahma created Shatrupa and they begat the first man, Manu, who waited ever so patiently until he found Ananti, with whom he begat more sons. In all these mythologies, the woman is created by/from the man. Versions of the story of Eve, the snake and the apple also appear in the myths of other cultures. But as long as we have the binary division, we also have the wish for bisexuality.

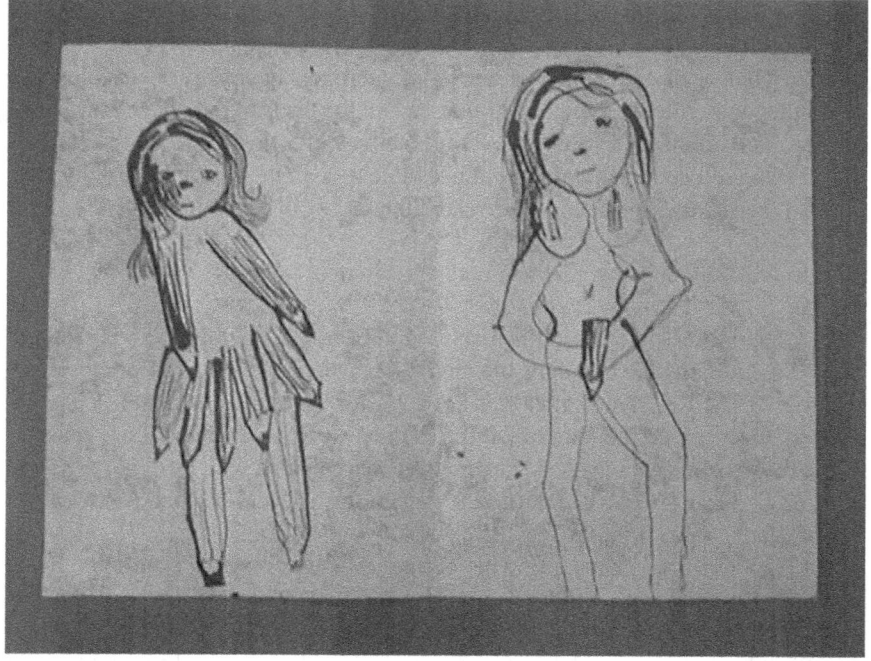

Figure 11.2 Body\Others\Pencil. Rakefet Viner Omer. 2012–2016.

Consider the expression of the wish for bisexuality in the work of art by Duchamp: Mona Lisa with moustache and beard. This also appears in Dali's Mona Lisa with moustache. Another example is a self-portrait of Dali with male organs and a woman's breast from which a baby is suckling. I was struck by the wish this painting appeared to be expressing – to be both male and female at the same time, to have a penis that can fertilize a woman but also milk with which to feed the baby.

Another contemporary example is Rakefet Wiener's (a famous Israeli artist) drawing of a woman with a penis, side by side with a woman with a dress composed of penises, some of which turn into crayons (Figures 11.2 and 11.3).

In her novel, *Orlando*, Virginia Woolf (1973) seems to play on this same notion of fundamental bisexuality. Orlando, her trans-historical hero-heroine, lives through some of the major cultural-historical changes in Europe, from the Elizabethan period to the 20th century. At first, Orlando is a nobleman and a favorite of

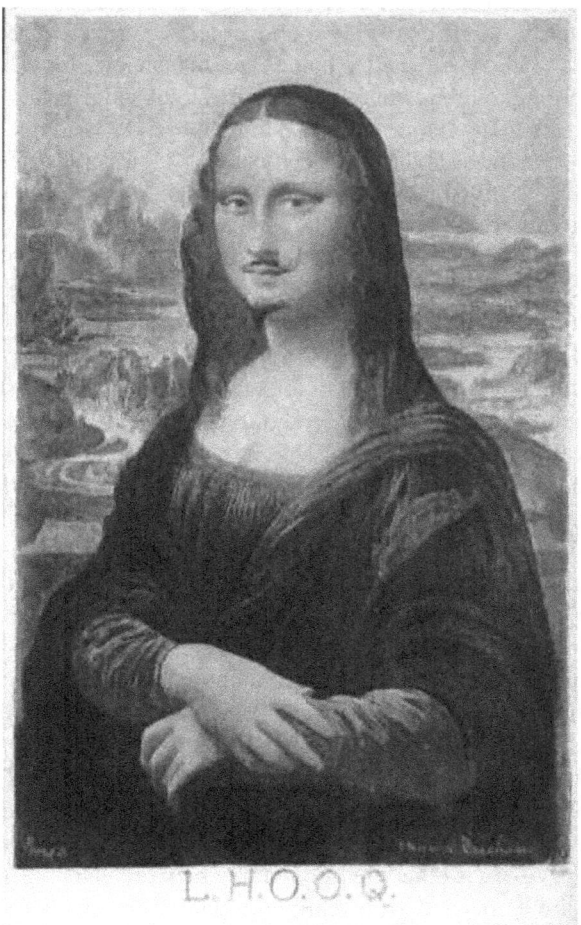

Figure 11.3 "L.H.O.O.Q.," Marcel Duchamp, 1919.

Queen Elizabeth. In the middle of the book, he becomes a woman – and lives the rest of "her" life as a woman, remembering that she once was a man. Although he becomes a woman halfway through his/her era-straddling existence, Orlando has not changed at all in other respects. Changing sex affects his/her future but not his/her core identity. Thus, Woolf implies that one's core identity is located beyond gender traits, which she regards as mostly stereotypical social attributes. She also implies that childhood identifications are the same multifaceted web for both girls and boys, and only later does society, with its determinations and stereotypes, enter the picture and create gender differentiation.

According to Freud, the ego is first of all the physical ego. One can say that the social unconscious also stems from physical origins. The same, he would argue, holds for gender – which begins with the body. Here again, I am not speaking about sexual attraction so much as about one's biological sexual identity – being male or female. This is in inherent in species aspects or elements of the foundation matrix as well as socially constructed. **Freud** believed that all humans were bisexual, by which he primarily meant that everyone incorporates aspects of both sexes, and that everyone is sexually attracted to both sexes. In his view, this was true anatomically and, according to Freud, therefore, also mentally and psychologically.

We can find the first reference to bisexuality in Freud's writings in his letters to Fliess (1896) where he says that he is convinced by Fliess regarding his thoughts about bisexuality. On 1901 he writes to him: "my next work will be called 'Human bisexuality'. It will go to the root of the problem and say the last word it may be granted me to say." This was never accomplished, but he mentions bisexuality a couple of more times. Later, Freud (1905) traces sexuality to the young child's discovery of the anatomical differences between boys and girls. He also asserts that "Anatomy is destiny" (Freud, 1925).

Yet, the asymmetry of Freud's thinking on the genders and his strongly differential evaluation of masculinity and femininity is obvious and reflects contemporary cultural values. In his paper on "The Ego and the Id" (1923), he argues that biological and psychic bisexualities are in fact the basis of the child attraction to and identification with both parents and this leads to the Oedipus complex. The fact that Freud did not develop further his theory about this issue might be contributed to the cultural atmosphere at his time which had an impact on his thinking. Although the concept of gender was not used by Freud, The asymmetry of his thinking on the genders and his strongly differential evaluation of masculinity and femininity is obvious and reflects contemporary cultural values. He traces sexuality to the young child's discovery of the anatomical differences between boys and girls. According to him, "Anatomy is destiny" (Freud, 1905, 1925). Both men and women are missing something, he claims. Both long for what they lack. But there is a crucial difference: women are missing the male sexual organ, an impossible longing that must therefore be renounced. Men, however, lack passive feelings vis-á-vis other men, something they dread to experience because such feelings are associated with femininity and castration. As far as Freud is concerned, men have all the organs they could possibly want; what they need to overcome are childlike illusory fears.

According to Elizabeth Young-Bruehl (1996), the term *gender* was first used in a psychoanalytic context in the late 1960s. It represented a move away from the early Freudian emphasis on the psychical consequences of anatomical difference, toward a more **active, constructive notion of sexual identity**. We could also regard this as **a move away from characterology to the study of identity,** or from essentialism (i.e., the attempt to define the essence of each sex) toward constructionism, or the assumption that **gender identity is constructed**. Young-Bruehl (1996) traces the current use of the term *gender* to Simone De Beauvior who, in her book *The Second Sex* (1974), writes:

> It is not the body-object described by biologists that actually exists, but the body as lived in by the subject [in society]....It is not nature that defines woman; it is she who defines herself by dealing with nature on her own account in her emotional life.
>
> (p. 42)

De Beauvoir was clearly saying that "anatomy is not destiny." From there, feminists took the direction of the gender-androgynous, and later to a non-binary sexual identity (Butler, 1995), the meaning of which could be that "gender is not destiny."

One could say that flexible movement between bigenderality and bisexuality is mentally healthier, a matter of what he termed "mental hygiene." However, Irene Fast (1990) argues that the trauma entailed in discovering sexual difference is the child's realization that she or he cannot be both male and female. This realization marks the end of omnipotence. Aron (1995) and Mitchell (1991) agree with Fast that awareness of sexual difference requires the recognition of limits, and that such a recognition is associated with feelings of loss, denial, envy and demands for restitution. However, they look at bisexual completeness not as something that needs to be overcome, abandoned or renounced, but rather as something to be integrated with other more differentiated positions. Aron discusses this possible movement as stemming from earlier phantasies of combined parenthood (1995). Sweetnam (1996) relates to the experience of being able to move between the two as reaching the depressive position. We can conclude that the fantasy of bisexual completeness continues to exist in everyone and plays a major, fundamental, and constructive role in creativity and in our capacity to think and symbolize. I argue that this fluid movement is possible because of the biological and societal parts of our foundation matrix.

Foulkes, in his wish to advocate group analysis, wrote (1964), "...what was thought to be biological, is often cultural inheritance. The task [is] to...do away with pseudo problems such as biological versus cultural, somatogenic versus psychogenic, individual versus group, reality versus fantasy" (p. 77). Thus, one can assume that Foulkes was advocating bisexuality and bigender flexibility. He (1964) emphasizes how important it is that group analysts have access to both our masculine and feminine dimensions and qualities. According to Aron, analysts

> need to have access to their bisexuality—to phantasies of themselves as male and female and to themselves as male and female, with both heterosexual

and homosexual desires—access to their own internal mothers and fathers, in order to make optimal use of the analytic process

(1995, p. 232)

The same applies to group conductors. Only if the group conductor can have the access to his bisexuality, can both paternal and maternal transferences directed toward the conductor be identified by him or her.

Here is a vignette about myself as a conductor which shows the impact of our current culture on our thinking, although we think that we are open-minded to fluidity of gender:

> A patient in one of my groups, a 32-year-old woman who was never able to form a meaningful relationship with a partner, told the group that the day before, she had slept with a man to whom she wasn't attracted, simply because he wanted to. Among other things, I told her that she did not respect her body. The patient was very hurt by what I said and the group supported her, arguing that I was too blunt and quite conservative. Several months later, a male patient in the same group, who also has difficulties in forming intimate relationships, told the group that he met a woman and later slept with her, despite not really knowing why and not really being attracted to her. The group members replied that this woman was toying with him and taking advantage of him. I said that in order not to feel castrated, he pushed himself into doing something he did not truly want.

In the following session, the woman patient mentioned above expressed her anger at me, saying that she had come to realize how "sexist" I was and accused me of telling her that she did not respect her body while I used completely different terms when talking to the male patient, without considering that it is actually the same kind of "disrespect of one's body."

Even though I see myself as an open-minded person and even though I have spent years teaching gender and sexuality, trying to show others just how much we are trapped in age-old social stereotypes, it appeared that I could not completely escape these stereotypes and images that dwell inside us, as part of our social unconscious. As forward thinking as we would like to be and as much as we would hope to control our unconscious rather than the other way around, we cannot deny this part of ourselves. Still, it is also important to acknowledge that my interpretations were directed to two different motivations behind the agreement of the female patient and the male patent: the first was to placate the other boy, whereas the latter was to prove to himself his virility.

The various derivatives of the binary categorization and the various ways of dealing with it are present in our foundation matrix to this very day, even when we are fully aware that the social construction of gender is just as powerful – and perhaps even more so, as the biological construction of it. Just as the binary division into males and females as well as the binary division of men and women, is present in the dynamics of our foundation matrix, and in the dynamics of our social unconscious, equally present is the primordial aspiration for omnipotence, the rejection of this division and, of course, the wish for bisexuality.

I teach courses on gender and sexuality and, in the first lesson, I usually ask my female and male students to recall their earliest childhood memories that represent their femininity or masculinity, respectively. Here are some of the memories that came up:

- Men's memories: his mother talks to him and complains about his father; he is standing on a porch facing the street, urinating on people; he is holding a stick in his hand, feeling that he is allowed to kill; a teacher is leaving him in charge of the classroom.
- Women's memories: she is walking in nice tight cloths, with a bra and with her long hair untied; her father is looking at her as if she were a princess; she is in love with a youth movement instructor and hiding it; she is wiping her father's kiss from her cheek; she is having her first kiss; she is going out with a new dress and new shoes, feeling like a princess.

We can see that the first memories that came up as inner representations of femininity and masculinity are very much in line with commonly held stereotypes, namely, those attributing power and activity to men, and dependence, passivity, seduction, intimacy, and also fear of sexuality to women. Still it is not possible to decide whether our sense of gender is biologically determined no less than socially. Or as Foulkes wrote (1964) this issue is not relevant.

In the analytic groups that I conduct, I hear similar responses. For example, in one of the groups, a woman said: "in my experience, all the men here feel as though they were undressing me. They would like me to take my clothes off. And the women - they laugh at me." Another woman says: "I would like to explore why all the women here took my side, stood by me, when I talked about my pain, while all the men attacked me."

Both women's perceptions of the other members in the group were in line with commonly held attitudes. They distinguished between the reactions they evoked in males and in females. It is worth noticing that the two women used different languages: the first one used the language of seduction and the second one used the language of pain. They felt that these two modes of behavior attracted different and contradictory reactions from the other males and females in the group. The male group members found it difficult to empathize with a female who expressed pain, but they reacted differently to seduction. The female members could immediately identify with expressed pain, but reacted negatively to the language of seduction.

I have seen various examples of the wish for bisexuality in the groups that I conduct. For example, the wish for bisexual completeness is evident in the way the men in one of my groups try to cope with the fact that they cannot conceive and deliver babies. Their solution for their feeling of being barred from that experience is by bringing out their feminine part through identification with the women in the group and with their wives in the delivery room (Ofer, 2016).

These stories are a way of dealing with this envy and dread (Chasseguet-Smirgel, 1984; Horney, 1932). Another recurring trope is that of the distinction between the good woman and the witch. This, also, is probably the result of dealing with a splitting of the mother figure, to whom one is sexually attracted. If all these stories, myths and folktales, which tell of good and bad mothers, of the prince who saves the damsel from the witch (the bad mother), are indeed a reflection of our social unconscious, then they are a way for society and for individuals in society to deal with envy of and attraction to the omnipotent mother. The binary categorization of men and women, the glorification of men, the belittling of women and the belief that woman is born of man, the splitting of the original woman into Eve and Lilith, to a merciful mother and a witch mother, all these are ways through which we try unconsciously to deal with these feelings. Roth (2007) and others (Elior, 2019) note that myths, stories and legends were all made by men. This may indicate that stories about woman being created by/from man are an expression of envy and a personal and social instrument for dealing with this envy. Similarly, the split woman-figure we find in many myths (e.g. the Amazonian women) is a defense against the conscious recognition of the seductive power of the omnipotent mother and wife.

Here is a vignette from another analytic group: Bruce attended the group for three years. He was both very sensitive and cynical at the same time. He was afraid of expressing his feelings – tender feelings as well as aggression. He is about to go abroad and leave the group. Rachel reads a farewell letter to Bruce and she also brings him a gift – a painted red heart in an envelope. In the letter, she writes:

> I hope you are leaving wholeheartedly and not just because you said you would leave. I also hope that you take along with you all the issues that we worked through together. I want to thank you for the gentle things you said, although you are not aware of the warm feelings that come through your words, from time to time. And last but not least, it is a pity that you cannot work together with us on what has been emerging in you with regard to femininity, I think this issue is crucially connected to your own masculinity.

Bruce: I really feel that Dan and Simon are much more masculine than I am. They are strong, muscular.

Dan: What is masculinity? What do you mean?

Simon: I think that Bruce really feels less masculine. For some reason you [addressing Bruce] see me as more masculine because I hit the man on the beach when he threatened me [this is an event Simon recounted a few months earlier]. I, on the other hand, look at it as an expression of weakness. I would not like this to happen to me again.

Rachel: I always arouse certain reactions in you, Bruce, and then you relate to me as if I was attacking you, while that's not the case at all. I feel that you are unable to be there when I am being tender towards you and want your warm feelings. You are afraid of your tender parts.

Analyst:	it is heartwarming[2] how all of you can see yourself as both masculine and feminine. But with Bruce we can see how sometimes it is difficult to accept our bisexuality, and we wish to have differences between men and women.
Bruce:	I guess I do have some serious problem with my manhood. I am not the typical masculine figure and I don't feel comfortable with it...Where I grew up the other children were always mocking me. I was the only Jewish child, weak, not good at sports, from a very poor family. I had nothing to be proud of...
Judy:	But you have so many good things in you. And you really attract me with your wisdom and empathy. Why do you have to be seen as such a strong man and not accept all parts of you?

Bruce was transfixed on some stereotype masculine traits, and was bothered by the existence of some so-called feminine traits in him. Images of masculinity and femininity were fixed within Bruce, rather than fluid. This was reflected not only intra-personally, but also in his interpersonal relations with men and women outside the group. The group saw through it and has tried in the past and in this session to help him achieve some gender fluidity (meaning psychic bisexuality). Members of the group were much more flexible than him with their gender identifications and wanted to help him with this.

Freud (1918) said that human beings share three narcissistic injuries, corresponding to the scientific discoveries made by Copernicus, Darwin and himself: the first is that the earth is not the center of the universe, the second is that we are descended from apes and the third is that we are not conscious of everything that happens to us, and are thus not in control of what happens to us and of what we do. The desire to eradicate differences, to erase this binary categorization, exists in our personal and social unconscious and is manifest, among other things, in drag shows; in the surfacing of people who consider themselves non-binary. Their use of language also *serves* to avoid any unequivocal determination of belonging to this or that gender; they try to create new linguistic terms for self-definitions that do not conform to this binary division. They thus alternate between using "he" and "she" or use the plural or neutral pronouns. Our unconscious contains no contradictions and so the wish to enforce differences and the wish to eradicate them can co-exist in us. More than that, both psychoanalysts and group analysts argue that accepting our bisexulaity is necessary to for creativity (Aron, 1995; Nitsun, 2006; Ofer, 2016; Winnicott, 1971; Raphael-Leff's (2007) concept of generative identity also applies here).

However, today, we can see how modern technology helps us to both erase differences and to perpetuate binary distinctions: sex change operations and the use of hormones allow people who want to alter their sex to do so and fulfil their wish. However, by the very act of seeking to become a member of the opposite sex, the transsexual[3] person perpetuates the binary nature of gender categorization.

The debate concerning gender and sexuality – between viewing gender as a definite binary category or as a fluid construction – this debate which is also expressed in mythology, philosophy, art, literature, and psychoanalysis, about whether our identity as man or woman is biologically or culturally derived – this debate is not merely theoretical. It is a debate that reflects *a central conflict in the human psyche, in our foundation matrix, and in our social unconscious: on the one hand there is our wish, and indeed our real need, to firmly establish differences, and yet on the other hand, we have an equally strong wish and need to erase or blur these differences, to mask their meaning, to be complete, with no deficiency or lack, and to fulfill our bisexuality.* This is the social heritage from generation to generation and that is still with us even in our very postmodern world.

Group analysis by the very existence of various participants, men and women, through resonance, mirroring, and exchange, through communicating the various voices of the group members can possibly bring with it more flexibility and less rigidity. Thus the movement between fluidity and fixity becomes more available for us. Fluidity then can inhabit both foundation matrix and our conscious self.

Notes

1 I owe this concept to Earl Hopper, personal communication.
2 The use of this word is indicative of my countertransference preference for gender fluidity.
3 Historically and medically, the term transsexual was used to indicate a difference between one's gender identity (their internal experience of gender) and sex assigned at birth (male, female or intersex). More specifically, the term is often (though not always) used to communicate that one's experience of gender involves medical changes, such as hormones or surgery, that help alter their anatomy and appearance to more closely align with their gender identity. Despite their similar definitions, many transgender people don't identify as transsexual.

References

Aron, L. (1995). The internalized primal scene. *Psychoanalytic Dialogues, 5,* 195–238.
Britton, R. (1989). The missing link: Parental sexuality in the Oedipus complex. In *The Oedipus complex today*, ed. J. Steiner (pp. 83–102). London: Karnac Books.
Butler, J. (1995), Melancholy gender—refused identification. *Psychoanalytic Dialogues, 5,* 165–180.
Chasseguet-Smirgel, J. (1984). The femininity of the psychoanalyst in professional practice. *International Journal of Psycho-Analysis, 65,* 169–178.
De Beauvior, S. (1974). *The second sex.* New York: Bantam Books.
Elior, R. (2019). Plenary lecture given in the IIGA conference "Wings and Roots", Jerusalem.
Fast, I. (1990), Aspects of early gender development: Toward a reformulation. *Psychoanalytic Psychology, 7,* 105–117.
Foulkes, S. H. (1964). *Therapeutic group analysis.* London: Karnac Maresfield Reprints.
Freud, S. (1896). Letter from Freud to Fliess, December 6, 1896. The Complete Letters of Sigmund Freud to Wilhelm Fliess, 1887–1904, 207–214.
Freud, S. (1901). Letter from Freud to Fliess, August 7, 1901. The Complete Letters of Sigmund Freud to Wilhelm Fliess, 1887–1904, 446–448.
Freud, S. (1905). *Three essays on the theory of sexuality (1905). The standard edition of the complete psychological works of Sigmund Freud, Volume VII (1901–1905): A case of*

hysteria, three essays on sexuality and other. Standard Edition (9, pp. 123–246). London: Hogarth Press, 1959.

Freud, S. (1918). *From the history of an infantile neurosis*. Standard Edition (17, pp. 3–123). London: Hogarth Press, 1957.

Freud, S. (1923). *The ego and the id. The standard edition of the complete psychological works of Sigmund Freud, Volume XIX (1923–1925): The ego and the id and other works* (pp. 1–66). London: Hogarth Press, 1961.

Freud, S. (1925). *Female sexuality*. Standard Edition (21, pp. 223–246). London: Hogarth Press, 1961.

Hopper, E. (2003). *The social unconscious: Selected papers*. London: Jessica Kingsley.

Hopper, E. (2018). Notes on the concept of the Social Unconscious in Group Analysis. *Group 42*(2), 99–118.

Hopper E. & Weinberg, H. (Eds.) (2011). *The social unconscious in persons, groups and societies: Vol. I: Mainly theory*. London: Karnac.

Horney, K. (1932). Observations on a specific difference in the dread felt by men and by women respectively for the opposite sex. *International Journal of Psychoanalysis, 13*, 348–360.

Mitchell, S. (1991). Gender and sexual orientation in the age of postmodernism: The plight of the perplexed clinician. *Gender and Psychoanalysis, 1*, 45–73.

Nitsun, M. (2006). *The group as an object of desire: Exploring sexuality in group Therapy*. London: Routledge.

Ofer, G. (2016). Gender multiplicity in group analysis: Bridging identities fluidity and fixity in group analysis. *Group, 40*(2).

Pearlberg, R. (ed.) (2018). *Psychic bisexuality: A British-French dialogue*. London: Routledge.

Plato's Symposium (360 B.C.). English translation by B. Jowett (1953). 4th edition, Oxford. Pp. 520–525.

Raphael-Leff, J. (2007). Femininity and its unconscious 'shadows': Gender and generative identity in the age of biotechnology. *British Journal of Psychotherapy, 23*(4), 497–515.

Rose, C. (2002). Talking gender in the group. *Group Analysis, 35*(4), 525–539.

Roth, B. (2007). Pan's Labyrinth, Loneliness and Tragedy. Intergroup Psychoanalytic Conference. Vancouver, British Columbia. Unpublished communication.

Scholtz, R. (2011). The foundation matrix and the social unconscious. In: *The social unconscious in persons, groups and societies, Volume 1: Mainly theory*, ed. E. Hopper & H. Weinberg (pp. 265–285). London: Karnac.

Seaglow, I., & Hopper, E. (1973). Some observations of gender identity in therapeutic groups. In *Proceedings of the fifth international congress for group psychotherapy, Zurich*, ed. Ambros Uchtenhagen, Raymond Battegay and Adolf Friedman. Bern: H. Huber, 32–39.

Sweetnam, A. (1996). The changing contexts of gender: Between fixed and fluid experience. *Psychoanalytic Dialogues, 6*(4), 437–459.

Winnicott, D. W. (1971). Creativity and its origin. In *Playing and reality* (pp. 76–100). London: Tavistock Publications.

Woolf, V. (1973). *Orlando: A biography*. New York: Harvest books/Harcourt Inc.

Young-Bruehl, E. (1996). Gender and psychoanalysis. *Gender and Psychoanalysis, 1*(1), 7–18. https://www.britannica.com/topic/Tiresias

12 Fear of envy and dispossession

The Evil Eye

Leyla Navaro

This chapter addresses to the relational dynamics of envy, the fear of envy and dispossession, and discusses the unconscious functions of the symbolic 'evil eye' talisman.

If malign envy is a toxic and mostly other-destructive emotion, the fear of covetous envy may turn to be quite an apprehensible and self-restricting one. Malign envy triggers imminent aggression accompanied by other-destructive thoughts and feelings that are acted out as covetousness and wish of annihilation. The envied part may counterattack, fight back and plunge into rivalry, or defensively pull back, hide or disappear. Both the acting out of malign envy and the fear of envy carry inherent gender differences (Navaro, 2007). This chapter explores the fear of envy, how it affects insidiously one's relationships and its consequent threat of physical and emotional dispossession.

Centuries of war, invasion and pitiless looting in the Middle East succeeded to seed a deep angst of dispossession from one's precious goods. Both official and personal histories have trans-generationally transmitted the lethal effects of pillage, looting and dispossession due to wars and social upheaval. This archaic fear coils in the background of our social unconscious and addresses to the angst of pillage and dispossession from one's precious goods. As a magical shelter against malevolent envy, the 'evil eye' talisman or 'hamsa' (a hand to stop malignancy) were created as symbolic protectors.

A case story

Visibility and stage fright were the main themes of our three-day marathon workshop, built on Marianne Williamson's quote: "Our deepest fear is not that we are inadequate. Our deepest fear is that we are powerful beyond measure. It is our Light, not our Darkness, that most frightens us". We were aiming to encourage participants to assert themselves, overcome eventual stage fright and not be afraid of being seen while displaying their potential and various talents. Twenty-four female participants registered, most were in their forties, a few in their fifties, all professionals, some married with kids and some single.

Self-imposed restrictions regarding self-promotion were voiced, as were matters of acculturation in gender roles, cultural and family values, etc. However, an

DOI: 10.4324/9781003425915-18

important dynamic seemed understated: the risk of attracting attention under the spotlight, risks of rivalry and competitiveness. The fear of attracting envy was in the air, unspoken. If this were an on-going group, we would allow the participants to explore and open up their thoughts and emotions around envy and competitiveness. However, this was a three-day marathon group and it required an intervention to accelerate the process.

As a team, we decided to introduce a competitive game: volunteers in the group would openly compete in order to win the first prize that was a scholarship for participation to our next workshop. The players were asked to promote themselves, their best attributes and achievements while convincing the jury (which was the whole watching group) why the prize should be given to her. The point was for participants to be assertive about their own attributes, promote themselves, experience rivalry, watch it in vivo and compete openly and experience the consequences of win or lose. The whole group watched and voted for the best competitor.

Three groups of four participants each competed by promoting their personal skills. Then the three semi-finalists competed for the final tour. They were given illuminated crowns that distinguished them from the rest of the group. At the final tour, the three finalists competed by trying to promote their own attributes on why the big prize should be given to them. The whole group kept watching the different styles of self-promotion and rivalry that were displayed by the various players, and voted for the best competitor. One finalist received the most votes from the whole jury. She was presented with a larger illuminated crown that distinguished her from all the others. She won the big prize.

After an intermission, the whole process was discussed within the large group of the workshop. The game had aroused very strong emotions such as anxiety, fear, shyness, shame, feeling frozen, confusion, excitement, playfulness and fun. However, a few participants voiced their disappointment and anger while criticizing the game. We turned to our small groups for further processing. Memories of open or stifled rivalries, the fear of being disliked and being outcast as the winner were among some of the shared anxieties.

The main theme was the fear of covert relational aggression from close friends and relatives.[1] A young woman confessed how she would not share her career successes with her mother. She did not wish her mother to compare her own stagnant housewife life with hers, and therefore feel unsuccessful in life. She was afraid of hurting her mother's feelings. Was she afraid of stirring her mother's unconscious envy? This was an emotional sting: she started to cry. Being protective toward her mother seemed more important than acknowledging mother's unconscious envy. Refusal of differentiation, separation, individuation, and consequently competition with the mother is mostly based on an unconscious 'oath of fidelity' in the girl's development (Navaro, 2007, p. 85).

Another participant could not share her happiness and success with her parents who had lived in difficult conditions. Being satisfied, happy, attractive, and successful might feel for them like a betrayal, forcing them to question their own lives. She was afraid of stirring in them some unbearable painful envy.

The winner of the game was confronted by a participant who tried to grasp her illuminated crown from her head: "You wear it too long and have already another one, let it be mine now". The winner mentioned being taken aback by this 'playful' aggression. She shared that she felt unable to respond. However, she defended herself by not allowing the person to grab her crown. Despite being professionals – and the winner was an attorney! – several participants confessed not knowing how to take success on the chin.

The group of only female participants was under the 'hypnotic power' of attributed gender roles in terms of modesty, femininity, fear of disapproval, and deep anxiety about covert relational aggression. Competing and winning while causing a friend's sadness and humiliation was difficult to endorse. Moreover, in case of winning, the fear of being secretly envied, therefore being attacked, worse being imperceptibly ostracized by estimated peers, was one of the most powerful impediments to their competitiveness. Unconscious anxieties were stirred up around the fear of being *dispossessed* from acquired closeness and friendship, acquired status and power within the group.

The lack of exposure and training in win/lose situations was obvious. For many participants emotional relatedness seemed more important than carrying the winning flag. Reluctance to acknowledge the victory because of fear from covert envy and rivalry was unconsciously among their main concerns. Many were afraid of losing closeness and friendship, of getting distanced or left out in the group. We had to reassure ourselves that the matrix was solid. Many group members knew each other from previous workshops, and their friendships were at stake in the win/lose situations.

For centuries, female competitiveness has been associated with loss of femininity, masculine attitudes, aggression and lack of sensitivity; it can even stir mockery and ridicule (women fighting 'ridiculously' against each other). Femininity has been constructed as if devoid of violence and destruction. The nourishing attributes assigned to women as mothers and caretakers do not allow them to kill overtly, win and to become 'heroines'. Female rage and aggressiveness go subterfuge; instead of overtly killing, women would rather *poison* their victim (Navaro, 2007). Sugarcoated venomous attacks, undermining behavior, secret coalitions, covert insinuations, change in closeness and distancing the relationship are familiar punitive experiences among females.

Envy in close relationships

Melanie Klein (1976) suggests that innate malign envy is directed toward the very fullness of the object, and is a way of spoiling it or attempting to do so. According to Klein (1976), the infant is angry that the mother possesses something (the breast) that s/he desires, and the infant tries to spoil and destroy the mother's creativeness by projecting badness, mainly bad excrements and bad parts of him/herself unto the mother, initially unto her breasts. However, if the capacity for love is adequately developed, then the infant can experience enjoyment, which is considered to be the basis for gratitude (Klein 1976). Klein's view of envy emphasizes its biological/organismic sources; she regards envy as the first mental representation of the so-called 'death instinct'.

The mother is likely to be an object both of survival, helplessness, frustration and hunger. She is regarded as a cornucopia in the land of plenty. The structures of the family and the society confirm the overarching importance of the mother-infant relationship and its instinctually laden qualities. Hopper (2003a) has emphasized the importance of helplessness and frustration with regard to the control of nourishment, whether it be milk or emotional nourishment. Deprivation, homelessness and hunger elicit poverty and powerlessness, accentuating deep humiliation and shame, especially when there is comparison, which maximizes envy, because comparison implies a 'better than me' reality. Thus, envy becomes relational. It is actually the aggressive response to profound feelings of dependency, helplessness and humiliation (Hopper, 2003b, p. 57). Similarly,

> malign envy is directed towards objects who are perceived as able but unwilling to help, and who are perceived as responsible for failed dependency, that is failed containment, holding and nurturing … (A)ccording to this perspective, malign envy is not innate, but develops as a defense against feelings of profound helplessness, which are a consequence of traumatic experience.
>
> (p. 57)

'Grenvy', as coined by Coltart (2020), is a combination of greed and envy.

Although envy arises prior to the formation of sex and gender identity and identifications, the acting out of envy and being envied are experienced differently by the different genders. Power struggles in duel, rivalry, gun wars and their various displays on the visual media are socially officialized grounds of acting out envious aggression: the winner turns to be a hero for both genders. While men openly experience pride in success, women are inclined to subdue their victory out of empathetic concerns for the loser or out of fear of malevolent backlash. Women tend to fear damaging close relationships, losing friends, being *emotionally dispossessed*, being excommunicated and especially being scapegoated: e.g. many women excelling in higher positions or earning higher income risk distancing, separation or divorce due to the unconscious envy and stifled rivalry in the couple. The promotion and success of the woman may be experienced as a 'power imbalance' in the traditionally attributed gender roles. It may backlash as emotional distancing, separation, physical and emotional aggression, or loss of sexuality and closeness.

Friendships, love, emotional ties and sibling rivalries among women repeat the same dynamic: suppressed rivalry in order to preserve attachment objects. A tacit gender-bound contract inhibits many women from openly competing with each other (Navaro, 2007, p. 85) especially within important relationships. Traditional gender development has demanded that women be mainly nurturing and not be involved in fights and competition. For centuries, women have been trained not to compete, and if they must compete, to be sure not to win (Alonso & Rutan, 1979).

Maguire (1987) claims that when women feel hostility and envy toward other women, it is usually denied or expressed in indirect ways, e.g. by consciously or unconsciously arousing envy in others, by idealizing the envied person and finally by being preoccupied with the fear of being envied by others, and, thus, hiding and devaluing one's own assets and successes. The intense fear of envious attacks may result from a projection of one's own unconscious envy as well as be a manifestation of one's relationship with a mother who envies her growing daughter. Due to gender differences in physical and aggressive strength, women are more vulnerable in situations in which they have to defend themselves. Women feel fear and pain in 'loneliness', whereas men have been taught to feel pride in 'solitude', despite experiencing the pain (Navaro, 2007).

In so far as they have been acculturated under male dominance, women are more sensitive to non-verbal cues, especially body language (tone of voice, silences, etc.). They are better than men at identifying a non-verbal emotion and decoding the implicit content of a dialogue (Bourdieu, 2001). Consequently, despite being unnamed or undefined, potential aggression, malignant envy, competitiveness are somatically felt and constitute the 'unthought known' (Bollas, 1987).

Fear of dispossession: emotional pillage

Unconscious envy is riddled with difficulties of the 'damned if you do, damned if you don't', thus creating a double-bind situation for the envied 'victim' with no escape from the inherent wrath of the envier (Safan-Gerard, 1991). When the venom is everywhere unpredictable, undefined and unnamed, the threat becomes even greater.

Unconscious envy involves what I would call *emotional pillage*. It is intended to *dispossess* the 'other' from her most precious pillars of psychological survival, such as closeness, friendship, intimacy, support, mutuality and empowerment. These notions are vital, especially in female relationships. In most societies, men learn how to live and survive with a lack of closeness and intimacy, whereas closeness and intimacy, especially with female friends, are vitally important in women's lives. Survival in a male dominated world is smoother with the support of female friends who share similar difficulties. Women sense where it mostly hurts in other women. *Dispossessing* the 'rival' from her psychological supports (friends, group, support system) is a pitiless weapon for dismantling her.

Emotional pillage is a bloodless form of covert aggression. The humiliation and rage associated with feeling envious is projected into the one who is envied. As an outcast, she is the one who now feels envious of the solidarity and continuing friendship of the group from which she has been excluded. She either disappears, that is physically leaves the place or position, or she subdues her success by making herself unseen, unnoticed. Moreover, the projection of these emotions is likely to be introjected by the 'victim' of the projection. Processes of projective and introjective identification prevail.

This is how the 'Ouroboros syndrome' functions (Navaro, 2007, p. 148). Ouroboros is the mythical serpent that constantly eats its own tail (http://www.gods-heros-myth.com). All power and forcefulness that are in the tail (phallus) are eaten up and consumed. The envied 'victim' eats herself up; she subdues her light, makes herself unnoticed and disappears. Leaving the position, self-imposed solitude, hiding, dimming one's lights, disappearing accompanied by inhibited anger and self-mutilation are only some of the painful consequences of *covert scapegoating*. It functions so insidiously that the victim unconsciously collaborates with the aggressor and contributes to her own self-destruction. This may be called self-scapegoating: by fear of being socially scapegoated, the victim scapegoats herself by disappearing. Instead of being exposed to the shame of open rejection, some women may opt to self-scapegoat, that is, dim their lights and disappear.

This entire process is quite familiar to women. For centuries, we have been confined solely to maternal roles that demand unquestionable self-sacrifice leading to permanent de-selfing. By being defined rather than defining themselves, women have been accustomed to adopt and introject these social projections. Women conceive and define themselves within the dominant masculine conception. It requires serious consciousness raising and personal awareness in order to be able to 'undress' oneself from those attributed social garments. That is why many women still feel embarrassment and threat in positions of being envied. "Making oneself unseen, like animals that feign death, staying immobile, paralyzed, changing color, adapting to the color of the surroundings like chameleons, are some of the female defenses used in facing envy, competitive aggression, and potential destructiveness" (Navaro, 2007, p. 142). In the classical child stories, e.g. 'Snow White' and 'Sleeping Beauty's 'deep sleep' is a powerful imago of a female defense mechanism in a fiercely envied position. Instead of becoming assertive and fighting back, those 'heroines' dim their lights, become quiet and 'sleepy' while making themselves disappear in order to be saved by the prince (designated hero) (Navaro, 2007). In fact, this is a gender-specific form of envy-preemption (Kreeger, 1992).

Classical gender roles are changing and evolving, however. Despite the classical 'glass ceiling', many women are competing for survival and promotion, although they might still be perceived as 'masculine' or as a 'bitch' by all genders.

The socially unconscious fear of envy: the Evil Eye

Freud has stated:

> One of the most uncanny and wide-spread forms of superstition is the dread of the Evil Eye.... Whoever possesses something that is at once valuable and fragile is afraid of other people's envy, insofar as he projects on them the envy he would have felt at their place.... What is feared is thus a secret intention of doing harm, and certain signs are taken to mean that intention has the necessary power at its command.
>
> (1916/1974, p. 240)

Concerns in social justice, equality and 'sensitivity to thy neighbor' may shade one's full enjoyment in one's plenitude. The envy of the watching eye of the less lucky ones may be felt, fantasized or projected. Thus, Freud points to 'projected envy' and to the intensity and power of this emotion that is intended to do harm and cruelty (Kilborne, 2008, p. 135).

According to spiritual or sometimes religious views, covetous glares foul up a person's spirit and may destroy his/her achievements. They badly affect health, deter success, and create discord in relationships. They are likely to bring misfortune, suffering or just general bad luck to the recipient of the look.[2]

However, envy is too painful and humiliating for conscious awareness. It stirs up confusion, anger, helplessness and destructive feelings. Therefore, there is a need to project those feelings unto the other. Malignancy and greed belong to the outside.

In various cultures the Evil Eye talisman is regarded as a protection from covetous envy. According to the Cambridge Dictionary, a talisman is 'an object to bring good luck or keep its owner safe from harm'. By being attributed with magical or protective powers, talismans are believed to protect the wearer from evil influences. The empowering of an object as a talisman is the result of an unconscious magical attitude that animates the object beyond its material reality.[3]

This millenary belief has been trans-generationally transmitted and is still alive in several Eastern Mediterranean cultures: Mesopotamian, Assyrian, Babylonian, Egyptian, Israeli and others. Amulets with the eye symbol are commonplace. So too are the hamsa (the hand with the Evil Eye) figure as a representation of the watching protective eye. Called also 'nazar' in Turkey (malicious glare), it is offered as 'good luck' to a new house, a starting office, a newborn baby, intended to magically bestow good luck, health and happiness to its beholder. In the Aegean Region and other areas where light-colored eyes are relatively rare, people with green or especially blue eyes are thought to bestow the curse, intentionally or unintentionally (Daniels' Encyclopedia of Superstitions). This might be an allusion to foreign invaders (i.e. Vikings) who come for the appropriation of coveted goods (Hopper, personal communication).

The eye might represent Mother's eye (Hopper, 2021). Mother's eyes are the first interactive object that the baby perceives while breast-feeding. The plenitude of the milk associated with the pleasure of the holding are the first experience of cornucopian protection that the baby experiences and gradually introjects. Mother's watching eyes combined with the plenitude of the feeding and holding give a feeling of solid protection. The mother-infant interactive gaze builds a tacit contract of vital protection and confidence. The 'eye' becomes the doorkeeper who watches the household and repels malevolency and covetousness. Similarly, the open hand talisman (hamsa, mainly in North Africa and Israel) represents a protective hand that is believed to magically repel malevolency as it usually carries a watching eye symbol.

Schaverien (2011, p. 161) argues that the talisman is a 'transactional object':

The word transaction implies a category where the object is used in exchange for something else; it is an object through which negotiation may take place. This may be thought to involve a conscious transaction but the process…is primarily unconscious.

(Schaverien, 2011, p. 166)

Consequently, beyond its material reality, the talisman becomes imbued with a magical power.

Amulets and talismans are used as disposal objects of feared and unwanted feelings. The disposed object is supposed to endorse the 'bad' energy and thoughts attributed to the outside. Thus the 'evil eye' talisman is supposed to endorse the malevolency of the surrounding covetous glares. Evil Eyes and protective talismans become a disposal outlet. They symbolize the greed of the surrounding envious eyes toward oneself.

An extensive use of amulets, talismans and similar superstitious objects involves a deep anxiety, fear and the wish to control life events while using an unconscious projective identification process. The desire to protect oneself from malignant destructive looks may be based on an unconscious projection of one's own envious feelings. It is a process of looking at oneself through the eyes of the other, and of imagining being malignantly envied. Thus, the need of prevention from malignancy by using 'protective' Evil Eyes.

The Evil Eye: meanings and functions

According to Kilborne (2008), the social dimension of Evil Eye experiences and their potential for communication, as well as culturally constituted defenses, collective experience and collective representations are blended with the dynamics of shame. "In societies where beliefs in the Evil Eye prevail, these can at once provide explanations for human misfortune and suffering and, because they entail shared values, actually reinforce human bonds" (p. 144). For example, Kilborne (2008) claims that the avoidance of facing envy in the United States is associated with the Horatio Alger's myth that everybody who works and strives well can and will thrive and become wealthy. By encouraging 'healthy competition' over conspicuous consumption, the basic feelings of envy are stifled within the legitimization of destructive rivalry.

> In this way, the predominance of materialistic values (represented, for example, by the importance ascribed to the gross national product) provides those who succeed financially with culturally sanctioned ways of defending against shame and vulnerability. In the process however, the American emphasis on competition and money undermines social responsibilities and human bonds.
> (Kilborne, 2008, p. 130)

Thus envy *per se* becomes unaddressed (as if non-existent) and conceived only as emulating legitimate competitiveness. It might also be a mechanism used by the powerful rich through which they try to maintain the status quo of the under privileged without the threat of their envious attacks (Weinberg, personal communication).

Influenced by religious norms, Western values consider envy as one of the primary sins, therefore untouchable, as if non-existent. Envy goes stifled and covetousness plays in only an indirect way. Envy is disguised under jealousy that seems more human and acceptable.

Eastern cultures in which the Evil Eye and hamsa are prevalent seem to be more aware of the existence of envy. Kilborne (2008) claims that the Evil Eye stands for illness, misfortune and secret shame. The functions of beliefs in the Evil Eye are "a part of an explanatory system designed to account for human suffering, uncertainty, and illness, and as a way of making human feelings recognizable" (p. 132). Thus, the collective representations of the Evil Eye alleviate feelings of anxiety, shame, powerlessness and misfortune while relying on shared belief system (p. 138).

The use of the Evil Eye in this socio-cultural region of the world is directed more widely than to only the fear of 'thy neighbor's envy'. Centuries of warship accompanied with pitiless looting must have sealed a '*ghost-emotion*' of the *fear of dispossession* in the population's psyche. Due to the past generations' inability and unwillingness to review and mourn losses of people, land and possessions, such traumatic events remain like dormant ghosts in our social unconscious. The mental representations of the tragedies that have befallen the group are dormant ghosts in the deep drawers of our stocked memories. The shared mental representation of the massive trauma suffered by our ancestors is prone to be reactivated in times of political unrest and social upheaval since the sense of basic trust and security have already been trans-generationally shaken (Volkan, 2001).

Ghosts of pillage and dispossession sleep silently in our souls. Oral history, family remembrances, confessions and silences are loaded with a gnawing fear of aggressive attacks and stake of dispossession. They create a deep sense of insecurity, chronic anxiety, angst, a feeling of helplessness, lack of basic trust, and a sense of uncontrollability about one's future. At the same time, the fear addresses to the lack of trust in one's government's safeguarding duties in times of conflict and war; it represents an unspoken anxiety about the lack of life preserving securities and governmental warranties.

Thus, the collective representations of the Evil Eye carry a placebo panacea in the shared wishful belief of magical protection against human misfortune. Moreover, by publicly acknowledging the existence of envy and greed and its painful humiliation, the Evil Eye contributes to commonly displace and project the sharp feeling of envy into anonymous others. As a conscience cleaner, it represents a common tacit understanding that envy is always outside, in the 'others', thus contributing to the tacit collective projection of the 'not me'. By creating a commonly shared illusion, it seems to publicly state that we all are in the same boat against the evil of envy that coils always 'in the others'. Thus, the Evil Eye represents a collective projective identification designed to soothe the shame and humiliation of tormenting envious feelings. Its twofold functions are to project the 'not me' while creating the illusion of some magical shelter. We may state that the Evil Eye has been created as a 'therapeutic' outlet against the deep anxiety of both internal and external malevolence.

Notes

1 'Relational aggression' involves the withdrawal of intimacy, of closeness and friendship. It includes covert bullying and manipulative behavior. Social exclusion, silent

treatment and spreading gossip and rumors through social media are some of the toxic weapons aimed at damaging the rival's social status or relationships. Relational aggression is essentially a stifled poison, imperceptible on the outside, yet enrobing the victim and hurting her basic trust in life and in her relationships. Prevalent among adolescents, 'relational disorders' accentuate the location of the disorder on the relationship rather than in the individual (Friedman, 2019).

2 In American street culture, covetous glares were called 'whammies' and even 'double-whammies'. Al Capp, the famous cartoonist, created a character who was famed for the power of his whammies. His name was Eagle-Eyed Flegel. He was not generally regarded as a middle-class Christian man (Hopper, 2021).

3 Superstitions have evolved to reduce anxiety and create a false sense of control over outer conditions. Superstitious beliefs are mostly transmitted within the family or community. According to Vyse (2013), if we have an internal locus of control, we believe that we are in charge of our fate and can make things happen. However, if our locus of control is external, things may happen outside our will, thus creating a lot of anxiety. Sometimes, the creation of a false certainty may seem better than no certainty at all. Carrying an object or wearing an item of clothing, an amulet that one deems to provide shelter or luck, may prove to be effective, and, thus, to provide security and confidence, but actually it may have a placebo effect connected to our belief system.

References

Alonso, A., & Rutan, S.J. (1979) Women in group therapy. *International Journal of Group Psychotherapy*, 29(4), 481–491.

Bollas, C. (1987) *The Shadow of the Object: The Psychoanalysis of the Unthought Known.* New York: Columbia University Press.

Bourdieu, P. (2001) *Masculine Domination.* Polity Press. UK.

Coltart, N. (2020) *Slouching Toward Bethlehem … and Further Psychoanalytic Explorations.* Phoenix Publishing House. UK.

Daniels, C.L. et al., eds, *Encyclopedia of Superstitions, Folklore, and the Occult Sciences of the World* (Volume III), (190 Honolulu: Univ. Press of the Pacific.

Freud, S. (1916/1974) *Introductory Lectures in Standard Edition* (Vol. 16). London: Hogarth Press.

Friedman, R. (2019) *Dreamtelling, Relations, and Large Groups, New Developments in Group Analysis.* London: Routledge.

———— (2003b) *Traumatic Experience in the Unconscious Life of Groups: The Fourth Basic Assumption: Incohesion: Aggregation, Massification, or ba I:A/M.* London: Jessica Kingsley Publishers.

Hopper, E. (2021) Personal communication.

Kilborne, B. (2008) The Evil Eye, envy and shame. In L. Wurmser and H. Jarass (Eds). *Jealousy and Envy: New Views about Two Powerful Feelings* (pp. 129–148). London: Routledge.

Klein, M. (1976) *Envy and Gratitude.* New York: Basic Books.

Kreeger, L. (1992) The 16th S.H. Foulkes lecture: Envy preemption in small and large groups. *Group Analysis*, 25, 391–408.

Maguire, M. (1987) Casting the Evil Eye: Women and envy. In S. Ernst and M. Maguire (Eds). *Living with the Sphinx, Papers from the Women's Therapy Center* (pp. 117–152). London: The Women's Press.

Navaro, L. & Schwartzberg, S.L. (Eds) (2007) *Envy, Competition and Gender: Theory, Clinical Applications and Group Work.* London: Routledge.

Safan-Gerard, D. (May, 1991) *Victims of Envy.* Paper presented at the Academy of Psychoanalysis 35th Annual Meeting, the 'Darker Passions', New Orleans.

——— (2011) Gifts, talismans and tokens in analysis: Symbolic enactments or sinister acts? *Journal of Analytical Psychology,* 56, 160–183.

——— (2019) *Ghosts in the Human Psyche.* Phoenix Publishing House Ltd.

Vyse, A. S. (2013) *Believing in Magic: The Psychology of Superstition.* Oxford University Press.

Section B

Addiction

13 Addiction in Egypt in the context of its foundation matrix

Mona Rakhawy and Nabil Elkot

Addiction is both a culturally and clinically determined phenomenon. Cultural values may differentially shape people's attitudes toward substance use and may influence their behavior in using drugs (Unger et al., 2004). Patterns of drug use can evolve from stereotypes, values, attitudes, and norms that a society assigns to any particular drug. One's specific culture plays a critical role in forming expectations about potential problems one may encounter with the associated drug use.

Cultural norms may either play a protective role or represent a risk factor for individuals. In every day clinical practice in addiction clinics, it is not uncommon to witness two different paths by two family members from different generations, as for a son and his father. Younger generations seem to be more prone to complications than the older one. Such phenomena may be attributed to the different sociocultural influences to which each generation was exposed; the older generation being more protected by the extended family and the inherited social regulations, which have been missed among the younger. As such, considering cultural differences is crucial for clinicians attempting to understand the underlying factors behind drug use, hence installing effective and appropriate interventions (Hobbs, 1989).

The perception of the addictive phenomenon in the Egyptian society ranges between a threatening malignant use that endangers longevity, and a harmless recreational use. This chapter will introduce a brief review of substance use and abuse in Egypt. A special emphasis on the social, cultural and clinical conceptions related to drug use will be presented from a historical background as well as from a present perception, including clinical considerations.

Historical perspective

Revisiting the history of substance abuse in Egypt is of significant value, especially when considering Hopper's (2003) argument that people re-live and re-enact what remains un-mourned both personally and societally and Weinberg's (2007) analysis of how this is rooted in the histories of particular societies.

Alcohol use and abuse dates back to the ancient Egyptian period. Different types of beer were described in the Egyptian papyrus. Lutz (1922) defined barley beer as the oldest drink known to man, originating in the ancient Egyptian era before 3400 BC. Over time, alcohol abuse became widespread in the society, and drinking beer

DOI: 10.4324/9781003425915-20

expanded rapidly to become the national drink of Egypt. Beer was often supplied by the state and has been mentioned as a part of almost every major festival in ancient Egypt. However, despite the ancient Egyptians first acknowledged the beneficial effects of alcohol and disregarded its possible harmful effects, eventually, the unfavorable effects of alcohol consumption were recognized. Concerns about drinking alcohol stemmed on an ethical basis, later on financial regulations were established. Heavy taxes were imposed on circulating alcoholic beverages and have represented a remarkable source of income for the country up to the present moment (Mark, 2017).

Alcohol and cannabis were the most commonly used substances in Egypt throughout its history. Cannabis was known since 4,000 years and was one of the most popular drugs (Nahas, 1985; Soueif, 1996). Its use was documented only during the 12th century. According to Ibn Al Bitar, a 13th-century pharmacist, it was planted and taken by Egyptians for its perceived positive effects. Furthermore, cannabis had its unique use among different religious populations. To illustrate, it was widely used at that time by the Sufis during their religious festivals (Soueif, 1996). The first scientific documentation that suggested an association between chronic cannabis and alcohol use with mental illness in the recent time dates to 1895. It was referred to Dr. J. Warnock, the medical director of Abbasiya Hospital, which is the oldest mental health hospital in Egypt. Warnock (1903) reported that 15% of the cause of all hospital admissions was due to hash use, and another 15% resulted from the use of the combination of hash and alcohol. As reported, there is evidence that chronic use of cannabis is linked to dementia and early death (Soueif, 1969).

The pattern of substance use/abuse was found to be related to the sociopolitical changes in the country. Following World War I, the first wave of heroin and cocaine use quickly spread in Egypt. They were not regulated by law and were sold by a burgeoning pharmaceutical industry looking for new overseas markets (Nahas, 1985).

After the 1952 Egyptian revolution, the problems related to cannabis use progressed. Severe penalties and anti-smuggling measures were imposed by the Revolutionary Council, which has restricted the consumption of hash. So, although the population expanded by five million between 1958 and 1967, the number of people using hash declined by more than 50% (Nahas, 1984).

In the seventies, and with the launching of "free market policies," the second wave of heroin use reached the country. At that time, Egypt shifted from a closed conservative social community to a liberal one. The rapid social change during this era weakened the defenses against drug addiction and was linked to personal and social transformation in the pattern of using drugs, leading to a new rise in the abuse of substance in the country. Drugs were mainly used in Cairo and other big cities, mostly by individuals with little earlier exposure to substance use; those who have not developed protective normative values. A sharp rise in heroin use was noted in the eighties and was seen as a "national disaster." It was attributed to the rapid economic superficial growth, the disruption of the established social and value systems, the creation of social uncertainty and the availability of the substance (Okasha et al., 1990). Another increase in the rate of substance use was reported at the turn of the 21st century. The prevalence of drug use in Egypt had increased from 6.2% in 1996 to 19.1% in 2016 (Hamdi et al., 2016; Rakhawy et al., 1996). This escalation may reflect the rapid social changes during this period, especially following the 2011 revolution.

Between approval and disapproval

The official attitude toward permission or prohibition of drugs dates back to early times; it has fluctuated along the history of substance use in Egypt and has been subject to different uncertainties. Efforts to stop cannabis use began as early as the 14th century. Individuals using hash were sometimes punished by having their teeth pulled out (Mills, James and Barton, 2007). In 1877, the Ottoman government, ruling Egypt at that time, commanded the destruction of all cannabis in the country. In March 1879, the Khedivate of Egypt banned cultivation, distribution and importation of the drug (Abel, 2013).

There was no legislation forbidding the sale and use of cocaine and heroin before World War I. Subsequently, people consumed the reasonably priced drugs openly. At that time anyone could purchase drugs with no requirement of a medical prescription (Nahas, 1984). In 1917, Russel Pasha, the English commandant of the Cairo city police at that time, inspired by the English policy in India, suggested governmental legalization on various substances. He described cannabis and opium as "black drugs" and cocaine, morphine and heroin as "white drugs"; the latter being described as a "major danger to the country." The Pasha stressed on the importance of ignoring the black drug traffic for focusing on the white drug one (Russel, 1949). He called for the legalization of cannabis, to be grown domestically and suggested licensing its intake, which would provide a source of income to the Egyptian government. However, this proposal was refused by the Egyptian authorities, which imposed similar penalties on all drug users (Kozma, 2011).

During World War I and after 1919 Egyptian revolution against the British occupation, the use of cannabis had shown a rapid growth, and cocaine and heroin spread in the whole country. The authorities became highly alarmed about the increasing number of young people who abused opium or cannabis, many of whom abandoning their families and quitting their jobs. As a result, in 1929, a counterbalancing movement against the widespread of drugs was boosted, and the Egyptian government created the Central Narcotic Intelligence Bureau (C.N.I.B.). Russell Pasha himself has headed the C.N.I.B. from 1929 to 1946 (Nahas, 1984).

In the 1930s, Dr. Ghalloush, the head of one of the Egyptian charities, organized a campaign in support of cannabis use and to deny its harm. He questioned the governmental allowance of liquor and prohibition of cannabis (Al-Nakkash, 1998). Despite Dr. Ghalloush's campaign and similar activities, the C.N.I.B., in addition to other non-official efforts, continued to prohibit the use of all kinds of drugs, and succeeded to lower the rate of drug abuse. Five years later, the rate of convicted addicts lowered from 5,681 in 1924 to 674 in 1934; and that of prisoners from 78% addicted to heroin or cocaine went down to 14%. The decline continued till 1946, when heroin and cocaine use had almost disappeared and hash consumption was decreased from 18.7 tons in 1927 to 2.1 tons (Nahas, 1984).

Although cannabis use is legally banned, alcohol has not been officially prohibited till the present time. Nevertheless, in some cases, alcohol is restricted for personal reasons such as the belief that its consumption goes against one's religious beliefs and practice. Even though alcohol is placed as the second or third substance used in the country, it still does not represent one of the major clinical issues.

From a religious perspective, the attitude toward consumption of alcohol and cannabis are not the same. Forbidding alcohol was clearly stated in Quran verses. The Coptic Church in Egypt bans alcoholic spirits. There is no equivalent scripture related to the use of cannabis, which is perceived by some as "benign" and "accepted." However, the general consensus differed with time. In 1982, the Grand Mufti of Egypt, who represents the main Islamic consultancy, issued a religious decree (fatwa) prohibiting the consumption of cannabis and other drugs, and equating them with alcohol. Nevertheless, some religious leaders unofficially expressed their belief that drug use can be graded with varying punishments, based on the degree of harm induced by the drug (Gutierrez, 2015). Interestingly, religious prohibition is inconsistent with the legislative regulations in the country as well as the degree of expansion of the drug. Alcohol, which is explicitly prohibited by religion, is not officially an illegal substance; even though it is less consumed relative to the other drugs. The opposite is found in the case of cannabis.

The phenomena related to the intake of alcohol in context of such ambiguous sociocultural situation is evident when we observe the pattern of alcohol consumption with Egyptian Muslims during and following Ramadan (the holy month of fasting). It is not uncommon for Muslims who indulge in alcoholic beverages to abstain from drinking alcohol during the holy month. In the following days, nevertheless, they typically have gatherings where they drink alcohol to celebrate their success in obeying religious orders.

Generally speaking, a concealed controversy exists between tabooing and untabooing cannabis and alcohol. The resulting challenges affect substance abusers in their representations and their healing journey as well. Boundary diffusion and oscillation between prohibition and permission of substance use in Egypt are unavoidably presented in clinical settings. Uncovering such deep social structures and understanding these tides can illuminate to clinicians the relationship between the two contradictory societal attitudes.

Drugs in everyday life

Despite drugs being illicit, there is a tendency to normalize cannabis among some Egyptians social strata (Gutierrez, 2015). As noted by a French adventurer and hashish smuggler, the Egyptian farmer relies on stimulating properties in hash to compensate for underfeeding and combat fatigue. It was also reported that the farmer uses hash with moderation; the "hashish drunkard" with his hallucinations and delirium is the exception (Monfreid and Treat, 1930).

In our practice, we have noticed that certain people in Upper Egypt, South Sinai and other regions of Lower Egypt consider cannabis as a basic need. Its intake has become habitually part of their everyday routine for many individuals. Tramadol and hash are sometimes distributed as an act of generosity in social occasions such as weddings and funerals. Drugs are not infrequently used for their claimed benefits. In addition to its pain killer properties, Tramadol is labeled as "the stimulant," for its ability to prolong work, spare energy and delay exhaustion. A driver who uses tramadol shares, "I work 15 hours a day. If I stop using tramadol, I won't be able to work or even get out of my house. Besides, everyone else working in the bus station is also using tramadol." Mothers sometimes give opium to their children in an attempt to calm them or end their diarrhea. Drugs have also been used to promote productivity and function.

The pattern of acceptance and rejection of specific drugs is considerably linked to the social background. Tramadol, which is a synthetic opioid, is relatively considered to be a socially accepted drug in Egypt. Thus, it is commonly used. However, people generally refrain from using other opioids, such as heroin for it is subject to more negative stereotypes throughout the cultural history in Egypt. Typically, people who abuse drugs try to assign moral, social or religious meaning to their addictive behavior. For example, a young man who has been using hash and tramadol for ten years expressed "I drink everything even 'cockroaches' (an antiparkinsonian drug causing tactile hallucinations) ... I use any substance and only avoid alcohol for my fear of God, and Heroine as it is for junkies."

In terms of popular culture, proverbs are often used among Egyptians. They provide opportunities for gaining sensitive insights. Based on Hopper and Weinberg's view that language is fundamental to the formation of the social unconscious (Hopper and Weinberg, 2012), revisiting the Egyptian proverbs would provide a valuable source for understanding the verbal expression of the Egyptian social unconscious. Drug use and abuse has been emphasized in some of the Egyptian proverbs, such as "A good life is either a good wife or a good water pipe." The mentioned proverb relates cannabis to marriage in bringing well-being. Proverbs were also used to warn against the undesirable consequences of using substances, and were even used therapeutically, to provide a culturally oriented insight into such associated negative effects (Rakhawy, 2017a).

Addiction and gender

The prevalence of addiction among men in comparison to women is higher all over the country (Hamdi et al., 2016). Nevertheless, the range of differences varies in different regions. The male to female ratio in Upper Egypt is 5:1 and in Cairo is 7:1, which are the highest female rate, when compared with the other Egyptian regions. The lowest Male to female ratio was found in the middle and north Egypt (13:1). This might be interpreted in terms of the openness of life in Cairo. Besides, women living in Cairo have less family supervision and protection, and they are more exposed to stresses than their counterparts in other Egyptian governorates. Although the culture in Upper Egypt is more conservative, the attitude toward drugs is permissive to some extent, which invites more females to use drugs than those in middle and north Egypt (Hamdi et al., 2016).

Likewise, culture and gender differences influence the pattern of use in the whole Arab region. In Yemen, for instance, Khat is widely used by both men and women in everyday social gatherings, with no specific differences (Al-Juhaishi, Al-Kindi and Gehni, 2012). The WHO considers Khat as a substance of abuse, and the drug does not exist in Egypt.

Colonialism and the conspiracy theory

Egypt has been colonized by many countries throughout history. The colonial system has inevitably shaped the pattern of substance abuse in the country. Generally speaking, colonization has influenced the lifestyle of African countries, including substance consumption. Before the European colonization, alcohol was moderately consumed as a source of contentment, as well as a part of social ritual. It was taken in its un-distilled form with limited cost and consumption (Obot, 2015). Following colonization, distilled spirits were offered as gifts to native Africans who became more accustomed/used to the stronger form of alcoholic beverages and the Western style of consumption. Thus, complications associated with high consumption of hard alcohol appeared in the society. The fluctuation between the social malaise and the wealth produced by alcohol has created the love-hate public image of drinking that is still seen in our present time (Pan, 1975).

Colonized countries did not get their full independence by the end of colonization; the countries were still influenced by economic, political, cultural and technological manipulations, a phenomenon known as "neocolonialism" (Sartre, 1964). Colonial rulers found such implicit ruling much easier compared to the direct one. They used the respect linked to traditional institutions as one of their marketing foundations of the alcohol industry. Seaman's Schnapps is an African drink that has been advertised as "the 'Original Number 1 prayer drink', a drink that fulfills the yearning of our valued heritage passed down through the ages" (Obot, 2015).

The "Iron Kina of the Hero" was one of the main drinks advertised in the 1970s Egyptian TV. It included 25%–35% alcohol and was branded for facilitating health and strength. In this regard, the WHO conducted a project on alcohol marketing and promotion in Africa and revealed that alcohol was often promoted for bringing cultural pride in five African countries (Obot, 2013). Alcohol legalization was viewed by some as a response to the British to promote the English wine in Egypt (Al-Nakkash, 1998). Additionally, cannabis expansion was commonly perceived as an American/Western conspiracy against Egypt, which has been exaggerated in the 1950s (Gutierrez, 2015).

Addiction, culture and creative arts

Addiction has been presented in many aspects when it comes to the Egyptian arts scene. This has provided a rich material for understanding the sociocultural perceptions and the underlying dynamics in a relatively conservative society, like the Egyptian one. A wide array of novels, songs and movies has depicted different perspectives of drug abuse in a variety of contexts. For instance, Egyptian songs have reflected the different and often contradicting attitudes toward drugs. Some support their prohibition, while others believe in compromising the harmful effects. A third party digs more deeply, trying to justify the underlying social and psychological reasoning and temptation of substance intake.

Many stories about drugs connect directly to some Egyptian celebrities. Sayed Darwish and Om Kolthoum are two famous singers of the early and mid-1900s. Their songs and concerts revealed the reality of the Egyptian society at that time. Darwish was also a composer. His songs have illustrated the rapid and unprecedented popularity of drugs during the early 20th century (Seth, 1966). For example, in the song "Alcocaingia," he empathically described the use of cocaine. Another song of his described the effect of cannabis use on their mind and social life. A third song evidently described the negative effect of smoking Cocaine. Sadly, it is well known that Darwish himself died by overdose (El Shahat, 2016). In the mid-20th century, Om Kulthum used to have a concert on the first Thursday of each month. It is well known that cannabis was not infrequently used in many of the family and friends' gatherings that used to happen regularly on such nights.

The Egyptian Nobel Prize winner, Naguib Mahfouz, depicted in his famous novel "A Drift on the Nile" the role of drugs at a time when the absurdity of life was dominant and the people were yearning for a meaningful existence (Wisner, 2011). The novel was first published in 1966. It was written following the 1952 Egyptian revolution, when a post-dependence authoritarian regime emerged in Egypt. In this period, a feeling of alienation was prevailing in the country (Farley, 2011). Most of the novel's inspiration events and ideas happened on a houseboat on the Nile where Anis, an Egyptian civil servant, spent his time preparing the place and smoking cannabis. Anis was called as The Prince of "Blessings" for the good quality of cannabis he brought to the group of intellectuals gathered on the houseboat to smoke, enjoy their time and discuss political issues (Al-Nakkash, 1998).

The novel included different representations of the middle-class society such as Anis, a famous journalist, a storywriter, an actor, a young female journalist, a house wife, a female student, and others. The guard of the houseboat was an ordinary man overwhelmed by contradictions between the moral and immoral. He was consistently present in the background of the gatherings.

The atmosphere inside the boat was generally gloomy. This isolated environment, surrounded by many water pipes, shed light on the role of substance use in the middle of political, existential, cultural and ethical dilemmas.

Despite being written since more than 50 years, Mahfouz' novel does not only reflect the dynamics related to drug use in the Egyptian society at that time, but also resonates with what is witnessed in our present clinical settings. The cry for help, "Hey, anything, please do something; we have been smashed by the nothing!" reminds us of the voices of the Egyptian revolution of 2011. It is worth mentioning that the 2011 which was followed uprising was followed by a rapid escalation of drug abuse.

Specifically, the houseboat represents a special alienated place such as the distant deserts where drugs are taken in Egypt. The houseboat was located in the Nile, at a line where land and water meet. This line can be seen as demarcating the subculture of the group of substance abusers, from the culture of the wider Egyptian society. The houseboat was a pseudo-protected environment that shielded against "the collapse of the belief ... the belief in anything." In the gloomy atmosphere, personal and collective anxieties were overshadowed by the effect of substance.

The relationship between drug abuse and the anxiety resulting from the personal, social and political confusions in the Egyptian society has been emphasized.

The group tried to cope with the failure, hopelessness and helplessness that dominated the society. For each of the group members, using drugs carried a differentiated role. For example, Anis tried to forget his miserable life, a young female shared her existential issues that were discussed within the group, and a married lady tried to escape the reality of her unhappy marriage by taking part of this gathering. With the facilitation of cannabis and alcohol, each member has developed his own defenses. Denial, nihilism, intellectualization, rationalization and cynicism were evident. This resulted in a state of euphoria within a context of pseudo-philosophical meaningless discussions. Earl Hopper referred to this phenomenon as retreatism and as alienation, as forms of "the instrumental adjustment," related to the failure to recognize social reality and the use of effective and efficient coping mechanisms, including collective innovation and even rebellion (Hopper, 1991, 1995). The in and out movement along the Nile border calls for further reading.

The peace and tranquility inside the houseboat changed after the incident when the group hit a lady with a car during one of their late night excursions. They fled back to the houseboat and started a kind of defensive intellectualization, arguing about topics like life, death, morality and others. Anis got excited, then the guard pushed the houseboat to drift into the Nile River with no destination, drifting into the unknown and putting an end to the novel and the complexity of the situation. The indefinite ending to the novel events brings out in the open the consequences of using drugs; however, some critics considered this drift as Mahfouz's foreseeing of the following era in Egypt.

Addiction and religion

Similar to the previously mentioned artists, Yehia Rakhawy has had a major contribution in representing the voice of people in the field of mental illness and arts. Rakhawy believes that addiction needs to be understood from an evolutionary standpoint. Addiction may control all areas of a person's life. Moreover, addiction is prevalent all over the world, which threatens human survival. Hence it can be understood in terms of evolution. In essence, addiction represents a negative rebellious international subculture as opposed to a disorder or a pattern of substance abuse.

Rakhawy (2000) has emphasized the lifelong positive impact of the creative aspect of religion. He believed that such positive effect might be achieved through authentic faith and practice. He suggested that some people have a fluctuating attitude toward religion, which can be attributed to denial, prejudice and fanaticism, and result in difficulty coping with the surrounding disharmonies. Therefore, some of the new religious movements (Lewis and Tollefsen, 2016) reflect individuals' trials to achieve intra-psychic harmony and an extended awareness with the universe and beyond. The trials result in varying degrees of success or failure.

Rakhawy considers the addictive phenomenon "…as a form of chemical substitute for religious commitment." (In greater detail, he has contrasted particular assumptions between religion and addiction, underlining the constructiveness of religion and the destructiveness of addiction.)

Religion provides solutions to various existential questions. Addiction, however, may appear to offer solutions to specific challenging issues, though not on a constructive level. In other words, Rakhawy's perspective can be summed up as "drugs are the religion of the abusers."

Moreover, all religions have their own structured performed rituals that typically occur within a set time, and group work is highly appreciated in religious practice. Analogously, the majority of addictive behaviors have their own rigorous rituals such as the timing and the place where the drug is taken, and group gatherings have their special value. Ultimately, almost all religions promise going to paradise and experiencing extreme happiness or ecstasy. Consistently, similar promises may be met along the different phases of addictive practice (Rakhawy, 2000). The comparable relationship between the role of drugs and that of religion is illustrated in a saying of a 21-year-old girl diagnosed with severe substance use disorder:

> Without drugs, I would have killed myself. Drugs helped me face my fears and overcome the flashbacks of my father and cousin's sexual harassments. At that time, I dressed in black, and painted everything in black: the ground, the wall and everything. I was distant from God, and tried to make a deal with the Devil ….

Her words seem to imply the protective role of drugs that she had associated with the Devil/darkness; as if using drugs was the rescuer from her trauma. This is one experience among many that emphasize the pattern of abusing drugs in response to trauma, despair, and helplessness.

Generally, it is observed that people experiencing drug addiction in our society oscillate between two polarizing extremes. Abstinence associated with exaggerated religiosity, hope and self-satisfaction, and pathological abuse associated with distancing from religion/God, despair and self-worthlessness. "I know that God will not forgive me, I'm guilty and he will never forgive me. Anyway my life is short; it's a matter of a year or two. I don't have time to repent." Said a patient under treatment for addiction. The link between religion and drugs has also been revealed in dreams of some individuals suffering from addiction: "I had a dream that I died on a mountain of Heroin and was resuscitated at the same place." From an analytical standpoint, Hopper views that the "mountain of heroin" might be a substitute for a breast, and certainly not a "good breast" for the patient (Hopper, 2020).

Therapeutic interventions

One of our work in the field of substance abuse is based on Rakhawy's view of the dose of information with respect to addiction. Rakhawy views that addiction is related to the level and expansion of awareness, especially in response to the exposure to current flooding of information. As addiction implies maladjustment to the overwhelming dose of information, Rakhawy suggests the optimal adjustment of the quantity (Dose) of information in addition to the level (Depth) of awareness, to be assimilated in creative re-patterning ways. The awareness expands beyond the mere cognition or alertness, to include the acknowledgment and the actualization of one's own creative reorganizing abilities. Practically speaking, our contracting with patients with substance abuse usually involves an agreement on down regulating the input of information, as by limiting the contact with the outside realities (such as work, friends and social media). Gradual re-patterning of such involvements is scheduled at a later stage. Rakhawy has referred to his postulation as the Dose-Depth-Awareness-Assimilation (DDAA) hypothesis. In our practice, we focus on awareness.

In this regard, Rakhawy challenges the pattern of our present practices that are based strictly on the use of medications and work through restriction of awareness, as opposed to positive reorganization of the pathological condition. He views that the current excessive reductionism in psychiatry and the abuse of the "medical/mechanical model" have faded the deeply rooted positive creative role of this branch of medicine. Consequently, DDAA recommends the revival of psychiatry in its original historical function (Rakhawy, 2000).

Treating addiction in a therapeutic community in Egypt dates back to 1973, with the foundation of Dar El Mokattam for Mental Health Hospital, the first milieu therapy in the region. At that time, patients with addiction were treated in the same environment along with patients experiencing other psychiatric disorders such as schizophrenia or mood disorders. They all followed the same milieu therapy principles where patients, psychiatrists, psychologists and other hospital staff work shoulder to shoulder within a common culture and therapeutic frame (Rakhawy, 2017b). Treating patients with substance abuse separately was a consequent step that took place in 1998, to offer a more specialized and focused care.

Along the evolution of the therapeutic interventions at Mokattam Hospital, cultural influences have evidently had an effect on the management strategies. Tailoring specific individual programs according to the client's own clinical and cultural background has been a necessary part of the treatment plans. This policy is highly supported in the literature. Rowan (2014) underlined the evidences that support the value of culture-based interventions in addiction treatment for promoting the client's general functioning and well-being. Rowan stressed on the continuous need for specific intervention programs to provide the corresponding practices given to a group of addicts with specific culture.

In our experience, sociocultural considerations strategically affected the management plans. Precisely, these considerations have shaped the training, supervision, and relatively guided the way of selection of therapists for working with specific patients. For example, therapists coming from high-middle- to high-class strata, and living in big cities like Cairo and Alexandria, were sometimes challenged when dealing with a client in a different sociocultural background or coming from smaller places. Some of these therapists used to be initially less flexible in compromising with clients having different cultures and value systems that accept drug use, even if socially permitted from the client's part. In other words, they disregarded and occasionally disrespected the specific values of clients coming from Upper Egypt and/or lower strata cultures. When individual cultural differences are not carefully considered, therapy risks being challenged and recovery may slow down. Accordingly, newly hired therapists were matched with client who fit with their distinct sociocultural background, which would facilitate acceptance, understanding and empathy at this stage. In order to maximize the safety of management process, therapists undergo appropriate training and supervision that addresses such cultural considerations.

On another note, importing the world's addiction treatment programs constitutes a significant part of the therapeutic practices in Egypt. The Alcoholics Anonymous (AA) and Narcotics Anonymous (NA) groups are well known to contribute to alcohol and drug abstinence all over the world (Kaskutas, Subbaraman, and Zemore, 2009). In Egypt, the Twelve Steps program was translated into Arabic in 1989 and incorporated into the already present therapeutic programs for addiction treatment. It has started as a small group in a little church in Cairo and expanded to include tens of thousands of people recovering from addiction that made up groups in almost every big city. Currently, hundreds of Egyptian treatment centers use the Twelve Steps program as the main recovery tool.

The Twelve Steps program has also been used in many Arab countries like Saudi Arabia and AL Bahrain. Initially, its main orientation was spirituality rather than religion, which is consistent with the original version. Many varieties were developed later to fit differentially with each country's cultural and religious background. Specific religious adoption started to appear as an orthodox Christian one adopted by some rehabilitation Christian centers, and an Islamic one implemented by some Salafi centers in Egypt and Saudi Arabia.

Moreover, in our clinical practice, the spiritual/religious dimension is sometimes used therapeutically as a harm reduction technique, particularly with people who have alcohol addiction, given that alcohol is known to be prohibited by Islam. For instance, some Muslim clients with alcohol abuse abstain from drinking alcohol during the holy month of Ramadan. Reinforced by different therapeutic approaches, this is sometimes used in a context that transcends specific time or conceptual margins. The same applies to pilgrimage that comes around two months later, and is sometimes considered in our management plans.

As for specific therapeutic approaches in Egypt, Rakhawy (2017a) has emphasized the importance of the therapists' consideration of the client's rights in the management of substance abuse. A person's rights involve the right to be wrong, the right to be different, the right to explore, the right to fear, and many other rights. Such rights were introduced in terms of understanding, assimilation and incorporation in the management of addiction and the training of therapists. The postulation is that abusing drugs tends to satisfy these rights quickly and efficiently, but in a deceptive, false and short-term way. Fulfilling these rights would play a preventive as well as a therapeutic role. While working on the right to be wrong, for instance, therapy provides a place that handles this right in a balanced therapeutic way. The acceptance of being wrong, and not necessarily making mistakes, may exempt those who enjoy it from the exaggerated rush toward serious problems.

The therapists' understanding of these rights is needed and should be considered in their basic training, as part of their practicing awareness (Rakhawy, 2017a).

It is to be noted that the strategies for therapeutic interventions for addiction in Egypt reflect to a great extent cultural transformation. Currently, the attitude of total prohibition of substance has shifted to the embracement of harm reduction programs by some, or the acceptance of a parallel existence of such programs by others. Simply put, a concealed or explicit permission of substance use with insightful consideration of safety measures is paving its way to the Egyptian society.

Conclusion

In conclusion, a broader vision of the use and abuse of substances in Egypt would shed more light on further understanding and exploration of the phenomenon. The intertwined attitude toward drugs, the degree of societal approval-disapproval, the equivalent official legalization-illegalization, and the normalization of drug use reflect many of the unconscious aspects of the foundation matrix of the Egyptian society.

Besides, addiction in Egypt relatively represents a micro-cosmos; the development of alcohol abuse as an addictive phenomenon in Egypt may represent a comprehensive pattern that reflects the history of the whole world. The dynamics involved in its evolution are highly influenced by the sociocultural background. Verbal, written and arts productions provide a rich pool for further exploration. The Egyptian views and practices in the field emphasize the evolutionary process, the culture and religion, the awareness, the stagnation and creativity, and the individual's rights.

So, can we understand and deal with addiction on deeper intrapersonal, interpersonal, transpersonal and transcultural levels? How much do therapists in Egypt and elsewhere collaborate for the sake of a better practice? If so, how much would this positively impact patients' treatment as well as therapists' training and practice? Contemplating on the process involved in this writing would provide some optimistic responses.

References

Abel, E.L. (2013) Marihuana: The first twelve thousand years. New York: Springer Science+Business Media. P.133

Al-Juhaishi, T., Al-Kindi, S. and Gehni, A. (2012). Khat: A Widely used Drug of Abuse in the Horn of Africa and the Arabian Peninsula: Review of Literature, Qatar Medical Journal, (2): 1–6.

Al-Nakkash, R. (1998). Naguib Mahfouz: Pages of His Diaries and New Lights on His Literature and His Life. Cairo: Al Ahram Center for Printing and Publishing (in Arabic).

El Shahat, S. (2016). One Day ... the Death of Sayed Darwish, the Imam of Composers under the Influence of Drugs. The Seventh Day, September 15 (in Arabic).

Farley R.J. (2011). Intellectual Space in Naguib Mahfouz' Thartharah Fawq al-Nil, CSULB McNair Scholars Research Journal, 15: 31–50.

Gutierrez, A. (2015). The Discourse of Drug Use in Egypt: An Interdisciplinary Exploratory Study. A Thesis Submitted to Middle East Studies Center in partial fulfillment of the requirements of Master Degree in Arts, AUC, School of Global Affairs and Public Policy.

Hamdi, E., Sabry, N., Sedrak, A., Khowailed, A., Loza, N., Rabie, M. and Ramy, H. (2016). Sociodemographic Indicators for Substance Use and Abuse in Egypt, Journal of Addiction & Prevention, April, 4(1): P34–41.

Hobbs J.J. (1989). Troubling Fields: The Opium Poppy in Egypt, Geographical Review, January, 88: 64–85.

Hopper, E. (1991). Encapsulation as a Defense against the Fear of Annihilation, The International Journal of Psychoanalysis, 72(4): 607–624.

Hopper, E. (1995). A Psychoanalytical Theory of Drug Addiction: Unconscious Fantasies of Homosexuality, Compulsions and Masturbation within the Context of Traumatogenic Processes, The International Journal of Psychoanalysis, 76(6): 1121–1143.

Hopper, E. (2020) Personal communication.

Hopper, E. and Weinberg, H. (Eds.) (2012). The Social Unconscious in Persons, Groups and Societies: Volume 1: Mainly Theory. Karnak: The New International Library of Group Analysis.

Kaskutas L.A., Subbaraman M. and Zemore S. (2009). Effective of Making Alcoholics Anonymous Easier (MAAEZ), a Group of Format 12-Step Facilitation Approach, Journal of Substance Abuse Treatment, October, 37(3): 228–239.

Kozma, L. (2011). Cannabis Prohibition in Egypt, 1880–1939: From Local Ban to League of Nations Diplomacy, Middle Eastern Studies, 47(3): 443–460.

Lewis, J.R. and Tøllefsen, I.B. (2016) The Oxford Handbook of New Religious Movements. New York, NY: Oxford University Press.

Lutz, H.F. (1922). Viticulture and Brewing in the Ancient Orient. Leipzig: J.C. Hinrichs.

Mark J.J. (2017) Beer in Ancient Egypt, Ancient History Encyclopedia, March 2017. https://www.ancient.eu/article/1033/beer-in-ancient-egypt/.

Mills, J.H. and Barton, P. (2007) Drugs and empires: Essays in modern imperialism and intoxication, c. 1500-c. 1930. London: Palgrave Macmillan P.172.

Monfreid, H. and Treat, I. (1930). Pearls, Arms, and Hashish. New York: Coward-McCann.

Nahas, G.G. (1984). The Escape of the Genie. A History of Hashish Throughout the Ages. New York: Raven.

Nahas G.G. (1985). Hashish and Drug Abuse in Egypt during the 19th and 20th Centuries. Bulletin of the New York Academy of Medicine, June, 61(5): 428–444.

Obot, I.S. (2013). Alcohol Marketing in Africa: Not an Ordinary Business, African Journal of Drug & Alcohol Studies, 11: 63–73.

Obot, I.S. (2015). Africa Faces a Growing Threat from Neo-Colonial Alcohol Marketing (Editorial), Addiction, 110: 1371–1372.

Okasha A., Khalil A. H., Fahmy M. and Ghanem M.H. (1990). Psychological Understanding of Egyptian Heroin Users, Egyptian Journal of Psychiatry, 13: 37–49.

Pan L. (1975). Alcohol in Colonial Africa. Helsinki: The Finnish Foundation for Alcohol Studies, Pitkansillanranta 3B, 00530. Helsinki. p. 22.

Rakhawy, Y.T. (2000). Addiction as a Chemical Religious Substitute, Egyptian Journal of Psychiatry, July 2000 (23).

Rakhawy, Y.T. (2017a). Some of What Is Going on Inside the Addict, and Glimpses of our Popular Culture. Cairo: The Association of Evolutionary Psychiatry and Group Work (Publisher).

Rakhawy, Y.T. (2017b). The Therapeutic Community and the Collective Consciousness. The 2nd Book. Series of Combating Addiction: Challenging and Confrontation. Cairo: The Association of Evolutionary Psychiatry and Group Work (Publisher).

Rakhawy, Y.T., Ewaida, M., El-Kott, S, Faheem, A., Abdulwahab, MM, et al. (1996). The General Secretariat of Mental Health - MOH: The National Research on Addiction (use, abuse, dependency and addiction) preliminary report, MOH.

Rowan M., Poole N., Shea B. Gone J.P. Mykota D., Farag M. Hopkins C. Hall L., Mush-zuash C. and Dell C. (2014). Cultural Interventions to Treat Addictions in Indigenous Populations: Findings from a Scoping Study, Substance Abuse Treatment, Prevention, and Policy, 9: 34.

Russel, T.W. (1949). Egyptian Service, 1902–1946. London: Murray.

Sartre, J.P. (1964). Situations V. Editions. Paris: Gallimard. English translation: Haddour, A., Steve Brewer, S. and McWilliams, T. (2001). Colonialism and Neocolonialism. London and New York: Routledge.

Seth, R. (1966). Russel Pasha. London: William Kimper.

Soueif, M. (1996). Drugs and Society. Kuwait: Aalam Almaarefa. P.41

Unger, J.B., Baezconde-Garbanati, L., Shakib, S., Palmer, P.H., Nezami, E. and Mora, J. (2004). A cultural Psychology approach to "Drug Abuse" Prevention. Substance Use and Misuse, 39(10): 1779–1820.

Warnock, J. (1903). Insanity from Hasheesh, Journal of Mental Science, January, 49(204): 96–110.

Weinberg, H. (2007). So What Is This Social Unconscious Anyway, Group Analysis. The Group-Analytic Society, 40(3): 307–322.

Wisner, G. (2011). Adrift on the Nile by Naguib Mahfouz, Words Without Borders, The Online Magazine for International Literature, WWB Daily, Published Mar 4.

14 Dangerous desire

Addiction, consumption and recovery

Martin Weegmann

Introduction

The starting point of this chapter is etymology and historical idioms of substance use and excessive consumption. Whilst all societies have intoxicants these are evaluated quite differently according to era, culture and place. As for the misuse of substances, 'addiction' often stands as a metaphor for wider social ills, as in the idea that the 'vice of drugs' is the ultimate violation of social norms, just as (presumed) good or healing substances can acquire a mythical status, as in the notion of a 'panacea'.

The chapter continues with clinical examples from a relapse prevention group, observations on the culture of substances from a group training event and an account of recovery as reported in group analysis. In all these examples, I hope to show how the relationships that people have with drugs are saturated by an intimate and extensive social matrix and that social unconscious models of substances affect their perception, use and misuse.

Idioms of excess

'Addiction' (*addicere*) traditionally signified being 'given over to something'. In Latin and Roman laws, the terms *addico* and *addictus* had positive as well as negative connotations, positive in the sense of, say, a person given over to civic devotion, or negative in the sense of, say, a person given over as a slave to a master or creditor. In English contexts, after 1500, addiction signified a form of 'surrender' – to a habit, penchant or occupation. 'Devotion' was a somewhat a somewhat similar word, then in circulation. As in ancient times, there were approved forms, such as spiritual or scholarly addiction or devotion to good fellowship, although they had downsides if carried to the extreme (Lemon, 2018). Surrender had positive connotations within specific contexts, Lemon (op. cit., p. 42), quoting Protestant sources, refers to those 'addicted to praiers', and to 'the meaneynge of the scripture'; as for their rival community, Catholics were blamed for 'addiction to superstitions'. By contrast to the positive, in Shakespeare's *Henry V,* the Archbishop of Canterbury refers to the King's misspent youth, where, "His addiction was to courses vain, His companies unletter'd, rude, and shallow, His hours fill'd up with riots, banquets,

DOI: 10.4324/9781003425915-21

sports..." (Shakespeare, 1970, p. 445). The theme expressed in this passage is about ruinous desire and the misuse of physical pleasures (and time), a familiar and repeating theme in the history of addiction.

We live in a culture of consumption where it is hard to draw the line between what is healthy and what is excessive. Addiction is extreme consumption or excessive appetite (Orford, 2009) and we refer to those who are *consumed* by an activity. *Con sumere* means to waste and destroy – as in 'riotous consumption' – and yet in modern societies we are invited into a vast world of consumption from the moment of our birth and brought into commerce with all those objects that promise satisfaction, until the time comes for their replacement by the next objects in the queue. One can propose the idea of 'promissory objects' that work by beckoning a new experience, but one already having a foot in the familiar (or the prototype) from which it is a departure, much like a variation in a theme of music. With respect to drug use, what is promised or anticipated in the 'fix', 'hit' or 'high' connects the user to a previous or an original experience. The term 'chasing' implies this kind of future-past, as re-seeking. Freud, for example in his early career, saw in cocaine the promise of a cure.

In neoliberal society, one can say that the 'ideal citizen' is a producer and consumer in roughly equal measure, but only if those goods are regarded as desirable objects and only if consumed in the right quantities. Prescribed ways of spending time and powerful inducements to do so (e.g. through advertisements) are all around. Pervasive and life-shaping, consumer culture plays upon the human balance sheet of past enjoyments, current, or creeping dissatisfactions, and incessant promise. The use of dangerous substances contradicts the model, cultivated citizen of neoliberalism (Giddens, 1992; Reith, 2004).

In summary, idioms are important because of their powerful, symbolic resonances. Words seemingly as simple as 'drug', 'drink' or 'intoxication' have layers of connotation travelling alongside with many implications for the understanding social unconscious life. Substances, and the disorders associated with them, readily function as metaphors and scapegoat terms standing for the ills and scourge of society as a whole (Levine, 1984; Room, 2003). This story is one of a complex choreography between such disorders and the broader rhythms of political, economic and cultural forces (Margolis, 2002).

Substances: fear and fascination

Substances can evoke fear and fascination. Ambivalence surrounds intoxicants as society continually defines and re-defines distinctions between proper and improper uses of the body, substances considered beneficial and those associated with horror. Included within this morbid interest are the places in which drug use occurs – the den, haunt, hang-out, the boozer, crack-house, and with the spoiled characters who use them – the fiend, junkie, inebriate, common drunkard, habitué, addict and many more. Interest in the use of substances is thus marked by fear aroused by the potential for deviancy, impropriety and sin. In Christian tradition, for example, if the body is regarded as a 'loan' during our time on here on earth, then the use of substances is potentially "an abuse of what is not our property" (Walton, 2001, p. 53). A whole history of 'sins of the flesh' is aligned to temptation and the likelihood that we can all 'wonder from the path'. Galatians 5, 19–21 (a Pauline Epistle) refers to 'acts of the flesh', to impurity and debauchery, and lists drunkenness amongst its examples. Sin and vice feature strongly in the historical register of addiction (Edwards, 2000). Alongside the familiar emphasis on what became known as the 'demon drink', Christian tradition also regarded wine, for example, as a gift, or, in the words of one puritan divine, the 'Good Creature of God' (Levine, 1978). There are many other instances and religions where the use of intoxicants and 'food drugs' (hallucinogens, stimulants) served positive spiritual and bonding purposes, as in ancient Central American civilisations. As times changed in England, religious conceptions and valuations were rivalled by those that emphasised liberty, including freedom of the body and disavowal of convention. The 18th-century figures of the libertine and rake, for examples, were often admired (men) precisely because of their ability to free sensual life from Christian asceticism and to flout oppressive conventions (Ashe, 2005). To be habituated to profligate and immoral conduct had an appeal of its own and the liberal notion of the body as one's sole property, with a corresponding right to use it as one wished, gained ground.

Derrida (1981, p. 20) suggested that the drug has, "Its power of fascination...... both beneficent or maleficent". The imagery of panaceas (from the Greek goddess *panakeia,* representing a universal remedy) and elixirs (with roots in alchemy) represent substances that are elevated, running alongside the converse of bad, malignant potions, poisons or drugs. Examples of such polarities can be found everywhere – including unexpected places. Take the extraordinary story of Freud's love affair with cocaine, the 'divine weed' as he called it, a curious footnote in the pre-history of psychoanalysis. Bernfeld's (1953) essay argues that Freud's forays into the uses of cocaine represented first efforts to achieve professional independence, to 'go his own way'. Freud also used cocaine personally over a number of years, enthusing about its qualities as a way of coping with dysphoria, social anxiety, fatigue and separations from his fiancé. Loose (2002, p. 199) suggests, "Freud believed he had found an ideal object, which would solve a lot of his personal, scientific and clinical problems". The consequences proved disastrous when Freud prescribed cocaine to supposedly cure his morphine addicted colleague and friend, von Fleischl, who subsequently died of cocaine poisoning. It was another addictive substance – nicotine – that led to Freud's painful demise and death.

Smoking is a striking example of a mass-produced substance that was glamorised and normalised up to its peak years in the mid-1960s when, in the US, a staggering 40% of the adult population smoked. Foulkes, I gather, enjoyed cigars (an identification with Freud, or a common habit of the era?) and smoked cigarettes in some of his groups in the early days (Malcolm Pines, personal communication). In the UK of the 1960s, as elsewhere, there was limited interest in the health consequences of smoking, with up to 70% of men and 40% of women smoking. People smoked everywhere, even in schools and hospitals, and, without doubt, the therapy room.

These reflections may at first sight seem remote or removed from clinical significance but have, I suggest, both contemporary relevance and great importance to understanding the social contexts in which people use or do not use substances. Patients – and their therapists – inhabit worlds that imbue substances with a wide range of meanings. Some are used so widely and are so integral to social life that we occlude their status as social commodities not to mention their economic centrality, as in the case of alcohol. An entire drink industry is built around constant efforts to invite and seduce us to use alcohol alongside injunctions to 'drink sensibly' and to enjoy 'in moderation'. It is important to acknowledge that not only do alcohol use disorders affect millions (including indirect effects upon the families of drinkers), but alcohol is everywhere and remains the nation's favourite drug. There is an entire anthropology of alcohol use in society, just as there is with that other everyday substance – sugar – with its many 'inside' and 'outside' meanings over the centuries, as Mintz (1985) put it.

Clinical

The following clinical examples derive from the author's former practice as clinical psychologist and group analyst working in the British National Health Service.

The relapse prevention group

The influential relapse prevention model of Marlatt and Gordon (1985) conceptualises addictive behaviours as maladaptive, over-learned behaviours whose short-term benefits seem compelling to the user. The use of a substance, at the time of use, seems to dissolve certain problems and to lift subjective feelings and becomes ingrained as a pattern or habit. For those embarking on change, relapse prevention approaches aim to interrupt these problematic, self-reinforcing patterns and build new, alternative skills of coping in their place. Unlike approaches that are mainly concerned with persuasion, motivation or challenging people to admit their alcoholism and to 'break down denial', relapse prevention is a social learning model that considers *how* people are addicted and the need to create an alternative repertoire of responses. The model offers a pragmatic and empirical explanation of addictive behaviours and seeks to build the confidence (self-efficacy) and skills required to forge a path of recovery.

I set up a weekly relapse prevention group as a slow-open group available to any client who could, if they found the group helpful, attend for extended periods of time. Based upon a social learning and a cognitive-behavioural model, I used group-analytic thinking alongside to guide its running. I incorporated creative group exercises to enhance dialogue and shared learning.

Mapping addiction

Amongst these creative group exercises was the construction of 'sketches and maps', consisting of a bird's-eye view of a person's living space, depicting their home, possible places of drug/alcohol use, areas of safety and other potential recovery resources (Weegmann, 2005a). Maps capture detail and those often messy and unobserved circumstances of a person's life space. Further, maps constructed in groups are seen by all and in group-analytic terms offer a rich, visual resource which adds an interesting dimension to the group matrix.

Consider two examples.

Julie's recovery map

Julie was in her first year of abstinence from substances and sketched a 'recovery map' resembling a spider diagram. As a regular group member, people knew Julie well but as she added detail to her map, we learned new aspects about her life and social connections. Not far from her home, which she depicted on the map as 'Safety', she drew a church and a group of people nearby-by, labelled 'Resource'. Julie was hesitant, worried that the group would not be interested to hear about 'private beliefs'. Confounding her worries, others were curious and Julie explained the centrality of church activities to her recovery, including a church walking group. Taking courage, she elaborated by sharing a parable of King David who sees the beautiful Bathsheba bathing from the vantage point of his palace. Julie explained that the King believed he could take anything – or anyone – he saw and so for her the story of Bathsheba was a tale of complacency, power and temptation. Julie used the parable as a self-reminder, saying, "I think of that story every time the thought of having a drink passes my mind".

In response, others in the group spoke of the complacency that creeps easily into recovery, marked by temptations to drink, nostalgia and distorted memories. One member said, "I can spot when the drinker in me starts to romanticise what I did and forgets that this got me into hospital". Another member added, "We all need good resources, like Julie".

Ian's drinking holes

By contrast to Julie, Ian struggled to remain abstinent from alcohol for more than a few weeks before 'falling off the wagon', as he labelled relapses[1] and was demoralised as a result. As Ian sketched his map in the group, populated by various pubs, one person commented, "your drinking is hidden in plain sight, it's all around you!" Ian rebutted the observation retorting that 'locals'[2] were 'common landmarks' but soon acknowledged how easily they became centres of his life. Ian entitled his map, 'My neighbourhood', but another group member suggested the alternative title, 'Ian's drinking-holes'.

There is a useful contribution for a sociology of drinking places (and other leisure spaces) conceived as 'third places' beyond home and occupation with distinctive conventions and opportunities for social bonding (Oldenburg, 1991). They are characterised by informality, playfulness, social contact and more. These were all relevant to Ian as pubs were his main option for spending time, rewarding himself, mixing in various 'regulars'. Giddens (1992) says that addiction is a form of 'time out' and if one's culture is centred around the idea that alcohol is, say, a reward, it is easy to understand the function and allure of pub life. Gusfield (2003) refers to 'rituals of drinking in society' and of drinking as a form of passage into play and informality. The ceremonials of drinking, as it were, construct this ideal, social activity. Adler (1991, p. 382), reviewing historical drinking patterns, notes, "through the giving and exchange of drinks social ties of obligation and reciprocity are established". Ian had little by way of an alternative notion of sociality and the pub provided a powerful, sensory familiarity with its 'homely sounds' and the positive anticipations of 'popping in' as he put it. Asked about the converse place represented by the relapse prevention group, Ian replied, "that's me looking for a new way". He was certainly looking for a different way but had little conception of what that could be. He wondered whether moving away from his neighbourhood could help, but another person said, "but you'll only take your problems with you, unless you do something about them". It proved a valuable set of explorations and challenges, with the presence of a map a life and depth to the group matrix which might not have been there through verbal dialogue alone.

In summary, the use of maps helps the group to trace the sites and territory of drinking and drug use and the social context of substance use and of stopping. They point to the importance of an 'ecological view' of addiction (Moos et al., 1990), including those positive resources that a person might not ordinarily notice. Addiction is a personal trouble and is staged in a social context. Such a simple statement could be taken as a definition of the social unconscious. Maps also help people to see tensions between realities and possibilities. As Schultz (1944) argues, everyday reality provides people with a sense of continuity and security, with its tacit recipes for action and the practical knowledge of what is likely to happen. What happens when a person embarks on a process of change, such as recovery from addition? "Through passage to a new status (e.g. ex-drinker) or a new social world (e.g. a recovery network), persons may find themselves on the threshold of unchartered territory whose customs, contours and inhabitants are unknown" (Pollner and Stein, 1996, p. 205). In this way, maps have relevance to group analysis given its commitment to understanding the lived social matrix. Substances figure large within the configurations of a person's life and circumstances and their social unconscious connotations are all around even if not quite seen. For Julie, it was spiritual convictions and commitments that provided her with an alternative world to that of substance use, whereas for Ian, his bearings were still tied up with the ceremonials and meanings of drinking. Maps brought it home, a reminder of the aphorism that 'a picture can tell a thousand words' (Dansereau and Simpson, 2009).

The training group

I conducted training in Belfast with colleagues from a Northern Irish addiction service. As part of the experience, I invited participants to explore (a) languages of intoxication and (b) substance use as social rite of passage.

As for the first question, the group delivered an impressive list of terms to signify intoxication (to alcohol), some of which they had used with others learned from their clients or teenage children. These included *smashed, blotto, plastered, hammered, pissed, legless, clobbered, shellacked, shot, bombed, wiped-out*. We noted similarities between descriptions of alcohol intoxication and that associated with other drugs – the sense of 'being out of it'. Some people recalled a former value, during an earlier era, on being able to 'hold one's drink', associated with masculine connotations of strength and prowess, contrasted with a newer generation who (in part for economic reasons) 'pre-load' with cheap alcohol and go out with the express motive ('on a mission') to get intoxicated. In Jack London's (1998) famous autobiographical account, he refers to his drinking as a 'badge of manhood'. Laddish, and increasingly ladette culture, were cited as powerful social influences over recent decades and the growth of 'binge culture'.

Others spoke about a contrast with a pre-intoxication state associated with respectable, moderate drinking, terms such as *merry, happy, jolly, relaxed*. Finally, some spoke of drink references as embedded within language and sayings, such as 'one for the road' (no longer heard as a result of drink/drive laws), 'hair of the dog' (i.e. using an alcoholic drink to cure a handover), 'hitting the grog' and countless others. Historical images of the 'drunken Irishman' were noted by the group, a colourful, genial character given to a love of tales as much as to love of drink.

The next question followed easily from the first. Turner (1969) sees rites of passage as transitions from one state to another, which traverse a betwixt and between or *liminal* period, which he defines as a movement, "though a cultural realm that has few or none of the characteristics of the attributes of the past or coming state" (p. 94). Rites of passage result in a (positive) change of status. There are obvious differences between formal, cultural rites of passage, such as those associated with religion, and its looser use as a common term, to apply to many formative experiences and psychosocial transitions. This is where initiation to drink (and the analogy with initiatory rites) and drinking to intoxication fits in and is in part related to an anticipated 'coming of age' linked to legal drink frameworks.

Members of the group thought that for males in particular, passages into drinking had the informal features of rites, such as the experience of first, serious occasion of intoxication. This might typically be seen as crossing a threshold and as a means of gaining credibility amongst a peer group. The excessive, silly or disinhibited behaviour that results – provided it does not go 'too far' for the group norms in question – marks the passage from a kind of 'novice stage' of drinking ability to a more serious one. Becoming violent is frowned upon in most social groups, whereas in a very different sort of social group, it might be facilitated through drink, in which case violence itself might be part of a rite of passage. A temporary reversal in status, such as a minor humiliation, may be the price to be paid for initiation, which shows an ability to let others 'have a laugh' or to 'take the piss' at one's own expense. 'Taking it on the chin' and sharing tales the 'morning after' is an important part of group bonding and of acquiring necessary drinking experience.

The other dimension was directly reflective of Northern Irish culture, in that two members of Catholic background (Protestant movements were however equally involved in temperance initiatives) explained that they had 'taken the pledge' as primary school children, a symbolic promise not to use alcohol until at least 18, unless a person commits to a life of teetotalism, which was not uncommon. 'Taking the pledge' has a wider history deriving from mid-19th-century temperance movements on both sides of the Atlantic; "I signed the total abstinence pledge, and resolved to free myself from the inexorable tyrant- rum", in the words of one famous reformed drinker (a temperance orator, known as the 'poet of the DT's'), writing his autobiography in 1845 (John B. Gough; in Crowley, 1999, P. 158). The 'Pioneers' were an early 20th-century Irish Catholic movement that sought to renew earlier temperance traditions and warn of the sins of drinking. Progress in life was only be made through Christian commitments and self-denial. The group added that whilst 'taking the pledge' may once have been a significant social promise – and remains so in a few quarters – 'breaking the pledge' is the power-reversing gesture for the young, in defiance or indifference towards traditional religious norms and frameworks for behaviour. Nowadays, much of that residual symbolism has gone and binge drinking and degrees of drug use are a norm for many.

Comment

We all have a relationship to alcohol and drugs, whether or not we use them, and this relationship is saturated by social unconscious connotations, those meanings that surround and precede us. The training discussion exercises proved an effective, evocative method of exploring meaning and locating aspects of cultural and personal history.

As a side-product, the training prompted me to think of my own culture, having been brought up in the North of England in a middle-class town with the message that drinking was a wasteful activity and that pubs were to be looked down upon. Drugs were acknowledged as being 'out there', somewhere, but in un-named or far-away degenerate places, like 'the city' elsewhere. My parents were not teetotal, but very moderate, occasional drinkers. They did not use religious reasons used to justify this, but I have come to interpret their attitudes (not unusual at the time in middle-class families) as a secular version of a Protestant work ethic, with value placed upon thrift, betterment and the productive use of one's leisure time. Their stance towards pubs had a strong class bias, with pubs regarded as suspect, wasteful places where 'common' and 'fickle' people spent their time and money; I shrink in embarrassment thinking about such attitudes now.

These examples, from the training context as well as the clinical maps, point to the importance of understanding how messages and models of consumption influence us. Arguably, the Eliasian 'civilising process' is not simply a question of etiquette, manners and other social presentations of the self but also about how we are supposed to act as *consuming* subjects. What, it must be asked, in a given society, constitutes our 'leisure life', the objects that we implored to use and enjoy and our relationship to relaxation or 'letting go'? Van Ree (2002) explores drug consumption from this perspective and the ambivalent messages about what is considered acceptable and what is considered problematic with respect to objects of consumption. Like Woultas and Denning (2019), he speculates on the intriguing role of 'controlled de-control' of behaviour and emotion when it comes to pastimes and the satisfaction of wishes. In the 1960s a new ethic of permissiveness (and other 'informalisations', as Woultas calls it) transformed social life and re-defined norms of living. The 60s was an era of 'sub-cultures' in which different social groups crafted distinctive languages and styles of conduct, including the use and valuation of different types of drug, such as in the UK booze amongst bikers and psychedelics amongst hippies (Willis, 2014). Wills (op. cit.) makes the important observation that, such groups were, "pioneers of cultural experimentation, the self-construction of identity, and the curating of the self, which, in different ways, have become so widespread today" (p. 3).

Narrative of recovery

Angie is an ex-patient who came into group analysis three years after establishing sobriety from drugs and alcohol. The excerpts are her own words, with permission to use (see Weegmann, 2004, 2005b, 2017b for further accounts).

Rock bottom or realisation?

Angie's family was from a heavy drinking culture and both her parents became alcoholic. An adult child of alcoholic parents then, in time she developed her own drug and alcohol problems, causing serious damage to self, relationships and hope. All in all, it took Angie two spells in rehabilitation, an addiction day centre and commitment to Alcoholics Anonymous to establish a secure sobriety, at which point she came into my psychotherapy group where she stayed for four years.

Asked to elaborate on what enabled her to change course – with the benefit of hindsight – Angie spoke of a 'moment of clarity' with the

> realisation that drink was more powerful than me. It was the destruction I had caused myself and others and I just knew the game was up. I didn't know where I was going but I knew I didn't want to be where I was or where I was heading.

She acknowledged that Alcoholics Anonymous grounded her sobriety and helped her to begin to heal herself. Their message, she said, was like the 'daily bread'. Group analysis, by extension, gave her time to explore her personal and family past and was, she said, a 'kind of special meal' that made sense only in terms of wider nourishment and grounding from elsewhere.

Experience and role of group analysis

Angie said that "3 years into sobriety I hit an emotional rock bottom" and wanted to work upon 'numb, very frozen' feelings she associated with past violence (partner violence) and a stultified relationship with her daughter. She confessed that the group was different from groups in the day centre and at first she found me a puzzle. In her words,

> I felt un-easy as I found him hard to read, I used to crack jokes about him and realise that I was testing him to see if he would react and hurt me. I projected

a lot of negative stuff I had around men onto him, as well as my own negative feelings I had about myself, which he pointed out. I felt very nervous attending this group as they were people from all walks of life, but the group helped me to challenge my assumptions about people, i.e. it's not just addicts that struggle in life. Slowly I began to sit with these uncomfortable feelings and began to trust the group and realised the psychotherapist wasn't this scary person I projected, and that he was a nice man. The group helped me grow, was a space where I first found my voice. I learnt that people can get angry but it doesn't have to end with violence, and I got in touch with some painful emotions....... The group expanded my life as I began to take risks, but positive ones. I went college.......

Mourning the childhood she did not have and re-evaluating the childhood she did have, were central to the work she did in the group. As she commented (after one year in the group), 'In these last few weeks, I've had so many feelings from when I was small, so many small things which make me angry to think about. It's like with everything they (her parents) always put drink first – like if we were on holiday, it would be the pub all day and if I was ill that was a problem because they might be too hungover to look after me. So, I had to look after me. They were always in some kind of mood-loud when they were drunk, feeling sorry for themselves the day after, or guilty when they were off it for a few weeks, and then I was given a lot of freedom, but punished when they were back on it again. I did not know whether I was coming or going'. As she spoke, Angie shook and would periodically glance at me. Because drinking was normalised, Angie had no evident means of 'seeing' the alcoholism at home during her growing up years. She did, however, recall a dawning sense that her family was not 'like others' and an awkwardness when the topic of family life was discussed at school. It was only when she managed to stop drinking and face reality that she was able to re-evaluate her parents and see the problems, which, to outsiders, would have been all-too apparent.

Angie was revisited by all those small details and patterns of family life, including sequences of behaviour, such as drinking parent – intoxicated parent – withdrawing/sick parent – dry parent. There were corresponding affective patterns, such as tension – disinhibition – moodiness – guilt. With the help of group discussion, Angie came to see how her own affective responses were tied in to the behaviour of her parents, as she learned the art of maintaining vigilance, scanning her parents for signs of the state they were in and, above all, maintaining safety. Her vigilance of me in the group, the nervous glance, was, I surmised, an expression of her need to maintain safety in the therapy and to anticipate my possible responses.

Comment

Initially, Angie experienced analytic group therapy as 'too spontaneous' and worryingly free of 'rules'; anxieties, such as these, were consistent with her experiences of a family life dominated by confusing priorities and inconsistent (liquid) rules. Her containers had not been reliable and much of the time, realities were simply drunken away. That was repeated with her own drinking.

Rey (1994, p. 457) wrote a notable paper, posing the question of who the patient brings with them into therapy. He speculates that patients bring with them a number of people and dilemmas, including an unconscious request to "bring about the reparation of important damaged internal objects without which the reparation of the subject's self cannot happen normally and happily". I agree with this, but would add that patients also bring with them wider transpersonal patterns and the implicit values they have lived around. For example, Angie had no stable concept of a 'sober household', as everything in her family had been distorted. There was, from the start at least, a fear and I and/or the group would not be a safe place and that 'anything could happen', and there was a reparative theme and a destructive aspect, struggling with each other. How could she engage in 'sober dialogue' and build an experience of a 'sober group' providing structure and clarity? Angie grew up with a negative model of what family life which she only questioned as she became a teenager and could make comparisons with other types of households, with different values or ideas of 'just' care. In her extensive empirical studies, Dunn (1988, p. 71) talks of children as akin to 'beginners' in the social world, who participate, "in the power politics of the family-withing-a-culture".

An understanding of recovery is of great importance if we are to support the Angie's of this world. For one, it is important not to see Alcoholics Anonymous and group therapy or analysis as rivals. Further, it is important that as therapists we appreciate something of the culture of fellowship groups, such as AA. Alcoholics Anonymous can be thought of as a natural form of group therapy without the group therapist, and as a 'narrative community' (Weegmann, 2004, 2017b). White (1997) uses another useful term, that of 'community of acknowledgement' to characterise a way of linking lives and supporting solidarity. The more the drug consumes a person's life, drawing them into narrow repertoires of behaviour, the greater the identity void, when (if) they decide to stop. People and things that used to matter increasingly become people and things that do not matter, as roles and relationships are lost and purpose eroded. As people get used to the freedom of non-using substances, they have to re-build themselves and carve a trajectory of living. Recovery is about a wholescale change of lifestyle. White (op. ct., p. 40) likens this to a, "migration of identity, an act of intentionally leaving one's life behind in order to make a new life for oneself".

Recovery is itself based upon pre-existing cultural models that are out there is a wider social matrix. Bellah's (1985, p. 153) account of community life refers to how communities,

> have a history- in an important sense they are constituted by their past- and for this reason we can speak of a real community as a 'community of memory', one that does not forget the past. In order not to forget that past, a community is involved in retelling its story, its constitutive narrative……..

In my own research (previously cited), and that of Swora (2001), Alcoholics Anonymous can be seen as a practice of building an alternative community, with the telling and retelling of stories of 'experience, strength and hope' and the building of a continuity of the self that was broken by years of drinking. Swora (op. cit.) sees it as also helping to heal memories and build hope for the future.

As people recover from substance misuse, they step into the unknown and this includes emotions, as Angie indicated. It is suggested that at a certain juncture in her recovery, group analysis offered a different type of small community. Angie needed to re-join a different kind of society and to appreciate similarities with others, 'normal people' as she put is, from 'all walks of life'. Group analysis provides a kind of 'college for emotions' and an opportunity to connect to self and others in new, sober ways and to take 'positive risks' in the words of Angie. From this vantage point, she was also better able to construct a clearer description of family life, re-evaluating 'lost time' as well as future possibilities. Recovery and therapy gave her the means to, and permission to have a story to tell and to figure out how to tell it.

Conclusion

I began by tracing some of the etymology of substances and excessive consumption and the in-built ambivalence that surrounds them. As Foulkes and Anthony (1957, p. 245) noted, *'words are old* and so *carry layers of meaning'*, but the question is not just about words but about how those words are embedded within the wider practices and discourses of social life.

The clinical and training event examples serve to demonstrate something of the social location of substance use, whilst the example of Angie in group analysis shows the importance of building adequate social resources, a narrative community, to support a process of recovery. I describe the construction and use of personal maps and how narratives in groups enable people to gain a better sense of where they are and where they wish to be, the cultural location of disturbance *and* progress. Cultures of consumption have a powerful presence in people's lives and alternative cultures of recovery are required if people are to find ways out of a chemical career.

Acknowledgements

Thank you to Silvia Angioi, Alistair Sweet and Angie for their generous comments. Thanks also to the editors of this volume.

Notes

1 In 19th century horse-drawn water carts or wagons were common and although it is hard to trace the exact origin of the term, 'off the wagon' it has come to be associated with a return to drink after a period of abstinence.
2 Jenkins (2007) provides an excellent social history of drinking establishments from the ale house to the modern pub. The terminology of the 'pub' is itself of interest, deriving, as Jenkins explains, from a compound: 'public' and 'house'. Watson (2002, p. 190) shows how drinking establishments are a kind of 'home form home', being, "important sites of social, political and economic exchange in almost every type of society".

References

Adler, M. (1991) From symbolic exchange to commodity consumption- anthropological notes on drinking as symbolic practice. Chapter 17 in Barrows, S. and Room, R. (Eds.). *Drinking: Behaviour and Belief in Modern History.* Berkeley, University of California Press.

Ashe, G. (2005) *The Hell Fire Clubs: Sex, Rakes and Libertines.* London, Sutton Publishing.

Bellah, R., Sullivan, W., Madsen, R., Swider, A. and Tipton, S. (1985) *Habits of the Heart: Individualism and Commitment in American Life.* Berkeley, University of California Press.

Bernfeld, S. (1953) Freud's studies on cocaine, 1884–1887. *Journal of the American Psychoanalytic Association,* 1, 581–613.

Crowley, J. (Ed.) (1999) *The Drunkard's Progress: Narratives of Addiction, Despair and Recovery.* New York, John Hopkins University Press.

Dansereau, D. and Simpson, D. (2009) A picture is worth a thousand words: a case for graphic representation. *Professional Psychology: Research and Practice,* 40/1, 104–110.

Derrida, J. (1981) Plato's pharmacy, in Barbara Johnson (Ed.). *Dissemination* (pp. 61–161). Chicago, IL: University of Chicago Press. Pp. 61-161

Dunn, J. (1988) *The Beginnings of Social Understanding.* Oxford, Blackwell Publishers.

Edwards, G. (2000) *Alcohol: The Ambiguous Molecule.* London, Penguin.

Foulkes, S. H. and Anthony, J. (1957) *Group Psychotherapy: The Group- Analytic Approach.* London, Penguin Books.

Giddens, A. (1992) *The Transformation of Intimacy.* Cambridge, Polity Press.

Gusfield, J. (2003) Passage to play: rituals of drinking time in American society. Chapter 3 in Mary Douglas (Ed.). *Constructive Drinking: Mary Douglas, Collected Works,* Volume X (pp. 73–90). Oxford, Routledge.pp73-90

Jenkins, P. (2007) *The Local: A History of the English Pub.* Stroud, The History Press.

Lemon, R. (2018) *Addiction and Devotion in Early Modern England.* Philadelphia, University of Pennsylvania Press.

Levine, H. (1978) The discovery of addiction: changing conceptions of habitual drunkenness in America. *Journal of Studies on Alcohol,* 15, 493–506.

Levine, H. (1984) The alcohol problem in America: from temperance to alcoholism. *British Journal of Addiction,* 79, 109–119.

London, J. (1998) *John Barleycorn: 'Alcoholic Memoirs'.* Oxford, Oxford University Press.

Loose, R. (2002) *The Subject of Addiction.* London, Karnac Books.

Margolis, S. (2002) Addiction and the ends of desire. Chapter I in Brodie, M., Farrell, J. and Redfield, M. (Eds.). *High Anxieties: Cultural Studies in Addiction.* Berkeley, University of California Press.

Marlatt, A. and Gordon, J. (1985) *Relapse Prevention.* New York, Guildford Press.

Mintz, S. (1985) *Sweetness and Power.* New York, Viking Penguin Inc.

Moos, R., Finney, J. and Cronkite, R. (1990) *Alcoholism: Context, Process and Outcome.* New York, Oxford University Press.

Oldenburg, R. (1991) *The Great Good Place.* New York, Marlowe and Company.

Orford, J. (2009) *Excessive Appetites: A Psychological View of Addictions.* 2nd Edition. Chichester, Wiley. *Pollner,* M. and *Stein,* J. (1996). Narrative *mapping* of social worlds: the voice of experience in Alcoholics Anonymous. *Symbolic Interaction,* 19/3, 203–223.

Reith, G. (2004) Consumption and its discontents: addiction, identity and problems of freedom. *British Journal of Sociology,* 55/2, 283–300.

Rey, H. (1994) That which patients bring to analysis. *International Journal of Psychoanalysis,* 69, 457–470.

Room, R. (2003) The cultural framing of addiction. *Janus Head*, 6/2, 221–234.

Schultz, A. (1944) The stranger: an essay in social psychology. *American Journal of Sociology*, 49/6, 499–507.

Shakespeare, W. and Henry V. (1970) In *The Complete Works of William Shakespeare*. 12th Edition. London and New York, Spring Books.

Swora, M. (2001) Commemoration and the healing of memories in Alcoholics Anonymous. *Ethos*, 29/1, 58–77.

Turner, V. (1969) *The Ritual Process: Structure and Anti-Structure*. Ithaca, NY, Cornell University Press.

van Ree, E. (2002) Drugs, the democratic civilising process and consumer society. *International Journal of Drug Policy*, 13/5, 349–353.

Walton, S. (2001) *Out of It: A Cultural History of Intoxication*. London, Hamish Hamilton.

Watson, D. (2002) 'Home from home': the pub and everyday life. Chapter 6 in T. Bennett and D. Watson (Eds.). *Understanding Everyday Life* (pp. 200–246). Oxford, Blackwell/Open University.

Weegmann, M. (2004) Alcoholics Anonymous: a group-analytic view of fellowship groups. *Group Analysis*, 37/2, 243–258.

Weegmann, M. (2005a) The road to recovery: journeys and relapse risk maps. *Drugs and Alcohol Today*, 5/1, 42–45.

Weegmann, M. (2005b) Dangerous cocktails: drugs and alcohol within the family. Chapter 9 in M. Bower (Ed.). *Psychoanalytic Theory for Social Work Practice: Thinking under Fire* (pp. 131–142). London and New York, Routledge.

Weegmann, M. (2017b) Alcoholics anonymous and 12 step therapy- a psychologist's view. Chapter 14 in P. Davis, R. Patton, and Jackson, S. (Eds.). *Addiction: Psychology and Treatment* (pp. 231–244). Chichester, Wiley.

White, M. (1997) Challenging a culture of consumption. *Dulwich Centre Newsletter, 2*, 38–47.

Willis, P. (2014) *Profane Culture*. Princeton, NJ and Oxford, Princeton University Press.

Woultas, C. and Denning, E. (2019) *Civilisation and Informalisation: Connecting Long-Term Social and Psychic Process*. London, Palgrave MacMillan.

Section C

Equivalence

15 The Brexit Referendum and the inability to mourn

Equivalence in a large group

Frances Griffiths

Introduction

In 2016, the British electorate, given a vote to "Remain" or "Leave" the European Union (EU), chose to "Leave", and in so doing changed the course of history. Events that led up to this agreement emerged in 2008 in connection with a global financial crash, but originated much further back to a time of Empire and colonisation. A collective memory of greatness serves to diminish the loss of Empire, which the Brits have never been able to mourn fully. However, the dilution – if not the shattering – of the myth of greatness has involved a massive social trauma of which the British people have been unconscious. This trauma is uncovered in an exploration of the socio-political culture of Great Britain, expressed in the language of the slogans "Brexit" and "Take Back Control", as seen in the proceedings of a large group whose primary task was to discuss and reflect upon the Brexit Referendum. I will offer some interpretations of, and associations to, the dynamics of the group in terms of the theory of Incohesion: Aggregation/Massification and of Pairing, the former as a consequence of failed dependency, and the latter as a consequence of the inability and refusal to mourn (Hopper, 2003b, 2022; Rosenbaum & Winther, 2012).

The concept of the tripartite matrix (Hopper, 2018, 2003a and this book) offers a template for perceiving and understanding the dynamics of groups, not only those who meet primarily for the purposes of clinical work, but also those whose primary task is to discuss a particular topic. Like most groups, "Theme-centred" groups are usually convened under the auspices of a sponsoring organisation. Therefore, I will consider the proceedings of the large group in question through the frames of reference of the foundation matrix of the contextual society, the dynamic matrix of the sponsoring organisation, and the personal matrices of a participant who personified some of the processes in question.

I would acknowledge my implicit bias. I am a citizen of the UK, and voted to remain connected to Europe. I am a member of the IGA and of the GASI. I co-convened the group with a senior colleague. This large group was sponsored by the IGA (UK), and it met in its building in London. In reflecting upon equivalence with regard to the tripartite matrix of a particular group, it is never entirely clear whether one is using the experience of the group as a source of further insight into

DOI: 10.4324/9781003425915-23

the foundation matrix of the contextual society and/or into the dynamic matrix of the sponsoring organisation, or vice versa; this question also arises in connection with individual participants in the group and with particular sub-groups who might develop within it. Of course, these are recursive processes. As a group analyst, I assume that insight based on experience will always be "negotiable".

One further proviso: all observations in our field – if not in life generally – are theory-driven, not only in terms of what is noted, but also in terms of what is ignored and what is not even seen. The best – if not the only – guarantee of neutrality and objectivity are observations from several observers, even if they are participant observers, and continuing open discussions, although safeguards must be established concerning the influence of sequential contributions to a developing consensus. Minority and supplementary reports are almost always a good idea.

Vignette

In July 2016, a large group for group analysts was convened in order for them to explore their thoughts and feelings about the Brexit Referendum. The majority of those who attended the group were seasoned group analysts. Most seemed to belong to the Remain camp (not wanting to disconnect from the EU).

There was an air of considerable disbelief at the outcome of the Referendum. The group began the discussion about the implications of the outcome for our relations with the rest of Europe. Within a few minutes, some conflicting opinions were expressed. The group began to polarise very quickly, perhaps even to form into several small sub-groups and contra-groups. People seemed to want to distance themselves from one another. Some tried to change the subject. People slightly shifted their chairs, and some avoided one another's gaze. "Eye rolling" could be seen. However, these indications of aggregation were very rapidly superseded by indications of massification. For example, participants started to nod in agreement with whatever was said. We became a large group of "noddies". We were group analysts who had much in common.

Suddenly, a well-respected member of the community of group analysts asked about the current display of photographs of the great men and women who founded psychoanalysis in the window of the nearby Karnac Bookshop, noting with disappointment and perhaps with dismay that the display did not include a photograph of S.H. Foulkes, the Founder of Group Analysis. The group became somewhat agitated about this. Various members began to ask questions and propose hypothetical answers to them about the display. Where was Foulkes? Had he been excluded deliberately or was this an oversight? Who left him out? Who was the culprit? Who was the perpetrator of this virtually violent act? Was he seen as not fitting in? Perhaps we needed to acknowledge that Foulkes himself had let us down? After all, had he not marginalised himself from the core of the psychoanalytical community? Clearly, it was necessary to find a new leader of the profession of Group Analysis. Since Foulkes had died more than four decades ago, the group might have considered who had replaced him. However, no one asked this question. In fact, it was opined that we no longer had a "leader".

A senior member of the community said that he would take it upon himself to sort out the "oversight" about the display of photographs with the Karnac people.

He worked with some of the men and women in the shop on manuscripts for books in *The New International Library of Group Analysis*, which was published by Karnac Books.

A discussion ensued about who might take the profession to a new and idealised space. Was a leader really needed? This discussion became a distraction – if not an obstacle – to the exploration of anxieties about the loss of our charismatic founding Father, the further loss of who had replaced him, the absence of a current leader, and the subsequent loss of identity and position within the broad field of psychoanalytical psychotherapy. This comment about what was not said is meant as an indication of what was said, in my opinion! People began to "chunter". The communication process seemed to become repetitive, without any deepening or clarifying communications. It was not acknowledged that following the death of Foulkes, the profession was characterised by complex dynamics of leadership, development, and regression, both nationally and globally. No sadness or mourning was expressed.

It was acknowledged that Foulkes was not only an immigrant from "Europe", but also a refugee from Nazi Germany. Our intellectual and professional parentage was "European". However, the group was not fully aware that ironically much of Group Analysis in Europe and elsewhere had been fostered by colleagues from the UK who initiated and pioneered training courses on the basis of the work of Foulkes. In some ways, The Referendum had cut us off from our children as well as from our parents and grandparents. Although these issues were briefly mentioned, they were not openly and explicitly addressed.

Towards the end of the group, one person suddenly identified himself as having voted Leave (and to disconnect from Europe). This person spoke of feeling that in telling us this there was a danger of being excluded by and from the group. Yet, he was determined to overcome what he took to be the power of these forces in the group against speaking out, talked briefly about how someone speaking out could be blamed for the marginalisation of Group Analysis within the wider professional community, and about various problems within the IGA. Issues of inequalities and elitism both within the wider society, within the profession, and within our professional organisations were mentioned. As anticipated, the group rounded on this seemingly lone voice. People were perplexed about how and why the large group had come so quickly to focus on a particular colleague. Although having brought a difference to our attention, what did this voice personify? What role had this person got sucked into? These questions were asked more or less as "asides" within several sub-groups. They were not asked loudly and clearly, and addressed to the group-as-a-whole.

Tension seemed to increase. The volume of conversation seemed to increase, as did the number of people who were speaking over one another. The babble of aggregation prevailed. However, the co-convenors stopped the group as scheduled.

The unconscious dynamics of the large group in terms of group regression, basic assumptions, and personifications

I would suggest that as usual for a discrete session in which people meet in order to discuss a theme about which they feel strongly and to reflect collectively on various aspects of this, the group regressed very quickly. This was seen in the loss of personal identities and in a sense that the group was not sufficiently cohesive for a cooperative rational discussion. Although many people knew one another and were in familiar surroundings, there was a sense of heightened anxiety, the usual complaints about being unable to see and to hear, problems with the windows being opened for fresh air but allowing too much noise from the outside, etc. There were complaints concerning the leadership and administration of the event. The leaders lacked authority, and the administration was inefficient.

In response to this sense of failed dependency, aggregation developed. However, there was a rapid shift towards massification in terms of "all for one and one for all" based on all of the participants being group analysts despite a myriad of other differences. They were reluctant to acknowledge differences in their points of view and/or interests. The massification was preventing the emergence of differences, which was necessary for discussion and debate. Debate was stifled. People seemed to be bored.

Rather than oscillate back into aggregation, the group shifted into basic assumption pairing as a manifestation of the use of sexuality as a manic defence against depressive anxieties. Perhaps this was associated with the inability/refusal to mourn lost but flawed objects, such as the EU itself as an overarching organisation and political idea, the founding parents and other leaders of our organisation, the prominence of the profession, the organisation itself, etc. In fact, this basic assumption pairing was seen in the emergence of the two-act play within a play involving the conception, gestation, and birth of a Messianic child (Hopper & Kreeger, 1980/2003). This often happens as a collective defence against the pains of loss and mourning.

In the first act of this nested play, the overt discussion was about the loss of Foulkes, the Founder of Group Analysis, and of subsequent leaders, and about problems in the organisation and the profession. However, this discussion was characterised by a collective disassociation from any affect of sadness or mourning. The discussion was performative.

The second act of this play involved another aspect of pairing, i.e. self-sacrifice in collusion with the emergence of a sub-group of "Roman Soldiers" who were prepared to carry out the act of ritual murder of the Messianic colleague who was a product of the pairing. Although it seemed as though this group analyst was trying to get the group to return to a discussion of Brexit, in fact he personified Messianic self-sacrifice. In effect, he was shut down and killed off. This sacrifice led back into aggregation.

The unconscious dynamics of the large group through the frames of reference of the foundation matrix of the contextual society, the dynamic matrix of the sponsoring organisations, and the personal matrices of several of those who personified key roles

The frames of reference of the foundation matrix of the contextual society

The denial of the pain and shame caused by the experience of Group Analysis having been "left out" and (for example, by not being included in the NICE guidelines for treatment, and by being excluded from the canon of great psychoanalytic literature) was unbearable. A narrative of greatness was called upon in order to try to "save face". This involved a basic assumption of aggregation in oscillation with massification, and a basic assumption of pairing leading to a search for a Messianic saviour.

"Great" as in Great Britain is based on the history of the nation as a coloniser and as an Empire. The British Empire existed for more than 400 years, from 1600 AD, spreading the country's rule and power beyond its borders through what is known nowadays as "**Imperialism**". The myth of a "shared reality" of greatness is based on its past identity as a coloniser and Empire builder.

Today, however, the nation no longer has an Empire, and no longer has favourable economic and political arrangements with its former colonies. Recognising the loss of status, power, and glory is painful. It requires a long period of authentic public mourning which was never fully achieved in Britain that has remained largely unchallenged in the foundation matrix and in the social unconscious. In the aftermath of social trauma, people rely upon dominant sub-groups who call for "greatness" in order to spare them the shame and pain of loss.

Mitscherlich and Mitscherlich (1967) have discussed a nation's inability to mourn with respect to post-war Germany: "The Federal Republic did not succumb to melancholia; instead, as a group, those who had lost their 'ideal leader', the representative of a commonly shared ego-ideal, managed to avoid self-devaluation by breaking all affective bridges to the immediate past" (p. 26). In a way, this is a manic defence against the pain and devastation experienced for the loss of "Fatherland". Ogimoto (2019, and this book) has applied this concept to Japan, arguing that after WWII the Japanese people lost the God Emperor and the Empire-motherland. As was the case for Germany and Germans, Japan and the Japanese avoided grief through their identification with the economic system and industrial achievements that followed the war.

The Brexit Referendum can be seen as a manic gesture that fused and confused a future identity with a return to the past. Any threat to a loss of position revives the desire for a narrative of greatness. This helps to relieve shameful feelings. This was the case in 1973, when GB became a member of the EU, which invoked shameful feelings about the need to belong. Membership was never fully embraced, which created powerful sub-groups of those who were for and those who were against the EU. There is of course much more to be said about this historic moment, but the sub-groups of those who were against membership of the EU were revitalised by the global financial crash in 2008. This massive and abrupt social trauma of financial collapse affected Great Britain most acutely. The making of great fortunes by some at the expense of the many was an echo of Empire building followed by Empire collapsing. The EU and Brussels bureaucrats were blamed for this. Membership of the EU was re-written as an error of judgement, and plans emerged which on the basis of the Referendum of 2016 would take GB out of the EU. GB would be great again!

The dynamic matrix of the sponsoring organisations

The dynamic matrix of the large group can also be seen in terms of equivalence with the dynamic matrix of the sponsoring organisations which involved processes of belonging, inclusion and exclusion, as well as power and the loss of power, and feelings of shame.

The death of Foulkes raised questions about the future of Group Analysis. Was there an heir or an heiress waiting in the wings? (Yair, 2017). The fear of annihilation was very powerfully resurrected in the large group with the exclusion of literature about Foulkes and Group Analysis in the Karnac window, not to mention a photograph of Foulkes himself. This was compounded by the experience of failed dependency on his successor. In fact, the search for a saviour coincided with the search for a perpetrator. In addition to the difficulty in mourning the dramatic death of Foulkes in a group of younger colleagues who he was conducting, the group-analytic movement suffered another failed dependency and loss when the ethical transgressions of his main successor were discovered. This created a split and a crisis in the organisation which prevented a proper mourning of the loss of him as a leader, and a thorough understanding of the failed dependency on him. Also, perhaps as a matter of contagion, several other senior figures were rumoured to have violated the ethical code.

The IGA in London also lost some of its international influence. The Institute had been involved in group-analytic training in several countries. However, it began to lose its hegemony as these countries developed their own training programmes and ultimately their own Institutes. The European Group Analytic Training Institutes Network (EGATIN) was both a story of its "greatness" and a story of the waning of it (Hadar & Ofer, 2001).

The Group Analytic Society International (GASi), the other sponsoring organisation of the large group, has also lost its British hegemony, starting with the election of GASi presidents from outside the UK (Germany, Italy, Denmark, and Israel), and continuing with moving its tri-annual symposia from England to other countries. The change of the name from GAS to GASi indicates this development: the "i" stands for "international", but the fact that this is indicated in small "i" reveals the ambivalence of the British about these developments. After all, the British still constitute the overwhelming majority of the membership of GASi, and these developments actually involve what was for them a loss.

The split between the IGA and GASi must also be acknowledged. The current President of GASi qualified at an organisation other than the IGA.

The personal matrices of several of those who personified key roles

The participant who ousted himself as someone who had voted to Leave spoke of his fears about not belonging to the IGA, and about not having full recognition of his qualifications as a "professional" group analyst. This was partly connected with differentiation between the two organisations, GASi becoming a "learned society" in the traditional British sense, and the IGA becoming a professional training and qualifying organisation. In other words, this particular participant became a personifier of the differentiation and the split. In some ways, this was connected with the inability to work through the failed dependency on the successor to Foulkes and the inability to mourn him, because after he was marginalised from the IGA on the basis of his ethical transgression, he took a more prominent role within GASi, which can be understood as a further source of certain conflicts within GASi and its internationalisation.

Conclusion

The group ended without returning to its primary task. The work group that had a clear identity at the start was upended by a basic assumption group that obscured its task and its capacity to function. The large group became characterised by Incohesion and Pairing, reflected in the inability to mourn. This was evident in the three realms of the tripartite matrix. It involved several losses: the British Empire and its "greatness", the hegemony of the hosting organisations, the leading figures of Group Analysis, and the failed dependency that followed.

Death and loss are inevitable, and mourning them is a life-long process. There is a continuing need for regular large group meetings for the discussion and working through of the various patterns of anxiety associated with these processes.

References

Hadar, B. & Ofer, G. (2001). The social unconscious reflected in politics, organizations and groups: a case of overseas group analysis training. *Group Analysis* 34: 375–385.

Hopper, E. (2003a). *The Social Unconscious: Selected Papers.* London: Jessica Kingsley Publishers.

Hopper, E. (2003b). *Traumatic Experience in the Unconscious Life of Groups.* London: Jessica Kingsley Publishers.

Hopper, E. (2018). The development of the concept of the Tripartite Matrix: a response to 'Four modalities of the experience of others in groups' by Victor Schermer. *Group Analysis* 51(2): 197–206.

Hopper, E. (2022). "Notes" on the theory of the fourth basic assumption in the unconscious life of groups and group-like social systems: Incohesion: Aggregation/Massification or (ba) I:A/M. In C. Penna (Ed.). *From Crowd Psychology to the Dynamics of Large Groups: Historical, Theoretical and Practical Considerations* (pp. 176–208). London: Routledge.

Hopper, E. & Kreeger, L. (1980). Report on the large group. In C. Garland (Ed.). Proceedings of the Survivor Syndrome Workshop (1979) *Group Analysis*, Special Edition, November. Reprinted in E. Hopper (2003) *The Social Unconscious: Selected Papers.* London: Jessica Kingsley Publishers.

Mitscherlich, A. & Mitscherlich, M. (1967). *The Inability to Mourn: Principles of Collective Behavior.* New York: Random House.

Ogimoto, K. (2019). The Inability to Mourn: WW2 and Nationalism in Germany and Japan. Unpublished presentation at the International Psychoanalytical Association 51st Congress.

Rosenbaum, B. & Winther, G. (2012). Traumatogenic processes in a psychiatric hospital: unconscious destructiveness of leadership change. In E. Hopper (Ed.). *Trauma and Organizations* (pp. 23–44). London: Karnac.

Yair, G. (2017). The national habitus: steps towards reintegrating sociology and group analysis. In E. Hopper & H. Weinberg (Eds.). *The Social Unconscious in Persons, Groups and Societies: Volume 3: The Foundation Matrix Extended and Re-Configured* (pp. 47–64). London: Karnac.

16 The manic defense of reconstruction and the inability to mourn in post-war Japan[1]

Kai Ogimoto and Tomas Plaenkers

Loss and defeat in World War II

In 1945, Japan accepted the Potsdam Declaration and was defeated. Most of the Japanese archipelago was then occupied by the U.S. forces until 1952. This was led by Douglas MacArthur,[2] a war hero and the Supreme Commander of the Allied Powers (SCAP). He used the Emperor as the speaker of the SCAP in exchange for absolving the Emperor of war responsibility. In the process, the emperor declared himself a human being, and the emperor, who had previously been a present god, was now considered a human being, not a god. His authority was diminished and the people's "emotional connection to the emperor" was lost (Katoh, 2019). In an earlier paper, we pointed out that the "mourning work" of the emperor's declaration of humanity, necessary to accept the loss of the emperor as a living god, did not take place as Japanese society pushed forward with economic activities in the wake of the Korean War after the defeat (Ogimoto & Plaenkers, 2022).

The inability to mourn in Japan

Osamu Kitayama and Masayuki Hashimoto tried to deal with the problem of guilt in the Japanese people by analyzing the Japanese myth "Kojiki" (Records of Ancient Matters), which was part of the Japanese education as authorized history until the defeat in WW2. In a book called "Nihon-jin no 'Genzai' (Japanese 'sins')" (2009). They pointed out that in order to overcome Japan's unending original sins, it is necessary to face the original sins described in the myth. We will summarize part of the myth includes a Japanese original sin violating a "prohibition of: 'Don't look'" based on their book.

Here, in Kitayama and Hashimoto's book, the myths described in the Japanese Kojiki are introduced as follows.

> According to the myth, there have been two gods who created Japan. They are a male god named Izanagi and a female god named Izanami who were a couple as well as brother and sister. In the Middle-Earth land, Izanagi and Izanami produced many gods, but just as the female god finally gave birth to the fire god, Izanami was burned and died and went to the Land of the Roots,

DOI: 10.4324/9781003425915-24

which was the underworld. The male god went to the Land of the Roots to revive the female god and pleaded for her to return. Izanami said: "Please wait because I will consult with the gods of the Land of the Roots." However, the male god could not bear that and broke the prohibition of 'Don't Look' and looked inside. Then, it was the female god who became a rotten corpse. The male god felt fear in "look and awe" and ran away. The rotten body of the female god chased angrily saying "You brought shame on me", but the male god ran away to the Middle-Earth land. Then the male god placed a huge rock between the Land of the Roots and the middle earth-land, and so the countries of death and life were divided. To reduce the affliction borne in the Land of the Roots, the male god entered the stream of the river and carried out a ceremony to wash off the dirtiness of what he had done. After that the male god started producing many other gods by himself

(Kitayama & Hashimoto, 2009)[2].

This myth, "Kojiki", has been taught as legitimate history, or fact, in the national history classes of Japanese schools since the Meiji Restoration in 1868, until the defeat in World War II, so that the people could strengthen their "ties" with the emperor (Furukawa, 2020). In other words, it is considered to be part of the Founding Matrix of modern Japan. Under the fundamental national policy Japanese children and adults were taught that the Emperor is a descendant of these gods.

In a previous study, we stated that the response exhibited by the Izanaki in the myth was repression of his own murderous aggression toward the primitive object. We then proposed that Japanese society shares this repressed murderous aggression. With the defeat of the war and the Emperor's declaration of humanity and the subsequent concentration on economic activities, the Japanese murderous aggression was again repressed after the war (Ogimoto & Plaenkers, 2022).

In this myth, the male deity has lost his wife and sister, the female deity. What the male deity witnesses when the female deity tries to see him and breaks the "don't look" prohibition is an ugly female deity. Here we can see the projective identification of the male god's strong aggression. The male god establishes and divides the boundary between the land of death and the land of life, between night and day, There is no inner spiritual mourning, and guilt is repressed. This is quite similar to the reaction after the loss of the primordial object as pointed out by Mitscherlich and Mitscherlich (1967, see below). By exploring this process, the work of mourning the loss of the primordial object can begin.

This myth can also explain some of the gender power structure in the Japanese society, in which men (especially in authority position) are unconsciously perceived as above women, and might exploit their power without feelings of shame or guilt. It can be said that the Foundation Matrix in Japan is deeply connected to gender imbalance and the oppression of women by authoritative men.

German psychoanalysts A. and M. Mitscherlich (1967) describe a collective defense against group melancholy. In post-war Germany, which had lost the representation of the common ego ideal, instead of an explosion of melancholy, the impoverishment of the self was avoided by breaking all emotional bridges to the immediate past. In particular, they prevented a rapid decline in self-esteem by refusing to engage internally in their own behavior under the Third Reich. In this way, the explosion of collective melancholy was defended. Since then, it has become difficult to find themselves in anything more than economic activity (Mitscherlich & Mitscherlich, 1967). They explain that three types of reactions were observed in post-war Germany in order to reduce the overwhelming guilt burdens. First, a pronounced emotional rigidity; second, an easy identification with the winners of war without any sign of wounded pride; and third, a manic undoing of the past and a total and collective effort at reconstruction.

All of those reactions, we believe, occurred in Japan (Ogimoto & Plaenkers, 2022). After the Emperor's Declaration of Humanity, there was an emotional void (Kato, 2019). And instead of collectively confronting the crimes of invading other countries, massacres such as the Nanking Massacre, the misuse of countless women (so-called military comfort women), the attack on Pearl Harbor, and the abuse of prisoners of war in the Asia-Pacific Rim, Japanese people quickly idealized Douglas MacArthur and the U.S. military, and identified with Article 9 of the Japanese Constitution, which prohibited war and arms maintenance, as they idealized the philosophy of non-war. By promoting reconstruction and identifying with the rising economic system, they seem to have succeeded in avoiding the loss of their own self-esteem (Ogimoto & Plaernkers, 2022). Focusing on industrialization and the economic system, it was a manic defense against loss in Japan (although controversial).

A clinical vignette

I am reminded of the first author's six years of psychotherapy with a member of the war generation. The female client (age 80) came to therapy complaining of insomnia and hypochondria. She was born into an upper-middle-class family in the Tokyo metropolitan area.

In 1941, during her second year at a prestigious higher girls' school in Tokyo, Japan attacked Pearl Harbor and declared war on the United States. The war soon became one-sided, and indiscriminate air raids on Tokyo by the United States intensified. In order to avoid this, she and her family evacuated to the Northeast, where her father was born. Her father, who had been a businessman before the war, lost his job. The client, who had attended a prestigious higher girls' school, transferred to a local girls' school, thereby losing the career and life she had been promised there. Life was very difficult at the evacuation site. Not only did she lose her career, the client also lost her father's authority and many young relatives in the war front in the South Pacific.

In August 1945, Japan lost the war. Because of her father's sluggish business, it was difficult for her to return to Tokyo, and she spent some time in an evacuated area. Immediately after the war, she met her current husband through her father's employer, who was working alone in Tokyo, and they got married when she was quite old for the time. However, she did not have a new house, but built a shack out of tin plates in the burnt ruins of her husband's house, and lived with her mother-in-law, who lost her husband early, and her husband's brother and his wife in a room of about six tatami mats. She spent the post-war years of Japan's rapid economic growth taking care of her mother-in-law and husband and doing housework. The couple had a daughter three years after their marriage, but she was unable to feel a solid emotional connection to her daughter. She threw herself too much into caring for her mother-in-law, husband, and daughter, as well as the housework. However, in her 60s, when her mother-in-law and her own parents died one after another in just a few years, her dedication to housework became unsustainable. She began to experience insomnia, dizziness, and tears when she remembered the past. After five years of these symptoms, she came to see a psychotherapist.

In therapy, she continued to talk about what she had lost during the war, and to express her sadness and regret. Five years later, she began to express regret and feel sorry for her daughter, saying that she had not been able to connect emotionally with her daughter during the period of rapid economic growth right after the war, when she was devoted to her mother-in-law and husband, and striving to do her housework. She began to express her regrets and apologies to her daughter.

Her immediate post-war focus on caring for her mother-in-law and husband seems to have been based on a denial of what she had lost during the war. She was not able to do the work of mourning until almost 70 years after the war.

It was difficult for her to discuss the Emperor or relate him to the predicament she had experienced. The only time she put it into words was when she told me about an episode when she was commuting to the girls' school and every time the cable car was approaching the main gate of the Imperial Palace, all the passengers would get out of their seats and bow graciously to the palace. She spat out that she thought bowing was "kind of silly".

She recalled the immediate aftermath of the end of the war many times, yet stated that she "didn't feel anything" when the Emperor broadcasted the news of the defeat to the people. The only thing she remembered was that when the U.S. military advanced on Japan after the defeat and a large number of U.S. bombers flew low over the city where she lived, she felt, "Oh, now I'm going to die".

For most citizens of the mid-war generation, the mourning of the Emperor, the living god, was taboo and repressed to unconscious.

This may be one of the reasons why Westerners who observe the Japanese say that the Japanese do not assert themselves. If they were to express legitimate anger or assertiveness, they would be touching a taboo within their psyche, and would risk isolation in interpersonal relationships. Japanese people do not express anger, but instead let their emotions of confusion and fear surface.

Repetition of inability to mourn and manic defense of rebuilding

The libido that had been cathected to the Emperor before and during the war was transformed and cathected to the economy and money or numbers in the high economic growth after the war. When there is a loss that affects the whole society, instead of mourning, there is a manic defense of reconstruction. This was repeated in the Great East Japan Earthquake of 2011. In the aftermath of the disaster, which claimed some 15,000 lives, the government spent huge sums of money on reconstruction projects rather than fully funding the mourning process. There was no social mourning. The guilt of not doing the work of mourning remained in the psychic structure of many people, and this was manifested in the phenomenon that many survivors of the earthquake reported seeing ghosts in the northeastern region. When a massive social trauma is not mourned and cannot be openly discussed in the public discourse, it is in high risk to become part of the Social Unconscious of the people of that society (see "Chosen trauma", Volkan, 2001) and to impact their behavior without awareness (Hopper & Weinberg, 2011).

So, here is Japan's response to COVID-19: Japan hosted the Olympic games in August 2021, during the fifth wave of the delta strain of COVID-19, which is the most deadly and most medically strained. The games in Tokyo were played without spectators. However, in the midst of the largest number of deaths and the greatest medical crisis in recent history, a large number of staff and players gathered for a sports festival. Although the Olympics were to be a celebration of the recovery from the Great East Japan Earthquake, the cause of commemorating the Great East Japan Earthquake was lost. Only the manic denial function of the celebration remained. The pattern of inability to mourn and manic defense was repeated in the general response to COVID-19. Individuals who are unable or unwilling to engage in such manic defense become isolated.

The manic defense in the form of a collective obsession with economic reconstruction meshes with neoliberalism and **evidentialism**[3] of our time. Evidentialism and positivism create a divide between subjective and objective experience (Sun, 2016). The qualitative, time-consuming, and invisible work of mourning continues to be socially repudiated and remains unable to take place. The inability to mourn and the manic defense continue to be upheld ideologically and culturally.

Engaging in the work of mourning is one way to mitigate those aggressive feelings which might lead to the next war. When we are psychologically overwhelmed by loss, we try to reassert our subjectivity by setting up a hypothetical external enemy and attempt to overwhelm it with violence and force. Attempting to overcome internal oppression externally through violence or force is pointless. We must turn to the work of mourning.

AUM Shinrikyo and the emperor system

Nishimura (2016) has discussed the impact of war trauma and social unconsciousness in World War II on AUM Shinrikyō, an emerging religion responsible for the sarin gas attack on the subway in 1995. Japan's **"fundamental national policy"** before and during the war was imitated by AUM Shinrikyō (Isomae, 2019).

On March 20, 1995, during the morning rush hour, five followers of AUM Shinrikyo, boarded three subway lines in central Tokyo and at about the same time sprayed sarin gas, a highly poisonous gas, into the crowded subways around the political hub of Kasumigaseki. Passengers and subway workers collapsed on the train and in the station. In the end, 13 passengers and station staff died, and thousands were seriously injured in what became an unprecedented case of indiscriminate murder in Japan. As the police investigation progressed, it was discovered that the crime was committed by the AUM Shinrikyo, which has as many as 3,000 followers under the leadership of Syoko Asahara, and Asahara and his followers who were hiding in the cult's facilities were arrested. The death penalty was carried out in July 2018 amidst ongoing debate about his "responsibility capacity".

The totalitarian features of the AUM cult included a snitching system, information blocking, corporal punishment up to the death penalty, and encouragement of assimilation into the totality. The obedience of AUM followers to Asahara was, to the followers themselves and to foreign researchers, reminiscent of the pre-war and mid-war Emperor system in Japan. AUM cult was a pseudo "fundamental national policy" of Japan that mimicked the Emperor system before and during the war.

Asahara planned to poison the Emperor and take his place as the new emperor, he dreamed to be a new living god of Japan. This desire denies that the Emperor declared himself a human being and ceased to be a living god due to his defeat and the defeat of the U.S. military. In Asahara's mind, the Emperor remained an incarnate deity, and he wanted to replace himself as the living god in the living place. Fifty years after the war, the mourning of the Emperor as a living god is still denied, and the totalitarian regime of before and during the war continues to play out in Asahara and his cult, resulting in indiscriminate mass murder. Asahara's utterance that he would kill the Emperor and instead become the "king of Japan" also shows that the present god was not mourned in Asahara, who was not even born at the time of the defeat, but was socially inherited.

The AUM cult still exists. Asahara, the pseudo-emperor, and his followers, the pseudo-citizens, have denied their own responsibility, and AUM itself has abandoned its right and responsibility to look forward and rebuild itself in society by proactively assuming responsibility for its crimes. This is similar to Japan's behavior toward atrocities in the Asia-Pacific rim.

The AUM cult incident, which harmed many people and became a social problem, was portrayed by the media and other parts of Japanese society as an aberration and a "crazy group". As Foulkes (1983) presented in his concept of "the location of the disturbance", we believe that the structure of groups and organizations such as AUM Shinrikyo is commonplace in Japan. This can be observed not only in the heads of public organizations such as the current Japanese government, corporations, universities, and foundations, but also at the level of small organizations and societies. Examples of leaders abdicating their responsibilities while continuing to violate human rights are unfortunately repeated on a daily basis in Japan. The violent acts they committed are then swept under the rug.

The relationship with the United States

Historian John Dower (2000) describes the complicity of Japan and the United States as "embracing [Japan's] defeat" after the war. Hence,

> Whenever the Japanese took political action to reject the security treaty under which U.S. troops would be based in Japan, the U.S., through the Japanese

government, would have thoroughly crushed the political movement. If so, then Japan's postwar period has been one in which it has avoided confronting the violent nature of human beings, in other words, one in which it has denied its own violent nature.

(p. 182)

This is a postcolonial state in Japan. The U.S. occupation of Japan continues in an invisible way (Katoh, 2015; Yabe, 2017).

To what extent did the United States anticipate Japan's inability to mourn and its manic defense? Gorer (1942) had been analyzing the role of the Emperor in Japanese society since the middle of the war, and had reported to the U.S. military that the SCAP, with Douglas MacArthur as its symbol, should replace the Emperor's role. The occupation policy went along with it in quite some domains. MacArthur played his role well enough, and the Japanese media and society repeated the discourse that seemed to put MacArthur in the position of the Emperor. Dower described Japan and the United States as embracing defeat together, but what was embraced and hidden was not only the defeat, but also the loss of the Emperor as a living god. By avoiding working through the mourning of the Emperor, who is the living god, Japanese society and organizations have fostered a group that unconsciously and consciously commits violence and yet denies responsibility for it.

Conclusion

Some of the difficulty to mourn this loss is the repression and denial of the disappointment in and subsequent aggression towards the Emperor, and the "failed dependency" process involved (Hopper, 2022). The avoidance of guilt and shame, deeply embedded in the Social Unconscious of the Japanese people, as shown in their foundation myth, supports their inability to mourn such losses.

Those voices hurt the Japanese to the bone. The post-war Japanese still fantasize and dream that there is a present god in the Imperial Palace, surrounded by greenery in the center of Tokyo. They continue to deny that they have lost their benevolent mother goddess, the Emperor. It is painful to work with the loss of a primal object. However, the post-war system of Japan and the United States embracing and repudiating this work has allowed the repudiation of irresponsibility and violence in Japanese institutions to continue unchallenged, and the human rights of the vulnerable in society to continue to be violated.

As a further challenge, it is possible that the manic defense of reconstruction as a social response to loss is not limited to the post-war period. From the Japanese mythology of *Kojiki*,[4] we can see that the defense against loss is to devote oneself to productive activities (Ogimoto & Plaenkers, 2021).

Reflecting on the inability to mourn may be a starting point for overcoming the neoliberal system, a system that produces large social disparities and social and organizational neglect in the name of "self-responsibility". Further study is needed.

Notes

1 A part of this chapter was presented at the International Psychoanalytical Association 51st Congress, 27th July 2019: "The Inability to Mourn. WW2 and Nationalism in Germany and Japan", Chaired by Maria Teresa Savio Hooke (Australia) to whom we express our sincere gratitude and respect. She has continued to support us both academically and emotionally throughout the project. It is no exaggeration to say that this paper was co-authored by the three of us. A part of this paper was also presented by the first author at the International Dialogue Initiative (IDI) Case Conference, 30th September in 2020, with thanks to Gerard Fromm, Regine Scholz and Harriet Wolfe.
2 (Wikipedia) General Douglas MacArthur officially accepted the surrender of Japan on 2 September 1945 aboard the USS *Missouri*, which was anchored in Tokyo Bay, and he oversaw the occupation of Japan from 1945 to 1951. As the effective ruler of Japan, he oversaw sweeping economic, political, and social changes.
3 Evidentialism: https://www.encyclopedia.com/humanities/encyclopedias-almanacs-transcripts-and-maps/evidentialism.
4 Kojiki: *Kojiki* is a text of Shintoism, which was the state religion of Japan from 19th century until the end of World War II. Kojiki consists of myths, scriptures, histories, and folk tales about creators called "Kami" and their millions of descendants and spirits.

Bibliography

Dower, W. J. (2000). *Embracing Defeat: Japan in the Wake of World War II*; New York: W W Norton & Co Inc.

Foulkes, S.H. (1983) *Introduction to Group-Analytic Psychotherapy: Studies in the Social Integration of Individuals and Groups*; London: Taylor & Francis.

Furukawa, T. (2020). *Social History of the Founding Myth: The Boundary between Historical Fact and Falsehood (Kenkoku-shinwa-no-Shakai-shi: Shijiysu-to-Kyogi-no-Kyokai)*; Tokyo: Chu-ko shinsho.

Gorer, G. (1942). Japanese character structure and propaganda; Institute of Human Relations, New Haven: Yale University Press.

Hopper, E. (2022). "Notes" on the theory and concept of the fourth basic assumption in the unconscious life of groups and group-like social systems: Incohesion: Aggregation/Massification of (ba) I:A/M. In: C. Penna, *From Crowd Psychology to the Dynamics of Large Groups: Historical, Theoretical and Practical Considerations* (pp. 176–208); London: Routledge.

Hopper, E. & Weinberg, H. (eds.) (2011). *The Social Unconscious in Persons, Groups and Societies: Volume 1: Mainly Theory*; London: Karnac.

Isomae, K. (2019). *Intellectual History of Showa and Heisei: "Never-Ending Post War" and "Happy Japanese" (Syo-wa Hei-sei Sei-shin shi: "Oaranai-sengo" to "Shiawasena-Nihon-jin")*; Tokyo: Koudan-sha.

Katoh, N. (2015). *Introduction to the Postwar (Sengon nyu-mon)*; Tokyo: Chikuma-Shobo.

Katoh, N. (2019). *Introduction to Article 9 (Kyu-jyo nyu-mon)*; Tokyo: Sougen-sha.

Kitayama, O. & Hashimoto, M. (2009). *Japanese "sin" (Nihonjin no "genzai")*; Tokyo: Koudan-sha.

Mitscherlich, A. & Mitscherlich, M. (1967). *The Inability to Mourn: Principles of Collective Behavior*; New York: Grove Press.

Nishimura, K. (2016). Contemporary manifestations of the social unconscious in Japan: post trauma massification and difficulties in identity formation after the Second World War. In: Hopper & Weinberg, *The Social Unconscious In Persons, Groups, and Societies. Volume 2: Mainly Foundation Matrices* (pp. 97–116); London: Karnac.

Ogimoto, K. & Plaenkers, T. (2022). *"The Inability to Mourn" and Nationalism in Japan after 1945*. Submitted Manuscript.

Pines, M. (2003). Forward. In: Hopper, *Traumatic Experience in the Unconscious Life of Groups: The Fourth Basic Assumption: Incohesion: Aggregation/Massification or (ba) I:A/M* (pp. 9–10). London: Jessica Kingsley.

Sun, G. (2016). *The Dilemma of Talking about Asia: In Search of a Common Space of Knowledge (Ashia wo katarukoto no jirenma: Chi no Kyodokukan wo Motomete)*. Tokyo: Iwanami-shoten.

Volkan, V.D. (2001). Transgenerational transmission and chosen trauma: an aspect of large group identity. *Group Analysis*, 34, 79–97.

Yabe, K. (2017). *Unknowable: Hidden Structure of Controlling Japan (Shittewa-Ikenai: Kakusareta Shihai no Ko-zou)*; Tokyo: Kou-dan-sha.

17 Social unconscious and group psychotherapy in Georgia

Revaz (Rezo) Korinteli

Hopper (1996) stressed that groups and their participants are unconsciously constrained by social, cultural and political facts and forces as well as conscious ones. He writes:

> The central theme in my work is the study of the constraints of social systems on people and their internal worlds, and, in turn, the effects of social systems on unconscious fantasies, actions, thoughts, and feelings. ......An analyst who is unaware of the effects of social facts and social forces cannot be sensitive to the unconscious re-creation of them within the therapeutic situation. He will not be able to provide a space for patients to imagine how their identities have been formed at particular historical and political junctures, and how this continues to affect them throughout their lives.
>
> (Hopper, 1996, p. 7)

According to him, the here-and-now is influenced by the there-and-then in ways that affect the group's functioning. Identifying this influence accents what is possible or not possible in the therapy group as a social microcosm or mirror of the society in which it is embedded (Hopper, 2003).

Singer and Kimbles (2004) developed the notion of a cultural complex from Jung's theory of complexes for the purpose of understanding the psychology of group conflict. Cultural Complex is a psychoanalytical term applied in a global anthropological context to describe the splintering of identity and resultant anger and conflicts. "Cultural complexes are highly emotional, function independently of the ego, and possess multilayered dimensions, their content being structured by archetypal, cultural, and personal elements". They also suggest that cultural complexes can manifest in the individual psyche as a collective inheritance, formed over generations. A cultural complex, then, is a psychological complex applied to the collective consciousness of a group, as well as its individual members. The authors have defined cultural complexes as tending "to be repetitive, autonomous, resist consciousness, and collect experience that confirms their historical point of view" (Singer and Kimbles, 2004, p. 7). Cultural complexes (see also Singer and Kaplinsky, 2010) actually resemble the social unconscious concept as described by Hopper and Weinberg in the introduction to the first volume of their series of

DOI: 10.4324/9781003425915-25

books about the social unconscious (2011). Hopper and Weinberg extended their understanding and analysis of the social unconscious in their series of books, bringing examples of the foundation matrix of different cultures in Volumes II (2015) and III (2017).

The inability to mourn is a concept that Mitscherlich and Mitscherlich (1975) developed to describe the defence against mass melancholia in postwar Germany. "The Federal Republic did not succumb to melancholia; instead, as a group, those who had lost their "ideal leader", the representative of a commonly shared ego-ideal, managed to avoid self-devaluation" (p. 26). Post-Soviet countries, including Georgia, seem to have difficulties in mourning loss and thus the Communist ideology unconsciously still influences the behaviour of the citizens of these countries (Weinberg, personal communication). They fail to realize this Communist ideology as a defence against the pain of their failed dependency (Hopper, personal communication).

These concepts will be used in order to give a brief overview of the psychotherapy in Georgia. I will start with a brief review of the phenomena that we in Georgia inherited from the Soviet Union.

Soviet mentality

Soviet mentality has had an important influence upon the development of psychiatry in Georgia. The Soviet Mentality included (1) materialistic world view, (2) authoritarianism, (3) intolerance for dissidence and (4) silence and secrecy.

Materialistic world view

During Soviet times, Psychiatry was based on the materialistic understanding of a human being. Disease was regarded as disordered brain functioning caused by distorted biochemical machinery. Many of the current concepts have been moulded by the neurophysiology of Ivan Pavlov, Vladimir Bekhterev and Alexander Luria (Corson, 1976; Gray, 1979). Psychic disturbances were only considered on a somatic level (Calloway, 1993); psychic organization meant nothing; psychodynamic approach and psychoanalysis were rejected and even forbidden as being bourgeois (Miller, 2001). Pavlov's theory remained as the sole "truly materialistic" basis for Soviet psychotherapy (Segal, 1977).

During the early years, there was a small psychoanalytical movement based in Moscow. In the 1920s, there was a Moscow section of the International Psychoanalytical Association. The Russian Psychoanalytical Society was disbanded in 1933.

Authoritarianism .The relationship between the State and the People can be characterized as one between the Master and the Slave (Hegel, 1807). The state power, especially the leader, has always been identified as a masculine human being – a strong, just, merciful father, who protects, supports and takes care of the people (Urbanovich, 1999). Yet, Russia was a closed and isolated political system. It was based on dogmatization of social life and society, with rigid norms to which one had to conform and obey (Chaadayev, 1970; Kliuchevskii, 1960). In this grey and oppressive atmosphere, people had to conform in order to survive. Such a system can give birth to a benevolent dictator or a "tyrannical omnipotent father". Russia has almost always created conditions favourable to the rise of such omnipotent and tyrannical leaders, violators of human rights and dignity, such as Ivan the Terrible, Peter the Great and Stalin. On the individual level, the internalization of such figures leads to the creation of a rigid and destructive super-ego that can easily degenerate into an internal totalitarian persecutor.

Intolerance for dissidence. In USSR, dissidents were treated as mentally ill. Snezhnevsky (1960), and Snezhnevsky and Vartanian (1970) widened the frames of Schizophrenia. People who were against Soviet regime could be treated as having personality disorders or psychosis with slow-flow Schizophrenia i.e. Psychopathic-like Schizophrenia. Thus, there was theoretical and legal substantiation for using compulsory, involuntary treatment of dissidents in psychiatric hospitals. Sane people were admitted to psychiatric hospitals and treated against their will (Calloway, 1993). Any defiant behaviour was considered a mental disorder.

On silence and secrecy

During Soviet times, there were two "truths". One was official, declared and the other one hidden and kept in secrecy. This secret truth was available through dissident banned literature and through more traditional Georgian banquets with friends, where, with the help of wine, polyphonic songs, and relationships, it was possible to get in touch with the hidden truth and ambiguities of Soviet reality. At the same time, the presence of two truths created favoured the rise of paranoia-genesis within organizations and paranoia among people.

Theory and practice of psychotherapy in the Soviet Union

The Leningrad and Moscow Schools of group psychotherapy

Personality theory based upon the theory of relationships ("otnoshenia" in Russian) was developed by Miasishchev (1960), who called his method "Pathogenetic psychotherapy" this was the only dynamically oriented psychotherapeutic approach within the Soviet Union. The aim of pathogenetic psychotherapy was the reconstruction of the disturbed system of relationships/attitudes.

Rehabilitation has a special place in Soviet Psychiatry. According to Kabanov (1978), systems theory is more helpful in rehabilitation than simple psychoanalytic or behaviour models.

Group psychotherapy in the former Soviet Union could be described as authoritarian, hierarchical, psycho-educational and directive. Psychotherapists did not necessarily have psychiatric training, although they were usually medically trained (Calloway, 1993). Therapy groups are led by doctors and psychologists.

Psychiatry and psychotherapy in Georgia

Georgian psychiatry differed from the Soviet one. The founder of the Georgian Psychiatric School and Institute of Psychiatry, Mikhail Asatiani, practised psychoanalytical treatment. In 1908, he met C.G. Jung. The outline of C.G. Jung's Analytical Psychology was published in Georgia (Asatiani, 2001). The tradition of psychodynamic approaches was continued by Serge Tsuladze who studied medicine, psychiatry, and psychoanalysis in Paris at the Sorbonne University (Miller, 2001). He was analysed by the famous French psychoanalyst Francoise Dolto. In 1961, he came back to Georgia and started to work in Asatiani's Institute of Psychiatry in Tbilisi Georgia. In 1978, a conference was held in Tbilisi dedicated to "the problems of the unconscious". This conference was attended by esteemed colleagues from all over the world (A Collective Monograph, Tbilisi, 1978).

Uznadze Theory of Set. It is worth mentioning the contribution of the Georgian school of Psychology and its founder Uznadze (1887–1950). He was the first among Soviet psychologists to acknowledge and experimentally "prove" the ontological existence of the unconscious mind. He elaborated the Theory of Attitude and Set (Uznadze, 1966). According to him the ontological nature of the unconscious is the Set/attitude, that cannot be conceived of in purely physiological or purely mental terms (Uznadze, 1966). The general structure of psychic reality implies not only consciousness and the unconscious mind taken together, but as a certain protopsychic state of integrity, underlying the realization of consciousness and unconsciousness, including a full realization of the personality. This resembles Jung's notion of psychoid pole. Sherozia (1973) has tried to develop the Uznadze's theory of Set, and suggested a tripartite system of psyche: consciousness, unconscious psychic activity and Set.

Clinical illustrations

When Georgia broke free from the Soviet Union in 1991 and became independent, these characteristics of the Soviet foundation matrix did not disappear, but continued to rustle beneath the surface, affecting the behaviour of the people of Georgia. I will bring a few case vignettes to illustrate the unconscious aspects described so far.

Master-slave mentality

Mr.D was a 55 years old man. He had long standing dysthymic disorder and constantly complained of sleep disorders, difficulty in making decisions, lack of energy and anxiety. He managed to show up at his job conscientiously, but he found it difficult to take any initiative when it was expected of him. In the group he initially presented himself as a rather submissive and passive "good boy" who was completely unable to express any anger within session .

In the group he revealed a lifelong pattern of anxious dependency. He shared with group members his concern that he had always experienced considerable anxiety at the prospect of doing something alone or upon initiating any plan of action without consulting others. He was unable to make decisions for himself; even everyday decisions depended on excessive amount of advise and reassurance from others. He was unusually submissive and always in need of others to assume responsibility for major areas of his life. His fear of loss of support and approval made it difficult for him to express disagreement with others. He went to excessive lengths to obtain nurturance and support from others to the point of volunteering to do things that were unpleasant to him. He was unrealistically preoccupied with fears of being left to take care of himself and could not function well without someone else to take care of him.

He was brought up in a very old fashioned family. The father was a high rank official in Soviet Government. He was also fascinated by the great dictators and was very strict in the matter of discipline. Mr D's mother never really wanted a child and had only produced him as a sort of gift to his father and she took little interest in him. She seemed hypnotized by his powerful and glamorous father who was idealized in the family, sometimes to the point of worship. Father held them in contempt and ridiculed their shortcomings. He turned Mr. D against his mother and in so doing he fed his own narcissism by ensuring that all of his son's love was directed towards him. The atmosphere of constraint, hidden existential dissatisfaction, fear, punishment, suspicion and basic lack of love for oneself and each other was reigning at home. The same was at school. People surrounding him told him how lucky he was to be son of such a wonderful father. The father forced him to become an "example" of a diligent child, well-bred in the communist spirit. The boy had to conform to these rigid norms.

His admiration of his tyrannical omnipotent father had never been total and there was also a strong wish to be free of it. He complained about his father's tyrannical character in the group. "I felt smothered and exploited by him. I always felt his strict eyes within me, controlling my every step. He controlled my life but if he didn't, my life would fall apart." Further group psychotherapeutic sessions led to uncovering anger at his father. Any independent action on his part seemed to reactivate feelings of painful anxiety, fear and guilt associated with early separations and punishment. He behaved as though convinced that he would be abandoned and punished for any autonomous behaviour.

This example illustrates that patient's internal world was dominated by his relationship to tyrannical father. The father was feared and idealized. The entire family was captured by the tyrannical omnipotent father. In his inner life, Mr. D was persecuted by a strict rigid Super Ego, which functioned like an internal tyrant. It is not only individual but also socially determined phenomena in Paternalistic Societies like Soviet Union. Society encouraged him to develop an attitude of worship towards his father. In his rigid dependent attitude towards authority he personifies the "master-slave" mentality described above. Although this example can be seen as representing an individual case (the personal matrix), we should remember that the social unconscious resides in each part of the tripartite matrix (Hopper, 2019).

Due to group psychotherapy, his harsh rigid Super ego structure gradually became softer. Interaction with members helped him to be more tolerant to himself and others. Group as whole provided him with a holding environment, secure space of good enough mother (Winnicott, 1967) and thereby strengthening his Ego structure.

Nostalgia for and idealization of the Soviet past

Mrs K, a 50-year-old woman with neurotic depression, suffered from sleep disturbance, fatigue, general weakness, lack of energy and bad mood. She believed that the main reason for her illness is the altered social-economic conditions.

MRS K: Doctor, how can you bear to live in such hard life conditions, where the corruption, lack of minimal possibilities for survival, instability, fear for future are reigning beside corrupted luxury?

DOC.:   I understand you very well.

MRS K: My family and all of us had better times, much better than now. I often have nostalgia for those happy days during the Soviet times under Soviet Government.

GROUP MEMBER ALEKO: Do you think that everything was O.K.?

MRS K: Almost everything, certainly everything, can be O.K. only in paradise. People were much kinder and the Soviet Government provided people with almost all necessary. The order was everywhere, in all spheres of life. Why was it to be destroyed?

GROUP MEMBER BEKA: They say, for freedom.

MRS K: I had freedom, I could freely go everywhere within the Soviet Union and it was also possible to leave for countries of the socialistic block and even for capitalistic western countries, by special permission of course.

GROUP MEMBER ALEKO: You lived without information you needed, which was available for the rest of the world. You could not choose your unique life style. There was no freedom in religious and political life. You did whatever you were told to do. The regime made decisions for you as if you were in a kindergarten.

MRS K: I didn't care, I felt safe.

GROUP MEMBER ALEKO: But they say that you were deprived of the most precious thing – sense of freedom: to make free choice, to take responsibility for success and failures, and for your life. We live when we create. In the free process of the creation the human being is awakened.

MRS K: This high minded philosophy is not for me. I prefer to live safe and in peace. I can't understand what is wrong when the Government made decisions for us. I was freed from making decision on important issues.

This fragment illustrates the denial of the horrible and negative sides of Soviet times: political repressions, concentration camps, conformism, empty shops without essentials and total lack of initiative and individualism (Solzhenitsyn, 1978). Social, political and economic crises caused by the collapse of the Soviet Union made people idealize Soviet time. It might also show how, in times of political-social turmoil, people prefer fulfilling basic needs such as food and shelter over more abstract higher needs such as freedom. Distorted patterns of relationships are associated with collective black holes (Doron, 2016).

The following sessions in the group continued with the conflict between independence and safety. Some members of the group attacked Mrs. K.'s denial. With some empathy and appreciation for Mrs K, I suggested that she was expressing feelings that others probably feel, but were suppressing. I tried to save her from being scapegoated by pointing out that group projected their disowned feelings. Some of the group members agreed. It helped integrate Mrs. K into the group.

In order to show one-sidedness of her position the leader and members suggested to Mrs. K. that she read A. Solzhenitsyn's book, *The Gulag Archipelago.* She did, and seemed to respond and feel better. Gradually her assumptions about the idealized past became less rigid and categorical and group responded by being less critical of her. Through membership in the subgroup, she explored one side of her conflict instead of denying it and she helped the group realized that she expressed their repressed feeling.

Unfortunately, denial creates fear towards everything new and anything that the future can offer. For some, Soviet times was a period identified with the archetypal dream of the Golden Age or Paradise, where everything is provided in abundance for everyone, and where a great, just and wise leader rules over a human kindergarten (Jung et al., 1970).

In ideal socialism, society has to be structured as one big family where the majority of the population are children or junior members of the family (Jung et al., 1970). They do whatever they are told to do and following the results of their assigned work, they are praised or punished. People feel safe as long as the responsibility for supplying their basic needs is fulfilled by their parents, which means members of the ruling class (Urbanovich, 1999).

Post-Soviet phenomena

The collapse of the Soviet Union gave birth to 15 independent states and dozens of expected and unexpected challenges that are described as Post-Soviet Phenomena (Strayer, 1998; Urbanovich, 1999; Watson, 1998).

Identity crisis

Compared to the big European Empires, the Soviet Union was unique. More than 100 nations, having different ethnic roots, languages and religious beliefs lived together for centuries, first within the Russian Empire and later within the Soviet Union. Russia never had overseas colonies. Russia did not have an identity independent from its colonies; there was never a clear division between Russia, as a nation, and Russia, as an imperial power. That's why policy of Russia tried to annihilate Georgian identity by Russification. In order to maintain their identity, Georgians strongly opposed this policy and were against it. It was the Christian

Church that played crucial role in preserving national identity. Unlike European countries, where Church sometimes repressed the independent way of thinking (for example Jan Hus, the Czech theologian), Church in Georgia had the function of an antidote against annihilation and massification.

Georgians may be rightfully proud of their ancient history, but their modern state has just passed a stage of infancy. Since the early 19th century, Georgia only existed as a part of the Russian Empire and later the Soviet Union, save for a brief intermission in 1918–1921. Thus, approximately a quarter of century ago, Georgia started to build a new nation and a new state.

Socio-economic-political traumas

I will first present a series of historical events that traumatized Georgia:

On April 9, 1989 mass meeting promoting independence was attacked by military forces of the Soviet Empire; 21 people were killed. April 9 has become a symbol of the innocent heroes sacrificed for independence of their motherland. A year later, on April 9, 1990, the parliament adopted and signed the Declaration of Independence of Georgia and "thus, mourning situation underwent metamorphosis and it was transformed into such a symbol of victory, which substituted the mourning by celebration of National Independence" (Sarjveladze 1999, p. 64). April 9 became the symbol of National Independence (*Baltic Assembly, 1989*; Sarjveladze, 1999).

At the time of the collapse of the Soviet Union, Georgia was ethnically diverse country, where about 70% of the population were Georgians. The Soviet Union created two autonomous regions within the Georgian republic: the Autonomous Region of South Ossetia and the Autonomous Republic of Abkhazia. These two regions considered by the Soviet regime as instruments of pressure to prevent the independence of Georgia.

1991–1992 ethnic conflict broke out in the Southern Ossetia between Georgians and Ossetians, more than 25,000 Georgians were expelled from Tskhinvali, and many Ossetian families were forced to abandon their homes in the Borjomi region and move to Russia. The traumatic wound is still open.

Civil War. The newly independent Republic of Georgia elected as its first president a leader of the nationalist movement, Zviad Gamsakhurdia, a famous scientist, writer and dissident. In December 1991 and January 1992, there was a civil war in Tbilisi. Enmity came from displaced communists and democratic intellectuals, who were frustrated by Gamsakhurdia's efforts to monopolize power. President of Georgia fled the country.

In 1992–1993, there was a war in Abkhazia between Abkhazians and Georgians. Because this war, both Georgians and Abkhazs were cruelly victimized and heavy casualties were reported. Supported by Russia (HRWAP, HRW/H, 1995), Abkhazia has achieved and maintained de facto independence from Georgia. More than 250,000 Georgians living in Abkhazia were ethnically cleansed by Abkhaz separatists and North Caucasians volunteers (Dale, 1996). They were incited by Russian State. Georgians lost the war, and as a result, there are thousands of Georgian IDP (Internally Displaced People) living in very hard conditions within the territory of Georgia and also out of its borders.

For the Georgian State, the loss of its territories and distortion of its territorial integrity was traumatic. The country got split, people became disconnected. The harshness of economic realities after the break-up also contributed to an identity crisis. Economy, very hard condition of life caused depreciation of idea of social justice and protection.

Thus, Georgia was involved in two ethno-territorial wars in Abkhazia and South Ossetia and lost both. This defeat consolidated after a short war with Russia in 2008, after which the entire territory of these two regions came under military control of the separatist authorities and Russia, which also recognized them as independent states.

But the trauma on the Georgian side is still felt by many, "who are aggravated by the Syndrome of Defeat and heartache for the lost territory" (Sarjveladze, 1999). The recurrences of hostile actions, hostage-taking, murders and terrorist acts were frequent in the region of Gali, which is part of Georgia and borders with Abkhazia. As a result, the neurotic traumatic reactions associated with post-traumatic stress disorders persisted. Time passes and no progress seems to be achieved in negotiations and uncertainty (Sarjveladze, 1999) makes the situation worse.

A clinical illustration of PTSD in the context of identity crisis

In the following example, Mr. N., a group member, is treated for PTSD.

Mr N. is a 35 year old refugee from Abkhazia, unemployed, who came to an outpatient clinic with a post traumatic stress disorder. He was suffering from insomnia with enduring repetitive nightmares and flashbacks. He was forced to watch his loved ones being tortured or murdered. He was a witness to how the tormentors emotionally tortured people by posing a moral dilemma to them- to betray their friends in order to save the loved ones.

Mr. N. was startled easily and described himself as constantly vigilant. He reported not feeling safe, having low frustration tolerance, being irritable and having explosive bouts of anger. During the war in Abkhasia he was arrested, later liberated and finally exiled from his home. During the arrest he was isolated from reliable information, material aid and emotional support from family, friends and community. The perpetrators tried to convince him that his closest friends had forgotten or betrayed him.

Mr. N.'s capacity for initiative and planning were diminished. His dissociative defence persisted after the trauma ended. He narrowed and depleted his quality of life and tried to protect himself from painful disappointment, which would create an even greater sense of desperation. He also deprived himself of new opportunities for coping that might mitigate the effects of the trauma. Disconnection from others and from society was characteristic to him as well. He and others had lost the capacity to trust people. He also felt that he no longer had confidence in his capacity to determine what is good and what is bad. The assumptions of his value system seemed to have been severely shaken by the war and the strong sense of betrayal was associated with it. Depersonalization as a subjective sense of being unreal, strange, and unfamiliar to one's self persisted long after the traumatic events. As the surviving witness he felt intense shame, defeatism and impotent rage. He told group members that the victims felt as if their tormentor has completely usurped their inner life and the core of their identity. He felt that the war changed his personality and identity.

In the group, Mr. N. dealt with mourning, despair, fear, and uncertainty. His suspiciousness could have been reinforced by widely held social attitudes about Russia's motivations in that region. His story resonated with group members personal stories, which helped to create the shared interactive, inter-relational field. With the help of the group, he experienced empathy and acceptance. The group tried to direct him to the future, helping him master a "maximal active life position".

The 21st-century transition

War with Russia

After shelling Georgian villages by Ossetian separatist Georgian government tried to put an end to these separatist attacks and restore order by military forces. Russia responded by sending military troops in South Ossetian and Abkhazian regions. After the war with Russia in 2008, approximately 20,000 Georgians were displaced who – in addition to the many thousands more forced into flight by the conflicts of the early 1990s – needed to be rehoused and provided with food and healthcare. The war caused severe destruction of roads, installations and army bases, and housing of approximately 20,000 ethnic Georgians.

Rose revolution

Massive political demonstrations (the so-called "Rose Revolution") were held in Tbilisi between November 20 and November 23, 2003. Many called the change of the government, a popular coup. After the Rose Revolution, bold measures to fight corruption were taken by Government. However, afterward, antidemocratic tendencies emerged and human rights violations by the government flourished. The judiciary was seen as the government's "appendix" (Amnesty International, Georgia, 2005; Humans Rights Watch, 2005). At the initial stage, the Rose revolution aroused hope, but soon the people felt disappointed and angry and it turned out that new government decided to rule based on dependency culture.

Current state of psychotherapy

Psychotherapy model

As said at the beginning, psychotherapy in Georgia is still unconsciously influenced by Soviet ideology, reflecting the Georgian foundation matrix (Hopper and Weinberg, 2015, 2017). Within the frame of the paternalistic model of psychotherapy, a psychotherapist is regarded as an Authority. Paternalistic psychotherapy model coexisted with the Saviour model. Most patients project the archetype of the Saviour or Inner Healer on to the psychotherapist; they do not take responsibility for their cure (Guggenbuhl-Graig, 1971). It obviously shows aforementioned master-slave relations. Patient cannot accept that a psychotherapist awakens, develops and promotes a person's own self-healing and capacities (Groesbeck & Taylor, 1977). As a result, any attempt to create an analytical working alliance in the form of individual or group psychotherapy can be experienced by some patients as a lack of therapeutic skill on the part of the psychotherapist. Although, the examples of group illustrate how some patients can make this psychic transition.

The following example illustrates a typical paternalistic model of the patient that a Georgian clinic might serve.

> A 50-year-old man came to the outpatient clinic with anxiety and hypochondria. He insisted on directive methods of treatment, namely hypnosis. The doctor tried to help him understand that the hypnosis can eliminate morbid symptoms for a while, but it can't remove the deep-seated cause of disease. The doctor suggested that the addition of long term methods would bring a more stable effect. When the doctor advised psychotherapy, including group psychotherapy, the patient was astonished. He asked : " How is it possible to cure neurosis without medicines and hypnosis and only by words and dialogues? How can words influence the brain ?" When he joined the therapy group, he continued his questions. "How can I become a participant of a treating process when I am not a doctor ?" "I can't understand how can I treat myself ?" One of group member answered that he was exaggerating the role of a physician –"A good and skilled doctor helps our inner nature and organism heal itself. The healing power and source are in you . You have inner drugstore and inner healer inside you." He answered : "I can't understand it . A politician must rule, a musician must play and a doctor must cure. Why do I need a doctor if I can cure myself and be treated by myself ?" As group treatment progressed, this patient became an active member. Over time, he came to believe in the power of psychotherapy. He got better without drugs.

It is not easy to tell whether this patient's resistance or character structure is due to Societal or family-of-origin influence. I presume they are a confluence of both.

Nostalgia for the past

The nostalgia of the past that was mentioned earlier, is a good example of the inability to mourn discussed in the introduction (Mitscherlich & Mitscehlich, 1967). It causes estrangement and aloofness from the present, strengthens rigidity of life stereotypes, conservative tendencies and leads to fear of novelty (Van Der Kolk & Van Der Hart, 1991). Psychotherapy is dealing with the breaking down of habitual stereotypes; it aims at the formation of a new orientation to the present and the creation of an awareness of the future and its possibilities. This all too often clashes with the patient's understandable fear of the future and novelty, with his or her idealization of the past and desire to cling to the security of the familiar.

Materialistic world view

Georgian patients seemed to prefer biological, medicinal treatment and consider it the main form of treatment; psychotherapy is secondary. Most patients do not believe in the psychogenesis of mental disorders. This world view presents a challenge for the psychodynamically oriented psychotherapist.

The future challenges

The most effective means for helping people in such conditions is to provide them with psychotherapeutic services. Among them, group therapy, I believe, is the most beneficial. In order to improve group psychotherapy services in our country and to bring them closer to modern standards, Georgian Group Psychotherapy Association collaborates with IAGP and AGPA. One of the outcomes of this collaboration is the project of the Training in Group Psychotherapy in Georgia (2015). This project has a great importance for Georgia for the following objective reasons:

I   Political – Group therapy is a product of Western civilization, and its development in Georgia is a small but significant contribution to the creation of democratic values.
II Economic – Group psychotherapy for patients is much cheaper than individual/ or drug therapy and covers a larger number of patients over a period of time.
III The cultural aspect – It also provides a good opportunity to study transcultural problems (cross-cultural study) in experimental groups, particularly in the post-Soviet space. Group psychotherapy as microcosm can influence the macrocosm-large group (political and cultural). By establishing within the members the capacity for free interaction, equality, tolerance to differences, assumption of responsibility group instils democratic values. It will function as an antidote against annihilation and massification, help to prevent the formation of false collective self and to create good enough society. We are not too grandiose in our intentions, but fervently hope that small-group processes will provide a useful model intervening in the social macrocosm.

This world view presents a challenge for the psychodynamically oriented psychotherapist.

References

A Collective Monograph. (1978). *The Unconscious Nature Functions Methods of Study.* Tbilisi: Metsniereba.
Amnesty International, Georgia. (2005). *Georgia and the European Neighbourhood Policy. Human Rights Watch* Briefing Paper. June 15, *2005*. Potential for Reform.

An Alternative Report on Economics Social and Cultural Rights in Georgia. Human Rights Information and Documentations Centre's Reports (2005). Next Stop – The Belarus Human Rights in Georgia. 37–38.

Asatiani, M. (2001). The Present State of Psychoanalysis Theory and Practice Matter According to Jung's View (In Russian). *The Georgian Psychiatry News.* 1, 26–29.

Baltic Assembly. (1989). Resolution of the Baltic Assembly on the Events in Georgia on April 9, 1989. *In Popular Front of Estonia* (15 pages). *Tallin: Valgus Publishers.*

Calloway, P. (1993). *Russian/Soviet and Western Psychiatry. A Contemporary Comparative Study.* New York: John Wiley & Sons, Inc.

Chaadayev, P. (1970). *Philosophical Letters & Apology of a Madman.* Knoxville: University of Tennessee Press. xi + 203 pp.

Corson, S. (1976). *The Psychiatry and Psychology in the USSR.* New York: Plenum.

Dale, C. (1996). Abkhazia and South Ossetia: Dynamics of the Conflicts. In: P. Baev & O. Berthelsen (Eds.). *Conflicts in the Caucasus*, PRIO Report 3, 96, Oslo.

Doron, Y. (2016). The Black Hole in the Social Unconscious: A Collective Defence against Shared Fears of Annihilation. In: R. Friedman and Y. Doron (Eds.). *Group Analysis in the Land of Milk and Honey* (pp. 75–88). London: Karnac.

Gray, J. A. (1979). *Pavlov.* London: Fontana.

Groesbeck, J. & Taylor, B. (1977). The Psychiatrist as Wounded Physician. *The American Journal of Psychoanalysis*, 37, 131–139.

Guggenbuhl-Graig, A. (1971). *Macht Als Gefahrbeim Helfer* (In English transl. *Power as a Danger in the Helper*). Zurich: Karger.

Hegel, G. (1807). 1967 *Phenomenology of Mind.* New York: Harper and Row Publishers.

Hopper, E. (1996). The Social Unconscious in Clinical Work. *Group*, 20(1), 7–42.

Hopper, E. (2003). *The Social Unconscious.* Selected Papers. London: J. Kingsley Publishers.

Hopper, E. (2019). The Tripartite Matrix, the Basic Assumption of Incohesion, Fundamentalism, and Scapegoating in Foulkesian Group Analysis: Clinical and Empirical Illustrations including Terrorism and Terrorists. *Group*, 43(1), 9–27.

Hopper, E. & Weinberg, H. (eds.) (2011). *The Social Unconscious in Persons, Groups and Societies: Volume 1: Mainly Theory.* London: Karnac.

Hopper, E. & Weinberg, H. (eds.) (2015). *The Social Unconscious in Persons, Groups and Societies: Volume 2: Mainly Foundation Matrices.* London: Karnac.

Hopper, E. & Weinberg, H. (eds.) (2017). *The Social Unconscious in Persons, Groups and Societies: Volume 3: The Foundation Matrix Extended and Reconfigured.* London: Karnac.

Human Right Watch Arms Project. Human Right Watch/Helsinki (1995). 7, 7.

Human Rights Watch (2005). Georgia and the European Neighbourhood Policy.

Jung, C., Von Franz, M. L. & Henderson, J. (1970). *Man and His Symbols.* New York: Doubleday & Company Inc., Garden City.

Kabanov, M. (1978). *The Rehabilitation of Psychotic Patients.* Leningrad: Medicina.

Kliuchevskii, V. O. (1960). *A History of Russia*, tr. C. J. Hogarth. New York: Russell and Russell.

Miasishchev V. (1960). *Personality and Neuroses.* Leningrad: Leningrad's University Publishing House.

Miller, M. (2001). *Freud au Pays des Soviets.* Paris: Le Seuil.

Mitscherlich, A. & Mitscherlich, M. (1975). *The Inability to Mourn: Principles of Collective Behavior.* New York Random House.

Sarjveladze, N. (1999). *Societal Trauma, the Phenomenon of Return and Aspiration for Re-Birth Society and Psychological Support.* Tbilisi: The Conference Proceedings. 63–65.

Segal, B. (1977). Soviet Psychotherapy: The Tasks and Methodological Problems. *Psychiatric Quarterly*, 49(1) 8–17.

Sherozia, A. (1973). *A Contribution to the Problem of Conscious and the Unconscious.* Tbilisi: Metsniereba.

Singer, T. & Kaplinsky, C. (2010). Cultural Complexes in Analysis. In: M. Stein (ed.). *Jungian Psychoanalysis: Working in the Spirit of C.G. Jung*, pp. 22–37. Chicago, IL: Open Court Publishing Company.

Singer, T. & Kimbles, S. (ed.) (2004). *The Cultural Complex: Contemporary Jungian Perspectives on Psyche and Society.* London and New York: Brunner-Routledge.

Snezhnevsky, A. (1960) (In Russian). On Peculiarities of the Course of Schizophrenia. *Journal of Neuropathology and Psychiatry*, 9, 1163–1175.

Snezhnevsky, A. & Vartanian, M. (1970). The Forms of Schizophrenia and their Biological Correlates. In: *Biochemistry, Schizophrenias and Affective Illnesses*, pp. 1–28. Baltimore: Williams & Wilkins.

Solzhenitsyn, A. (1978) *The Gulag Archipelago*. New York: Harper& Row.

Strayer, R. (1998). *Why Did the Soviet Union Collapse? Understanding Historical Change.* Armonk, NY: M. E. Sharpe.

Urbanovich, Y. (1999). *Psychodynamics of Post-Soviet Phenomena -Russian Case.* Tbilisi: The Conference Proceedings. 67–68.

Uznadze, D. (1966). *The Psychology of Set, Ed. Joseph Wortis*, trans. Basil Haigh, New York: Intern. Behaviour Science Series. Consultants' Bureau.

Van Der Kolk, B. & Van Der Hart, O. (1991). The Intrusive Past: The Flexibility of Memory and the Engraving of Trauma. *American Imago*, 48, 425–454.

Watson, E. (1998). *The Collapse of Communism in the Soviet Union.* Westport: Greenwood Press. 200p.

Winnicott, D. (1967). Mirror-Role of the Mother and Family in Child Development. In P. Lomas (Ed.), *The Predicament of the Family: A Psycho- . Analytical Symposium*, pp. 26–33. London: Hogarth.

Part V

Working in the tripartite matrix

18 The Trilogy Matrix Event (TME)

A setting for collective reflection on social system dynamics of the tripartite matrix

Richard Morgan-Jones

Background context to this chapter

This fourth volume edited by Hopper on the social unconscious begins with a description and an exploration of "The tripartite matrix in Foulkesian Group Analysis" (Chapter 2, this volume). This introduction traces the moves from the development of Foulkes' idea of the matrix to describe the web of conscious and unconscious communications that shape group interaction. Hopper then explores the "realms and dimensions" of the tripartite matrix as an "essential characteristic of the social system of any human grouping". He describes the personal, inter-personal and trans-personal dimensions of the matrix and mentions developments in Foulkes thinking described as the *foundation matrix*, the *dynamic matrix* and eventually the *personal matrix*. Additionally, he describes the use of the term *equivalence* in group analysis to explore the relatedness between these different dimensions, along with rich clinical examples.

By contrast, this chapter comes from a different "stable". Although the author has been much influenced by group analytic thinking and practice and in his clinical practice ran two long-term slow-open group-analytic psychotherapy groups and one long-term couples' group, in fact the design of the large group event described in this chapter derived from the practice and thinking of Tavistock group relations and the founding inspiration of Wilfred Bion.

The fact that Earl Hopper and Haim Weinberg have welcomed this contribution illustrates a point made in a commentary Hopper co-authored with Carla Penna, on papers collected a special edition of the *European Journal of Psychotherapy and Counselling*, of which I was a co-editor with Robert Snell, focused on psychoanalytic and group-analytic developments in Field Theory. Their commentary review was sub-titled: "…field, systems and silos. From electromechanics to the matrix" (Penna & Hopper, 2022: 127). This piece acknowledges the significance of Kurt Lewin's field theory in the development of psychoanalytic, group-analytic and group relations thinking and practice and points to the experiments at the Northfield Hospital as the "cradle" through which these ideas were embodied and conceived anew. However they point to the risk that this watershed ended up creating silos where people from different schools do not share common languages,

DOI: 10.4324/9781003425915-27

trainings or indeed cultures of practice, and thereby miss out on enriching each others' ideas through appreciative enquiry and critique (see Penna, 2022).

This is the professional and theoretical background for describing a new approach to structuring a large group experience where reflection on experience and the development of new communicational networks can be forged across the three realms described in Chapter 1.

Introduction to the Trilogy Matrix Event

Exploration of large system dynamics, in the TME, seeks to provide an experience through which to integrate reflection and learning across three overlapping perspectives:

1 The embodied role where what is personally physical and what is emotional meet in a social role.
2 Group and system dynamics with sub-groups, shared unconscious basic assumptions, struggles for identity and moves between effective collaboration and defensive collective mentalities.
3 Forces from the wider context in which the group lives, including trans-generational culture, bequests and trauma.

We can think of these three realms as force fields of dynamic experience and energy, with attraction and repulsion, with fragmentation and solidity, with change and resistance. This chapter seeks to describe methods that explore and learn from experiencing these dynamics and the ways in which different nested circles of enquiry shape each other. Part 1 describes this new design as a force field. Part 2 outlines how this framework has been applied for different purposes in different contexts with examples. Part 3 describes its rationale and potential for developing new dimensions of experiencing and exploring large group dynamics.

The Trilogy Matrix Event (TME) as a force field

A matrix is a womb that shapes the growth, birth and new life of an infant. The metaphor of a *matrix* describes the way this conscious and unconscious field is shaped by the multiple intersection of forces which are made available to be discerned. It seeks to *frame* the questions relevant to this field of study as a *life space* (Lewin, 1948/1997). These include how to create the setting for enquiry and how to support these enquiries through focused and distinct tasks for studying experience.

The diagram below provides a schematic overview of such a force field. In addition to the three realms of experience that the *TME* explores, the boundary between each is described using the idea of the internal and external pressure points that represent internal developmental thrusts, on the one hand, and the need to adapt to an external wider sphere of influence, on the other. This provides a semi-permeable boundary that can be described using the bodily metaphor of a skin that is more or less porous or opaque.

Describing an approach to studying organisational and societal dynamics, this chapter seeks to structure the understanding of these three different embedded

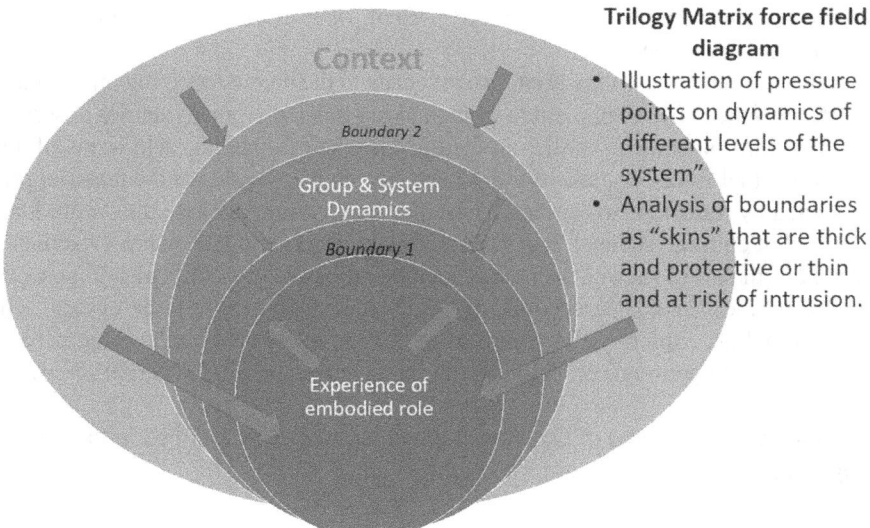

Trilogy Matrix force field diagram

- Illustration of pressure points on dynamics of different levels of the system"
- Analysis of boundaries as "skins" that are thick and protective or thin and at risk of intrusion.

Figure 18.1 Diagram of the Trilogy Matrix as a Force Field.

dimensions in a way that can make them apparent while working through the emotional realms and inter-related psychodynamics of each. These are the perspectives studied through the application of psychoanalytic ideas and experience to social settings that is often described as "systems psychodynamics" and engaged with through group relations learning experiences. These are applicable to groups, working teams and organisations and applied in multiple settings.

The basic model and three examples of using the Trilogy Matrix Event

The TME and the *trilogy approach* are designed for running workshops and groups to engage with wider and deeper organisational and societal psychodynamics. They began as a way to provide an experiential design for workshops on the theme of my book: *"The Body of the Organisation and its Health"* (Morgan-Jones, 2010), which seeks to relate bodily experience with organisational dynamics and the way the organisation as a social system is embodied in the effectiveness and *socio-somatic* health risks of its work force. The TME has been used to explore thematic workshops, career development workshops, Balint method work discussion groups and as part of a group relations conference providing reflection and gathering of here and now group experiences for learning and application within this tripartite model. The *trilogy matrix (TM)* is a way of describing the theoretical framework that supports the search to understand this complex field.

a The **basic model** of the TME is for a large group to meet in three concentric circles. The innermost first circle works for a set period of time reviewing its experience around a given theme. This is therefore a "here and then" event: *here* in the sense of making experience present, *then* in the sense of reflecting on previous experience.

b The second circle is then invited to associate to the theme reflecting on the material produced by the first circle while making links to group dynamics observed.

c The third outer circle is then invited to associate to the theme in terms of any contextual forces or dynamics linking them to observations of the material provided by the inner two circles. These perceptions may include the whole force field of cultural, societal, racial, economic, political and leadership dynamics.

d A fourth part of such an event may include reflective space in which to generate hypotheses linking perceptions of the dynamics across the three circles. This can include exploring the nature of the boundaries between the three perceptions and how porous or rigid they might have been around different forces.

Examples of this model of experience-based learning are described in the following three examples:

Example 1: A TME to explore the theme of shame and shamelessness[1]

One of the themes taken up in these workshops was the development of the trilogy method of reflective learning around the experience of shame.[2]

The questions used for each of the circles were as follows:

1 The inner first circle's task was to explore experiences of shame and shamelessness.

2 The second circle's task was to make observations on and to reflect on how they perceive the dynamics being discussed and were enacted in the exchanges in the inner circle.

3 The third, outer circle's task was to observe the discussions of each of the other two circles and to reflect on wider social dynamics.

During this workshop, in a second round of this TME there were the same three nested circles with people able to choose a different circle to work from. While the inner circle reflected on personal experiences of shame and shamelessness, the two other circles observed. Within the inner circle there were three empty chairs, which members from the other groups could occupy to comment on the dynamics they observed from the perspective of either group dynamics (second circle) or contextual dynamics (third circle). This method of working was used for 30 minutes followed by a review of the entire experience of both TMEs.

Using the trilogy approach to reflect on their experiences produced a significant dynamic. By exploring their personal and bodily experiences of shame, the outer two circles witnessed revelations of the pain of being shamed or people being shameless. This was experienced acutely. It was as if there was something infectious about the shame experience by being cast in the role of a voyeuristic observer in the outer two circles that belonged not just to being a witness, but by the structure of the event itself. For the first circle, this felt like being stripped of a skin or having the experience of another shamelessly stripping one of a skin as in cases of racism, gender identity prejudice, and phobia of difference (Morgan-Jones, 2017, 2022a).

Example 2: Poland on the Couch

In 2014 I was invited to work in Warsaw at the inaugural "Poland on the Couch" conference by Halina Brunning and Anna Zajenkowska. This included introducing Polish professionals including a good number of group-analysts to the TME methodology alongside a social dreaming experience (Lawrence, 1998; Morgan-Jones, 2019), inputs from representatives of Polish institutional life including politics and the media, psycho-social perspectives on Polish history and large group reflections.

There were two spaces for TMEs which I introduced and managed with my colleagues Halina Brunning and Olya Khaleelee. The theme of the conference was explored with tasks of the sub-groups being described as follows:

- Inner "Experience" group, the first circle: "to share experiences of what it means to be a Polish citizen in the present moment and have a Polish identity".
- Second circle, the "Dynamics" group: "to observe the experience group and then reflect on how they perceive the dynamics been discussed and enacted in the experience group".
- Outer circle, the "Context" group: "to observe the discussions of each of the other two groups experience and dynamics and to discuss wider social dynamics being revealed in the room".

The second session of this TME took place on a second day and, like the shame and shamelessness workshop described above, included chairs in the inner circle for members of the outer circles to occupy to offer observations or consultations about the dynamics observed from either of the other perspectives, dynamics or societal.

The experience of the first TME was fraught. The conference had stimulated many histories, personal and collective about Polish citizens exposed to humiliating invasion, persecution, genocide of three million of its Jewish population and a heritage of asset stripping of culture, language, identity, land and morale. These experiences were added to in the experience of the three nested circles with feelings of being watched, judged critically and even mocked.

By the second day, the social dreaming events and the focus of the presentations and discussions had moved on. People were more deeply in touch with feelings of tragedy, loss and pain that belonged in the inter-generational legacy from the past. This was linked to profound internalised suspicion and fear of criticism between Poles that risked undermining the extra-ordinary resilience, developmental capacity and courage to have survived horrors of past wars. It was as if the TME, alongside other elements in the conference had enabled expression and working through of internalised social and emotional attitudes that were both painful but sobering as the event began to map out the journey that Polish citizens had traversed, and which faced them in building a collaborative future. To some extent, the two-day container appeared to provide a chance for working through towards a more hopeful engagement with opportunities for the future.

In reflecting on regular gatherings that sprung from this foundational event, Zajenkowska explores key questions:

> Are we aiming to "analyse" the country, are we putting ourselves in the position of interpreters of the social processes or perhaps we have a different goal? After few years of organizing the projects now the aim became clearer. The purpose of the reflective citizens workshops, which are the core activity of Poland on the Couch, is not to "play the psychoanalysts" of the whole nation but to create transitional spaces for past and current traumas and other important events to be externalized, and to establish connection between citizens.
>
> (Zajenkowska, 2020)[3]

This reflection suggests that the event, marked by its title, could be described as a piece of "Sociotherapy", bringing to mind and working through trauma down the generations as a resource for motivating change in a social system as Kurt Lewin had proposed (Lewin, 1948/1997).

Example 3: Exploring the Meaning of Brexit and Trump in the UK

In February 2017, the Organisation for Promoting the Understanding of Society (OPUS) organised a day-long workshop under the theme of *"The UK on the Couch: Exploring Brexit and Trump"*. In many ways this echoed the Warsaw experience. During the day's event a Presentation was made by Simon Western on the theme while, he, Olya Khaleelee and I managed the two TMEs. This event was designed to *"join the task of OPUS to understand at a deeper and wider level the psychodynamics of society as a large group"*. The event was designed specifically to provide a reflective space through which *"one level of experience, reflection and analysis impacts on another to generate new hypotheses, leading to new possible action"*. It was also suggested that the event *"provides a kind of systems event familiar to group relations conferences but focused on 'work group' mentality using experience as a source of information rather than just discovery, expression and impact"*.[4]

During the two TMEs it was clear that the 50 members of the workshop were relieved to have a venue to share their dismay, anxiety and even despair alongside their fury and frustration at the twin shocks of the election of Donald Trump as the US president the previous year for the UK, to leave the European Union. Losses included rolling back the Welfare State that many had been involved in through their careers and the loss of social status as citizens who no longer carried respected authority for their contribution and vision of society, that was no longer respected.

Nevertheless, this psychodynamically sophisticated group of professionals were eager to explore their own projections and hatred of those who had voted against what they wished for. This elicited some misgivings about the European

Union which many felt had lost its way as a body to keep peace after a century of traumatising warfare. This failed dependency revealed old scars down generations of suffering in families and communities exacerbated by the economic divide between wealthy and poor that had not abated since the 2008 banking credit crisis and financial crash despite subsequent attempted cures to the financial system.

One hypothesis sought to gather the role of the UK as a unique centre of tolerating conflicts around differences of identity in a post-colonial world. The Brexit campaign had deliberately mobilised divisive anti-migrant feeling, racial prejudice and hatred of the intersectionality of gender diversity. These were chosen as focus for ills felt by traditionalists hankering for a by-gone age of imagined certainties. This also involved oscillation between primitive fears and excess excitement, masquerading as disapproval about mixed race and same gender partnerships. This contrasted with the values of international liberal ideals expressed in metropolitan populations seen by some as elitist that coalesced around the wish for independence from Europe.

Significant hypotheses were also voiced about attempts through gift work, care work and research to repair damage that felt at once like a body blow in attacking much needed dependency on the state by disadvantaged communities (inner circle), an attack on inter-dependency collaborative work (second circle) and failure in political leadership and followership (third circle).

The TME as a "new practice"

In the wider field of studying group dynamics in society and at work, there are many approaches to defining three "nested" circles of embedded domains where linked reflections on experience may be explored. These include:

- The person-role-system approach from the Tavistock Institute (Obholzer & Roberts, 1994).
- The Foulkesian *Tripartite Matrix* approach to the personal, the inter-personal and the trans-personal (Hopper & Weinberg, 2011, 2016, 2017, and especially as Hopper points out in the Introduction to this book, in chapter 1, giving priority to inside-outside could easily be reversed as does Foulkes' move between the *Foundation Matrix*, the *Dynamic Matrix* and the *Personal Matrix*. Alternatively, Group Analysis gives crucial priority to the Dynamic experience of the here and now group experience through which three other matrices intersect.
- The *Transforming Experiences in Organisations* approach of the Grubb Institute describing person, context and system overlapping in role experience, resourced by a larger transcendental "Source" of beliefs and values (Long, 2016).
- Agazarian's Systems Centred Theory (SCT) of exploration of three nested domains of person, system, group-as-a-whole focusing especially on sub-group formation and conflict resolution (Agazarian & Gantt, 2011).

Description of each of these well tried and developed schools of thought and ways of creating thinking, let alone comparison of similarities and differences lies beyond the scope of this contribution. Each approach provides different ways of reflecting on and experiencing these complex inter-relationships of different dimensions and perspectives with different emphases and purposes.

This locates the TME as a new practice (Morgan-Jones, 2022a) theoretically within the fields of group relations, group analysis and psychoanalysis and including their application to societal and cultural phenomena.

So why begin with the body and its means of seeking connection through the senses? This question relates to the way we take for granted, tacitly and unconsciously, aspects of the functioning of the main senses along with the main organs of the body. We take them for granted and are largely unconscious of them until such time as they make their presence felt in the form of sensations or our behaviour unconsciously seeking stimulation. The model being explored here is how the body is not just the source of sensation, feeling and experience. It also provides a container for experiences and emotions that we cannot digest. Even using such a metaphor, as did Bion (1963), suggests the physicality from which emotions appear. This is a two-way street across what Bion described as the *contact-barrier* (Bion, 1962). It is the body that generates, enjoys and suffers what belongs to the person, intertwined as we are with the group and the wider context. For this reason, cogent and significant as the structuring of ecological context may be through social sciences, the source and burden of their structure is experienced as sensation seeking meaning across the body-mind-group-context interfaces. We can also reverse this perspective and explore how the person can experienced as the embodiment of group and context, experiencing these other dimensions consciously and unconsciously inscribed on our unwitting behaviour.

That said, reflecting on experience as bodily experience is to be found in the mind. Language is involved as one channel along which communication is made, not least to the speaker who finds themselves through their mouth. Yet along with spoken language comes another channel, sometimes described as the "music behind the words". By this, I mean the non-verbal expression of senses, the use of metaphor to create images in the mind and the energy and forcefulness that communicates the temper of what is being said, the physicality, social role and significance of who and what the speaker is in the minds of others. With language we are already in the realm of the social, with non-verbal messages even more so. This second channel communicates across minds and penetrates unconscious elements of individual and group experience, which the emphasis on the body's sense experience reveals.

The three concentric circles can be seen as the creation of a framework within which members can wander around an experience exploring it from a fuller range of perspectives that do not just prioritise observation through sight. Bodily senses also include sound, smell, taste, touch, the kinaesthetic sense of movement and the proprioceptive sense of positioning of the body in space. Each of these encompasses unconscious and non- or pre-verbal communication. Each also includes developing the capacity for grouping of persons, thoughts and ideas as well as the shaping of conceptual frameworks born of cognitive learning across diverse domains developed as a means of describing and analysing experience. This bringing together, or linking discrete dimensions of experience, provides a chance to locate the experiences being mapped across a wider and deeper field without inhibiting the flow of new ideas.

Behind these elements is also the influence of Gordon Lawrence's development of Tavistock approaches in using *social dreaming matrices* as a way of mobilising the collective experience of the unconscious to develop new experiences, and new thinking that belongs to what Bion, in his later work, described as "thoughts waiting for a thinker" (Bion, 1967; Lawrence, 1998). What is particularly significant about this approach is the shift from the idea of the unconscious mind as a veil of repression behind which prejudices, motives and preconceptions remain hidden towards including the idea of mobilising the unconscious experience of dreaming and creative waking dream thinking to create new thoughts and hypotheses about complex social and organisational systems (Lawrence, 2000).

Across the bedrock of theory that underpins the TME are Bion's two theories of relating minds to bodies. The **first** is his theory of groups (Bion, 1961) and the way people instinctively and unconsciously form emotionally bonded groups which he developed in his *protomentality* through *basic assumption* and *work group* observations of group dynamics. The **second** is his *theory of thinking* (Bion, 1967) derived from Freud's idea that thinking was primarily unconscious and embodied in the intolerance of frustration. This made the capacity for thought as a relief from the burden of the need for others upon whom to evacuate toxic experience. This model of thinking begins from the mind's encounter with what Bion described as the *beta-elements* of raw sense experience that demand to be transformed through the *alpha-function* of maternal-like emotional recognition and containment, to create a differentiation between the conscious and unconscious elements of the mind (see Morgan-Jones, 2022b). In this way, external reality can be faced without the interference of primary processes and defences against them. Additionally, unconscious dream-like thinking can be mobilised to create imaginative links to give new meanings and to generate new ideas to be elaborated. The TME seeks to relate these two approaches and I now want to explore their integration before later turning to the **third** dimension of the context.

Research for integrating these ideas and their application draws heavily on *The Body of the Organisation and its Health* (Morgan-Jones, 2010) where I explored Bion's ideas of the body-mind inter-dependence and the desire to belong to a *group body larger than one's own* (Morgan-Jones, 2016). In Bion's early work on groups (1961), he makes sense of how to investigate the body-mind link through the social dimension. This he calls *protomentality*, the matrix from which all *basic assumption* group dynamics emerge. A key characteristic of protomentality is that what is physical and what is emotional cannot be distinguished. They are two sides of the same coin.

In Bion's (1967) theory of thinking, sense-impressions were transformed into emotions through the internalising presence of maternal-like reverie and attention. He described this as the way *beta elements* impacting the senses were transformed into emotions through *alpha-function* (Ferro, 2005). However, the idea first appeared in the form of a *protomental matrix* that encompasses the "groupishness" he suggests is at war with the desire for individual independence. For Bion, the *protomental matrix* was characterised by the fact that whether it was emotional or physical could not be distinguished as these aspects were opposite sides of the same psycho-social phenomena (Bion, 1961).

So far, we have established Bion's theories of group life and how it relates to the transformation of sensations into emotional experience. Now we come to the **third** circle to explore the way current societal trends and political and economic factors are seen to shape bodily senses, emotional experience and group dynamics. In developing Bion's thoughts about societal dynamics, my own work has been shaped by his references to links between *basic assumption mentalities* with the fields of both epidemiological and economic speculations (see Bion, 1961: ch 5; Morgan-Jones, 2010, 2011; Morgan-Jones & Torres, 2010).

Within a TME the task is not to surface unconscious dynamics so much as to mobilise unconscious dream-like thinking that is intuitive, metaphorical and imaginative in order to approach societal realities in a new way (see Armstrong, 2005). A further dimension in a Tavistock approach is the way organisations can be seen as open-systems exchanging goods, services, working lives, careers, trades and ideas with wider society in an inter-dependent way. From the Foulkesian group-analytic perspective, the context includes the *foundation matrix* for any group or person, which is so widely explored across this and the previous three volumes in this series.

This field can be studied around the capacity of what Bion (1967) described as the *contact- barrier* which protects the conscious from the unconscious mind and vice versa. This reversible perspective is key in addressing thinking that belongs to the realm of waking dream thoughts that are intuitive, symbolic and characterised as unconscious-to-unconscious phantasy. Where the *contact-barrier* breaks down, the inability to wake up and the inability to sleep risks producing the confused world of psychotic and delusional experience that Hopper describes associated with the traumatised group (Hopper, 2003). The boundary between the first and second circles (boundary 1 in Figure 18.1) and the boundary between the second and third circles (boundary 2 in Figure 18.1), can be thought of as semi-permeable membranes analogous to the human skin as a lax, rigid or flexible container as it deals with the forcefulness of managed and unmanaged intrusions and the porosity of the boundary (Morgan-Jones, 2023, 2010: ch 4).

Boundaries as semi-permeable and integrating membranes

In forging links between the three domains of the TME, a key idea is the investigation of what both distinguishes the different realms on the one hand and what joins them on the other. For Bion, a key idea was to describe the boundary contact-barrier that internalises containing capacity for delayed gratification and encouraged transformation of the threat of sense based and emotional overwhelm towards capacity for thought. In conceptualising the TM and using the diagram in Figure 18.1, this involves exploration of the two boundaries.

For this purpose, I have found invaluable use of the metaphor of skin as a semi-permeable membrane. This draws on the work of Anzieu (1984, 1989, 1990),

Bick (2002), Turquet (1974, 1975), Tustin (1986), Ogden (1992), Raufman and Weinberg (2016) and Ulnik (2007). It develops Bion's idea of *protomentality* as the key dimension of bodily experience that shapes emotions and groups them in the way he described the basic assumption mentalities. Basic assumptions can be seen as skins that permit the feeling of a bonded group that will assist in support- ing threatening emotional conflicts. (These dimensions are explored in my *The Language of the Group Skin*, 2017 & 2022.) Interpretation of these metaphorical skins as part of a force field can also be linked to the group-analytic approach of Pichon Riviere's concept of "el vinculo", the *link* (Losso et al., 2017). Such links can be seen as forged across the flow of the many, boundary crossing, internalised and externalised objects of relationships to be discovered through a TME among other settings across our psycho-social fields.

One area more exploration and mentioned above, is the nature of the thickness or thinness of these boundaries with more or less rigidity or permeability. Persons may be shaped by identifications that defy the demands of groups, or else that personify group membership (Hopper 2003; Turquet, 1974, 1975). Groups may also be shaped by becoming at the mercy of contextual forces they enact or else held together in rigid isolationism. By the same token leaders may hold societies to ransom or else be at the mercy of collective forces they ignore at their peril. Such dynamics might be enriched by understanding the nature of traumatised boundaries and the oscillation Hopper has described between aggregation and massification dynamics (2003), however this exploration will demand greater elaboration per- haps in a collection on large group dynamics. Suffice to say the TME might be able to provide interesting evidence about these processes.

Additionally, it aims to open up dialogue between different voices across groups and across internalised experiences that broaden and deepen the field as a container for hitherto unrecognised and unvoiced dimensions of large group dynamics. This dimension echoes Bion's final autobiographical work (Bion, 1974/1991) and the group internalised in individuals. This echoes developments in clinical psychoa- nalysis that develops field theory.

> Getting in touch with primitive mental states and with the origin of the self is strived for, not so much for discovering historical truth or recovering uncon- scious content, as for generating motion between different parts of the psy- che, for transforming barriers within the mind into caesuras (i.e., breaks after which there is continuity), and for incorporating and integrating different parts of the Self, even those seemingly inaccessible ones.
>
> (Bergstein, 2013)

This suggests that the purpose of the TME is not so much to analyse what are described as equivalences, as to free up communication between the three realms of the matrix. The TME moves beyond the application of Bion's initial application of psychoanalytic thinking in groups to incorporate his later thinking that includes container/contained (Bion, 1970), the transcendent and truth revelatory aspect of what he described as transformations in "O" (Bion, 1965, Grotstein, 2007), and his model of thinking (Bion, 1967, Lawrence 2005), his theory of waking dream think-ing and his autobiographical "Memoir of the Future" (Bion, 1974/1991) represen-tation of the internalised group epitomising Foulkes' *personal matrix*. Particularly significant in developing the TME has been developments in psychoanalysis of field theory and especially the *post-Bion Field Theory* developed around a num-ber of Italian psychoanalysts including, Ferro (2005), Civitarese (Morgan-Jones & Snell, 2022) and Neri (1998) and integration of their work with artistic expression (Snell, 2021).

To do justice to the matrix this suggests that we need to move beyond the work of Bion who described the essential body-mind-group inseparable combination as a *protomental matrix,* and of Foulkes whose pioneering work in developing group analysis using the concept of a *matrix* to describe the unconscious organic bedrock of shared dynamic experience and of its fundamental meaning as the womb from which new life is generated through words that evoke deeper and wider experience. Such ideas deserve poetry:

Matrix

A mass of fine-grained rock
in which gems, crystals or
fossils are embedded.
Something within or from
something else originates,
develops, or takes form.
We are a matrix
we souls who seek communion or
that which we call connection.
What is within us or from us
that will take form?
what gem, what crystal,
what fossil?

(Michelle Seligson[5] 2021)

Like much fine poetry, physical metaphor and language meet in creating a new shape for an old idea, while the language forges links between body, mind, society and meaning, unknown and yet to be searched for. Poetry is embodied, generated and could be explored through the lens of a TME.

Conclusion

In this chapter, I have described a framework for structuring reflection on, and observation of experience that forges links between the internalisation and exter-nalisation of conscious and unconscious forces. I have outlined developing a set-ting through which this approach can be applied to discover and work through the psychodynamics of complex inter-lacing fields. In the theoretical section I have explored some of the underlying theories particularly from Bion's thinking and from psychoanalytic developments in field theory to explore each of the three major dimensions of the TME. In ending this chapter as a contribution to understanding the social unconscious, I want to underline the methodology of this setting as a means of learning for reflection on the experience of what it means to belong to the large group which is humanity in its many dimensions.

Notes

1 This event was a regional meeting of the International Society for the Psychoanalytic Study of Organisations held in London 2015.
2 As John Steiner (2011) suggests in his book on "Seeing and Being Seen", Kleinians have majored in guilt and been slow to take up the socially based interactional experience of shame and shamelessness.
3 A striking development in this work is the collection of essays edited by Anna Zajenkowska and Uri Levin from Israel entitled, "Europe on the Couch: A Psychoanalytic and Socio-cultural Exploration of a Continent" (2020).
4 The quotations in *italics* are taken from the publicity for the event, written by this author.
5 Inspired by Gordon Lawrence's *social dreaming matrix,* two colleagues, Michelle Seligson and Kathy Cain, ran a new idea for a poetry matrix where, in place of sharing dreams, associations and meanings, we members of the workshop brought poetry for associations and meaningfulness. This poem was inspired by the poet's attendance at a TME.

References

Agazarian, Y. and Gantt, S. (2011). The group mind, systems-centred functional subgrouping, and interpersonal neurobiology. Ch. 5. Kindle Edition. In: Hopper E., & Weinberg, H. (Eds.), *The Social Unconscious in Persons, Groupsand Societies: Mainly Theory* (The New International Library of Group Analysis Book 1). London: Karnac.

Anzieu, D. (1984). *The Group and the Unconscious*. London: RKP.

Anzieu, D. (1989). *The Skin Ego*. New Haven, CT: Yale University Press.

Anzieu, D. (Ed.) (1990). *Psychic Envelopes*. London: Karnac.

Armstrong, D. (2005). *Organisation in the Mind*. London: Tavistock Clinic Series.

Bergstein, A. (2013). *Transcending the* caesura: Reverie, dreaming and counter-dreaming. *IJPA* 94(4), 621–644.

Bick, E. (2002). Collected papers. In: Briggs, A. (Ed.), *Surviving Space: Papers on Infant Observation*. London: Tavistock, pp. 55–59.

Bion, W.R. (1961). *Experiences in Groups*. London: Tavistock.

Bion, W.R. (1962). *Learning from Experience*. London: Karnac (1984).

Bion, W.R. (1963). *Elements of Psychoanalysis*. London: Karnac (1984).

Bion, W.R. (1965). *Transformations*. London: Karnac (1984).

Bion, W.R. (1967). *Second Thoughts: Selected Papers on Psychoanalysis*. New York: Jason-Aronson.

Bion, W.R. (1970). *Attention and Interpretation*. London: Karnac.

Bion, W.R. (1974/1991). *A Memoir of the Future*. London: Karnac.

Civitarese, G. (2013). *The Violence of Emotions*. London: Routledge.

Ferro, A. (2005). *Seeds of Illness, Seeds of Recovery: The Genesis of Suffering and the Role of Psychoanalysis*. London: Routledge, 35–36.

Ferro, A. (2019). *Psychoanalysis and Dreams: Bion, the Field and the Viscera of the Mind.* London: Routledge.

Grotstein, J.S. (2007). *A Beam of Intense Darkness: Wilfred Bion's Legacy to Psychoanalysis.* London: Karnac, 114–120.

Hopper, E. (2003). *Traumatic Experience in the Unconscious Life of Groups.* London: Jessica Kingsley.

Hopper, E. & Weinberg, H. (Eds.) (2011). *The Social Unconscious in Persons, Groups, and Societies: Volume 1: Mainly Theory.* London: Karnac.

Hopper, E. & Weinberg, H. (Eds.) (2016). *The Social Unconscious in Persons, Groups, and Societies: Volume 2: Mainly Foundation Matrices.* London: Karnac.

Hopper, E. & Weinberg, H. (Eds.) (2017). *The Social Unconscious in Persons, Groups, and Societies: Volume 3: The Foundation Matrix Extended and Re-Configured* (The New International Library of Group Analysis). London: Karnac.

Lawrence, W.G. (ed.) (1998). *Social Dreaming @ Work.* London: Karnac.

Lawrence, W.G. (2000). *Tongued with Fire.* London: Karnac.

Lawrence, W.G. (2005). Thinking of the unconscious, and the infinite, of society during dark times. *Organisational & Social Dynamics* 5(1), 57–72.

Lewin, K. (1948/1997). *Resolving Social Conflicts and Field Theory in Social Sciences.* Washington, DC: American Psychological Society.

Long, S. (Ed.) (2016). *Transforming Experience in Organisations.* London: Karnac.

Losso, R. et al. (Eds.) (2017). *The Linked Self in Psychoanalysis. The Pioneering Work of Enrique Pichon Riviere.* London: Karnac.

Morgan-Jones, R.J. (2010). *The Body of the Organisation and Its Health.* London: Karnac.

Morgan-Jones, R.J. (2011). The attempted murder of money and time: Addressing the Global Systemic Banking Crisis. pp: 74-88 In: Long, B. & Sievers, B. (Eds.), *Towards a Socioanalysis of Money, Finance and Capitalism: Beneath the Surface of the Financial Industry.* London: Routledge.

Morgan-Jones, R.J. (2016). Belonging to a body larger than one's own: The pair in the group, organisation and society. Ch. 9, pp. 165–191. In: Novakovic, A. (Ed.) (2015). *Couple Dynamics: Psychoanalytic Perspectives in Work with the Individual the Couple and the Group.* London: Karnac.

Morgan-Jones, R.J. (2017). *The Language of the Group Skin: How Teams Are Shaped by the Experience of Belonging to a Body Bigger That One's Own.* In an edited version of the on-line Italian Journal: Group: Homogeneity and Difference with special guest editor Martin Ringer.

Morgan-Jones, R.J. (2019). The dreaming body yearning to belong to a larger social body. Ch. 3, pp. 41–54. In: Long. S. & Manley, J. (Eds.), *Social Dreaming Philosophy, Research, Theory and Practice.* London: Routledge.

Morgan-Jones, R.J. (2022a). The Trilogy Matrix Event: A new practice for the study of group and organisational dynamics. *Socioanalysis* 23, 41–60.

Morgan-Jones, R.J. (2022b). The language of the group skin: What gets under the skin, attacking the capacity of teams to think. Ch. 7, pp. 99–113. In: M. Ringer, R. Gordon & B. Vandenbussche. *The Collective Spark: Igniting Thinking in Groups Teams and the Wider World.* Gent: Grafische Cel.

Morgan-Jones, R.J. (2022c). Ranging across Tavistock Approaches. In: *Organisational and Social Dynamics* 22(2): 187–204. London: Phoenix.

Morgan-Jones, R.J. & Snell, R. (2022) Guest co-editorial: "We Step into the Field". *Journal of Counselling and Psychotherapy* 24(1): 5–14. Special Edition on Field Theory.

Morgan-Jones, R.J. & Torres, N. (2010). Individual and collective suffering of organisational failures in containment: Searching for a model to explore protomental dynamics. *Socioanalysis* 12: 57–76.

Morgan-Jones, R.J., Brunning, H. & Khaleelee, O. (2016). *"Poland on the couch"* – with: Chapter 15. in Recenzja książki „Polska na kozetce" pod redakcja Anny Zajenkowskiej (Poland on the Couch) (pp. 269–278).

Neri, C. (1998). *Group.* London: Jessica Kingsley.

Obholzer, A. & Roberts, V. (1994). *The Unconscious at Work. Individual and Organizational Stress in the Human Services.* London: Routledge.

Ogden, T. (1992). *The Primitive Edge of Experience.* London: Routledge.

Penna, C. (2022). *From Crowd Psychology to the Dynamics of Large Groups: Historical, Theoretical and Practical Considerations.* London: Routledge.

Penna, C. & Hopper, E. (2022). Commentary on the special edition on developments in field theory of the European Journal of psychotherapy and counselling: Fields, systems and silos. From Electromechanics to the matrix. *EJPC* 24(1), 127–147.

Pichon Riviere, E. (2017). The theory of the link. Ch. 7. In: Losso, R. et al. (Eds.), *The Linked Self in Psychoanalysis. The Pioneering Work of Enrique Pichon Riviere.* London: Karnac.

Raufman, R. & Weinberg, H. (2017). Living in her skin: Social skin-ego and the maiden who enters others' skins in fairy tales. Ch. 3. In: Raufman, R. & Weinberg, H. (Eds.), *Fairy Tales and the Social Unconscious: The Hidden Language.* London: Karnac.

Snell, R. (2021). *Cezanne and the Post-Bionian Field.* London: Routledge.

Steiner, J. (2011). *Seeing and Being Seen: Emerging from a Psychic Retreat.* London: Routledge.

Turquet, P. (1974). Leadership: The individual in the group. In: Gabbard, G.S., Hartman, J.J. & Mann, R.D. (Eds.), *Analysis of Groups.* San Francisco, CA: Jossey-Bass.

Turquet, P. (1975). Threats to identity in the large group. In: Kreeger, L. (Ed.), *The Large Group: Dynamics and Therapy.* London: Constable.

Tustin, F. (1986). *Autistic Barriers in Neurotic Patients.* London: Karnac.

Ulnik, J. (2007). *Skin in Psychoanalysis.* London: Karnac, p. 302.

Zajenkowska, A. (2020). Group Analysis in Practice – Poland on the Couch Project. Unpublished Personal communication.

Zajenkowska, A. & Levin, U. (2020). Europe on the Couch: A Psychoanalytic and Socio-Cultural Exploration of a Continent. London: Routledge.